W9-DGG-508

The
Healing Power
of
Whole Foods

BETH LOISELLE

Introduction by WALT STOLL, M.D., A.B.F.P.

The Healing Power of Whole Foods

© 1993 by Beth Loiselle
All rights reserved. No part of this book may be copied or reproduced in any form without prior written permission of the author.

Library of Congress Catalog Card Number: 93-91693
ISBN 0-9637478-0-0

Publisher's Cataloging in Publication Data

Loiselle, Beth
  The healing power of whole foods.

  Index included.

  1. Cookery (Natural foods) 2. Natural
foods   I. Title

  [TX 741]   [641.3]

Cover photograph by Linda Henson
Cover design by Debbie Graviss
Illustrations by Matthew Focke

Healthways Nutrition
93 Summertree Drive
Nicholasville, KY 40356-9190
(800) 870-5378 or (859) 223-2270

www.wholefoodsforlife.com

Printed in the United States of America

Third printing, revised 2001
10 9 8 7 6 5 4 3

ACKNOWLEDGMENTS

Special thanks and appreciation to everyone who has helped, especially:

Walt Stoll, M.D., without whom this book would never have been written. His wisdom, knowledge, and inspiration have been invaluable to me.

My husband Jim, for his willingness and support many years ago when we totally changed our family's diet, for his insight in buying a home computer before I realized the need for one, and for his continued confidence.

My daughter Heather, for her humorous ways of encouragement.

My son Keith, for his endless help in desktop publishing.

Jim, Heather, and Keith, for eating most of my cooking experiments, the successes and the failures.

Friends, family, clients, and others for their recipes, suggestions, motivation, and recipe testing; among these are: Beverly Adams, Michelle Anderson, Robert Barnes, D.C., Nancy Bell, Kathy Brown, Leslie Bruner, Jennie Bryan, Donna Caldemeyer, Claire Carpenter, Rosemary Carter, Sonia and Lee Carter, Georgia Chase, Michael Clark, Anita Courtney, Maria DeMatteo, Anita Carol Drane, Margie Duncan, Melinda Duncan, Pat Durr, Barbara Eagleson, Carol Elkins, Kathy Farley, Rhonda Ferrero, Kerry Fluhart, Sheri Focke, Bernie Fritz, Leslie Goff, Debbie Graviss, Brad Grissom, Emmalene Hall, Rita and Louis Hardman, Gale Hartman, Linda Henson, Anne Hopkins, Donna Hottinger, Nicholas Howe, Helen Ison, Lena Jones, Betty Kendrick, Paula King of Great Harvest Bread Company, Ann Kirtley, Michael Lerner, D.M.D., M.S.D., Dorothy Loiselle, Mildred Lovins, Sandy Lyon, Susan Mason, R.D., Lauren McKee, Chuck Miday, Marty Morguelan, Martha and Ballard Morgan, D.M.D., Cindi Nave, my parents, Ann and Ray Oakes, Susie Oldham, Stella Prewitt, Rona Roberts, Marilyn Ryavec, Mary Seelbach, Leon Sharp, D.C., Beth Straub, Christine Stump, Nancy and Charlie Uhl and family, Pauline Vanover, Loretta Virgil, Carol Wathen, Tom Webb, Lora Wells, and Pam and Adam White.

Thanks also to the staff, management, directors, and members of Good Foods Co-op in Lexington, Kentucky, for their support and encouragement.

Joyce Gilmore, who edited my manuscript and offered much valuable advice.

The hundreds who bought my first book, *Whole Foods Cooking*, until it was completely out of print and so made it really inescapable that I write this book.

This cookbook is not intended as medical advice. It has been written for educational purposes only and provides information on improving your health by eating better. Cooking techniques and hundreds of whole foods recipes are included.

Please consult your physician before making any major changes in your diet, especially if you have medical problems.

Warning: If you have diabetes or if you have been eating a typical American diet consisting of large amounts of sugar, white flour, caffeine, or alcohol, it is very important that you begin the **Perfect Whole Foods** diet under the direction of a physician who can provide guidance and medical monitoring. Diabetics may have reduced insulin requirements. A sudden, total elimination of refined carbohydrates may result in withdrawal symptoms. The author and publisher accept no medical or legal responsibility for any problems caused or alleged to be caused either directly or indirectly by information in this book.

Individual books and quantity discounts are available from the publisher:
Healthways Nutrition
93 Summertree Drive
Nicholasville, KY 40356-9190
Telephone (800) 870-5378 or (859)223-2270
Or order online at www.wholefoodsforlife.com

CONTENTS

INTRODUCTION

Walt Stoll M.D., A.B.F.P.

The importance of diet in the area of human nutrition and well-being was dramatically demonstrated to me in 1977. This was after I had practiced conventional medicine as a Board Certified Family Physician for fifteen years.

At that time I was still teaching my patients that, and living my own life as though, diet had nothing whatsoever to do with disease or how people felt. Of course, at that time, I was experiencing a number of chronic medical conditions common to citizens of civilized countries. None of those conditions were truly curable by conventional medical approaches even though we had many effective treatments for them.

In 1976 I reopened my private practice of medicine, having just finished teaching medicine for three years at the University of Kentucky. As is usual with a newly opened practice, I was not very busy and had time to take some community education classes, one of which, Dr. Lerner's class, had been highly recommended to me by one of my patients.

Mike Lerner, a well known dentist practicing in Lexington, Kentucky, was teaching an introduction to Applied Kinesiology. The term meant nothing to me then but I know now that it opened the door to my practice of Holistic Medicine. Dr. Lerner, Dr. "Mike" to his patients, and now Mike to me, as he has become a good friend, showed me that one grain of sugar on my tongue caused a sudden loss of 90% of my muscular strength.

Since this experience could not be explained on the basis of my training and experience, I did not *want* to believe it. I later went to his office several times to experience Applied Kinesiology personally before I was sufficiently convinced to be ready to follow advice based upon the results of Applied Kinesiology testing.

Mike suggested I stop eating refined carbohydrates and caffeine (a diet I now know as a whole foods diet). To further test the validity of Applied Kinesiology, I resolved to follow the diet with the purity of a laboratory experiment. Consequently, I *totally* eliminated refined carbohydrates and caffeine from my diet with the single-minded focus I had seen previously only in my obsessive-compulsive or paranoid patients. I resolved that if one grain of sugar could make my body react so strongly, the diet might need to be perfect to work (at least in the short period of time I was willing to try it).

As it turned out, quick and dramatic results rarely occur until the practitioner has been compulsive about the diet for five to seven days. Even then, the changes are significant, but not nearly complete—most results occur over a period of three to six months. Even if you're not perfect on the diet, just moving in the direction of the whole foods diet will eventually improve anyone's health and feeling of well-being. The problem with not being perfect is that you will continue to suffer the symptoms of withdrawal for weeks or months that would normally be gone in three or four days if perfect.

I don't want to bore you with a list of my diseases, but I would not have believed the effect of diet on health had I not experienced it in my own mind, body, and spirit: On the day I started my diet my blood pressure was 160/110 and my cholesterol over 300. I was wearing a steel brace for ruptured discs in my back and had just been told I either had to stop jogging or I would need my knee caps surgically replaced with plastic ones. I always wore shirts with two pockets because I needed one pocket for nose drops for chronic sinus problems and the other for antacids for my chronic acid stomach. My previous ten years had been marked with several visits to the emergency room where one of my colleagues would surgically incise one of my severe hemorrhoids which had become thrombosed. I also suffered from a number of minor problems which included a life long battle with depression and obesity (at that time 263 pounds).

Within two weeks my stuffy nose and acid stomach were gone for the first time in more than ten years. Within six months all of the problems I mentioned were gone. In addition, I now had a soft stool every day shortly after arising. For twenty years I normally had a constipated stool only every seven to ten days.

The changes were so dramatic that my patients began to ask me what I was doing for my health. Sharing that information was what started my career in Holistic Medicine. I now routinely see these same changes in my patients who are willing to give the whole foods diet a try.

The problem has never been what to tell people to do but to help them to be able to do it. That is what this book, *The Healing Power of Whole Foods*, is all about. It not only gives you the tools to get the job done but also assures reliable and quick results.

Withdrawal symptoms are possible for three to four days after *total* elimination of refined carbohydrates. From then on you will begin to feel better than you have in many years. So long as you avoid re-contact, you should notice improvement in your health on a weekly basis for several months. Some of the symptoms of withdrawal include:

Fatigue	Sweating	Tingling of lips or tongue
Weakness	Hunger	Chilliness
Nervousness	Dizziness	Unsteadiness
Anxiety	Nausea	Drowsiness
Trembling	Visual disturbances	Mental confusion
Headache	Cravings	

There is only one situation in which the whole foods diet can be a risk. Any diabetic taking insulin must do the diet under medical supervision because their diabetic condition will improve so rapidly they will have to dramatically reduce their insulin dosage, frequently even to the point of stopping insulin completely.

Anyone who is *perfect* on this diet, and is not getting some positive results within one to two weeks, should go to the appendix of this book and read the information about the *four-day rotation diet* (p. 320) and combine it with the other information in this book.

I have now practiced medicine for more than thirty years, equally divided between being limited to conventional medicine alone and practicing the complementary addition to conventional medicine called Holistic Medicine. There is no comparison between the health and well-being of my patients I saw the first fifteen years of my medical practice and the patients in the last fifteen years who follow a whole foods diet. All of the latter patients' chronic illnesses either disappear or are much easier to treat.

The whole foods diet is not a complete solution to everyone's chronic problems but it will improve anyone's condition dramatically. This overall improvement in general health always makes management of any chronic disease easier, more effective, and less expensive. People who follow the whole foods diet carefully for a few months are much more likely to start exercise and stress reduction programs which then magnify the effects of the diet they are already on.

Only your own personal experience will ever let you find out if the results are worth the effort. *The Healing Power of Whole Foods* gives the most practical set of tools I know of to learn that for yourself.

You are more than you think!

A MESSAGE ON IMPROVING YOUR HEALTH

You are about to make important discoveries that can change your health and life. Although I originally wrote this book (previously called *Whole Foods Cooking*) to help Dr. Walt Stoll's patients follow his recommended diet, I have found that almost everyone can benefit from it.

Medical research continues to prove that a poor diet (like the typical American eats—high in fat, sugar, salt, and protein, and low in fiber, vitamins, and minerals) contributes to disease far more than was previously thought.

Poor diet → Disease

The focus of this book is on what I call the *Perfect Whole Foods* diet which *totally* eliminates *all* refined carbohydrates, all alcohol, and all caffeine. The *Perfect Whole Foods* diet is not for everyone—just those wanting to improve their health and willing to put forth some effort to do so.

This diet can help correct or prevent a variety of diseases and symptoms. If you have health problems that are puzzling your doctor or if you have gone from one doctor to another in search of help but to no avail, then the perfect diet may very well prove to be useful to you. You'll get the best results if you work with a medical practitioner who can make appropriate recommendations about exercise, supplements, relaxation techniques, and medications.

Perfect Whole Foods → Health!

In my work at Good Foods Co-op in Lexington, Kentucky, I often see Dr. Stoll's patients whom I have previously helped with the perfect diet. Most of them are simply amazed at how well they feel and how their health has improved. My personal experience with the *Perfect Whole Foods* diet made me a whole foods convert many years ago. Hearing so many others praise Dr. Stoll's diet confirms my belief in whole foods' special healing power.

If you don't follow the diet exactly, then you won't get the dramatic results of the *Perfect Whole Foods* diet; however, your health should still improve.

Remember

The more nearly perfect you are with the diet, the sooner you'll realize positive results. The less than perfect you are, the longer it will take for you to get results.

After you follow the diet and improve your health, you may want to go to a liberal whole foods diet. Use a more liberal diet also if you choose not to be so strict with your diet or if your health is already excellent. A liberal whole foods diet, although based on whole foods, doesn't totally eliminate refined foods.

If you haven't yet read Dr. Stoll's introduction to this book, please go back and do so before beginning the *Perfect Whole Foods* diet. It's critical that you be aware of the information he gives about withdrawal symptoms and his warning to diabetics.

Before you discover the healing power of whole foods, I want to give you a glimpse of what this book is about by sharing with you a recipe for improving your health.

A RECIPE FOR IMPROVING YOUR HEALTH

Recipes usually include a list of ingredients as well as instructions, and this recipe for improving your health is no different. Ingredients are listed below. Although I'm giving you here a simplified list of ingredients and brief instructions, the complete recipe will be found throughout the book. As with all recipes, the better you follow the instructions, the better the results will be.

Fresh or frozen vegetables
Whole grains, exclusively
Well-cooked dried beans
Unsweetened, fresh or frozen whole fruit
Nuts and seeds, in moderation
Unrefined oils and butter in moderation
Farm eggs
Mostly low-fat and nonfat dairy products
Lean and fresh meat, poultry, and fish (optional)
Pure water

Combine ingredients to create colorful and tasty meals. Add small amounts of optional ingredients, if desired. Choose a variety of foods, not the same ones over and over. Select organically-grown foods when possible. Avoid all foods to which you are allergic or sensitive, or which aggravate your particular health problem. Prepare foods simply, seasoning with herbs and spices and totally eliminating all refined carbohydrates, alcohol, and caffeine. Avoid excessive fat (20 to 30 percent of total calories as fat is a good maintenance diet) as well as artificial foods and additives. Drink plenty of pure water throughout the day.

Serve in a health-promoting lifestyle: take time to relax during the day, exercise regularly according to your own ability, and eliminate toxic chemicals from your environment. Be thankful for your food, maintain a positive outlook, and watch your health improve! Serves all.

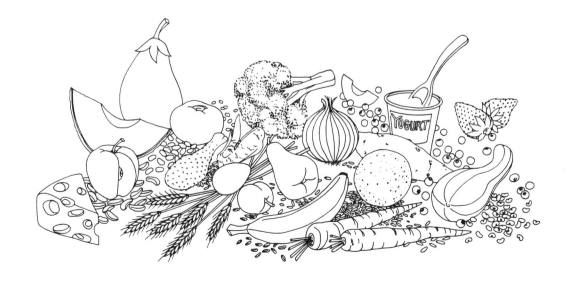

BASIC QUESTIONS ANSWERED

If you are not sure what whole foods are, or why you should eat them, this section will answer your questions. It will also show you how to determine which foods are whole and which are refined, what foods to eat, how long to stay on the perfect diet, and how to liberalize your diet.

What Are Refined Carbohydrates?

First of all, I'll give you some background information about carbohydrates and then, specifically, refined carbohydrates.

Carbohydrates are the body's preferred form of energy. Simple sugars or monosaccharides are the smallest units of carbohydrates. These sugars combine to form other simple sugars, called disaccharides. Units of glucose join to form starches, still another type of carbohydrate called polysaccharides. Cellulose or indigestible fiber is a polysaccharide also.

Classifications of Carbohydrates

Monosaccharides (Simple sugars)	Disaccharides (Simple sugars)	Polysaccharides (Complex carbohydrates)
Glucose	Sucrose	Starches
Fructose	Lactose	Cellulose (fiber)
Galactose	Maltose	

Whole or natural carbohydrate foods, as found in nature, contain sugars, starches, and fiber. They are also important sources of vitamins, minerals, protein, and essential fatty acids.

Typical Whole or Natural Carbohydrate Foods

Whole Grains	Dried Beans and Peas
Brown rice	Pinto beans
Whole wheat	Black beans
Whole rye	Kidney beans
Hulled barley	Split peas

Vegetables	Fresh Fruits
Corn	Apples
Potatoes	Pears
Yams	Grapes
Green peas	Pineapple

Now for the answer to the original question. Refined carbohydrates are those whole or natural carbohydrate foods that man has processed, changed, or fragmented. Vital nutrients are removed when man changes natural carbohydrate foods into refined carbohydrates.

Typical Refined Carbohydrates

White sugar	White rice	Peeled potatoes
White flour	Cornstarch	Apple juice

Some people use the term *complex carbohydrate* to refer to unrefined carbohydrates. That's not correct. Complex carbohydrates actually are starches and cellulose (polysaccharides) as opposed to simple sugars. By adding the adjectives *refined* and *unrefined* to the term *complex carbohydrate*, we can differentiate between refined starchy foods and whole, natural foods.

Examples of Complex Carbohydrates

Refined Complex Carbohydrates	Unrefined Complex Carbohydrates
White flour	Whole wheat flour
White rice	Brown rice
White flour pasta	Whole wheat pasta
Pearled barley	Hulled barley
Degerminated cornmeal	Whole grain cornmeal
Peeled potatoes	Potato with skin

Refined complex carbohydrates provide mostly starch and protein whereas unrefined complex carbohydrates provide starch, cellulose or dietary fiber plus all the trace nutrients the body needs to metabolize that carbohydrate.

Why Should I Eliminate Sugar?

Many people are aware that whole grains are nutritious, mostly because the importance of fiber has been emphasized by the media. The average person, however, doesn't know much about sugar other than it tastes good, causes tooth decay, and is usually eaten in excess. The body does not need refined sugar. While it is true that the body uses glucose as a source of energy and for proper brain function, plenty of glucose is available from unrefined carbohydrates like whole grains, dried beans, and whole fruits.

Occasional small amounts of refined sugar won't do much harm to a healthy body. However, at 130 pounds a year (the amount of sugar—white sugar, corn syrup, and high fructose corn syrup—the average American consumes each year), a healthy body won't stay well for long. One hundred and thirty pounds of sugar per year is equivalent to 40 teaspoons of white sugar per day! That's equal to 600 calories from sugar daily! Since many people, myself included, have eliminated or drastically reduced their sugar intake, the 130 pound estimate is likely too low and may be much higher among those who still eat sugar.

When you discover the damage sugar can do to the body, you will realize that sugar is not so sweet after all:

- As a result of over-consumption, sugar causes unstable blood sugar in many people. Being quickly absorbed, sugar makes the blood sugar level rise rapidly, causing the pancreas to over-produce insulin. Excessive insulin in the blood then rapidly lowers the blood sugar level—often lower than it was before sugar was eaten. The adrenal glands step in here with a hormone that releases glycogen (sugar stored in the liver) to help return the blood sugar to normal. This release triggers the pancreas again to produce more insulin which continues the blood sugar's roller-coaster ride. Unstable blood sugar can cause many physical and emotional symptoms. Low blood sugar or reactive hypoglycemia can cause one or more of a host of symptoms, especially during withdrawal or when the blood sugar drops as a result of eating sugar. In addition to Dr. Stoll's list of symptoms in the **Introduction** (fatigue, weakness, nervousness, anxiety, trembling, headache, sweating, hunger, cravings, dizziness, nausea, visual disturbances, tingling of the tongue or lips, chilliness, unsteadiness, drowsiness, and mental confusion), there can also be emotional instability, nightmares, insomnia, forgetfulness, depression, antisocial behavior, addictions, plus many more.

- Sugar lacks essential nutrients (vitamins, minerals, fiber, protein, and essential fatty acids) yet provides calories. For this reason, sugar is often called an empty calorie food.

- In order to metabolize or use sugar to produce energy, the body must draw from nutrient reserves provided from other foods. Many of these nutrients cannot be stored in the body so they need to be present every time sugar is consumed. Nutrients needed for sugar metabolism include thiamine, niacin, riboflavin, vitamin B-6, vitamin B-12, biotin, pantothenic acid, phosphorus, magnesium, potassium, manganese, zinc, copper, and chromium. Sugar, therefore, not only provides empty calories but creates a nutrient shortage.

- Sugar depresses the immune system. A specific way is that sugar weakens the conversion of essential fatty acids to hormone-like substances called prostaglandins. One function of these substances is to regulate white blood cell activity. Dr. Stoll says that the average lymphocytic index (how many bacteria a white cell can eat in an hour) is 13.6. The amount of sugar eaten in the average American evening meal lowers the lymphocytic index to 1.3 within an hour. This depression of immunity lasts four to six hours! Frequent doses of sugar throughout the day makes the body more susceptible to colds, viruses, bacterial infections, fungal infections, parasites, and even cancer.

- Sugar encourages the growth of *Candida albicans* in the intestinal tract, especially when the friendly bacteria have been destroyed by antibiotics, oral contraceptives, or steroids.

- Sugar increases dental plaque which promotes cavities and gum disease.

- Because it lacks fiber, sugar increases the time it takes for food to pass through the intestinal tract. Sugar therefore contributes to intestinal disorders like constipation, hemorrhoids, diverticulitis, and even colon cancer. Sugar also causes an increase in gastric acidity which leads to indigestion and possibly ulcers.

Terms and Sources for Refined Sugar

Amasake	Fruit sugar	Powdered sugar
Barbados sugar	Glucose	Raw honey
Barley malt	Grape sugar	Raw sugar
Beet sugar	Granulated cane juice	Ribbon cane syrup
Blackstrap molasses	Honey	Ribitol
Brown rice syrup	Kleenraw sugar	Rice syrup
Brown sugar	†Lactose	Roasted malt
Cane sugar	Lemon powder	Sorbitol
Cane syrup	*Malt	Sorbo
Caramel coloring	Malted barley	Sorghum
Caramel flavoring	Malted grain syrup	Sucanat
Caramel malt	Maltose	Sucrose
Corn sugar	Mannitol	Sugar
Corn syrup	Mannose	Syrup
Date sugar	Maple syrup	Toothpaste, most
Dextrose	Milk sugar	Turbinado sugar
Dried fruit	Molasses	†Whey
Dulcitol	Muscovado sugar	White sugar
†Fructose	Natural flavor (can be juice)	Words ending in "ol"
Fruit juice	Polydextrose	*Words ending in "ose"
Fruit juice concentrate	Orange powder	Xylitol

*Diastatic malt (sometimes called wheat malt) and cellulose are not refined carbohydrates.

†An Important Note About Fructose, Lactose, and Whey

Foods that naturally contain fructose, lactose, and whey are permitted on the perfect diet if the foods have not been refined. Two examples are milk and fresh fruit. The sugars in these foods (lactose in milk as well as fructose and glucose in fruit) are naturally present in the foods and are okay in moderate amounts since their accompanying nutrients are present. When fruit is juiced, however, the process removes the fruit's fiber, thus making juice refined. Also, any food that has the ingredients lactose, fructose, or whey added should not be used on the **Perfect Whole Foods** diet since pure lactose and fructose are refined carbohydrates and do not provide the nutrients that are needed for their metabolism; whey, when separated from milk, includes some lactose and should, therefore, also be eliminated. The removal of fat from milk is not considered a refining process.

If you are being treated for Candida, you should eliminate all fruit for the first three months of treatment or until all symptoms have disappeared. See **Appendix A** for complete instructions (p. 316).

Why Should I Eliminate Fruit Juice?

Because fiber is removed in making juice, fruit juice is a source of refined carbohydrate. Just like other refined sugars, the fruit sugar from juice is more quickly absorbed into the bloodstream than is the sugar from a fresh piece of fruit with its fiber intact.

If you compare how long it takes to eat a small fresh apple and to drink ⅓ cup apple juice (these two have approximately the same number of calories and grams of fruit sugar), you'll further understand why fruit juices are eliminated from the perfect diet. A fresh apple, because of its fiber, takes much longer to eat and digest and is more filling and satisfying than juice.

All fruit juices should be totally eliminated from the perfect diet. Even lemon and lime juices should be eliminated. Not all people are sensitive to the trace amounts of refined carbohydrates in lemon and lime juice, but since we don't know whether or not you are sensitive, it's best to eliminate it for a while—until your body gets healthy enough not to react. (The lemon or lime with its pulp can be used unless you are being treated for *Candida* yeast infections. See the **Appendix A** on page 316 for complete information about diet during this treatment.)

Raw, freshly squeezed vegetable juices (like carrot juice or celery juice) are okay on the ***Perfect Whole Foods*** diet. These raw juices are very concentrated in nutrients and, compared to fruit juice, contain relatively little carbohydrate. Because carrot juice has a greater concentration of carbohydrate than other vegetable juices, limit your serving size to 1 cup per day while on the perfect diet. It's also okay to use fresh or canned tomato juice and *V-8 Juice* diluted in foods like soups, stews, or salad dressings. Just don't drink the canned juices as beverages since you are likely to fill up on these rather than more nutritious foods.

Juices on the *Perfect Whole Foods* Diet

You Should Totally Eliminate	You May Use
All fruit and vegetable juices other than the exceptions listed to the right.	Raw, freshly squeezed vegetable juice (limit fresh carrot juice to 1 cup servings per day). You may also use fresh or canned tomato juice or *V-8 Juice* for cooking, not as a beverage.

Why Should I Eliminate Refined Complex Carbohydrates?

When the germ and bran are removed from whole grains to make refined grains (like white flour and white rice), at least thirty-six nutrients are either partially or almost totally eliminated. Most of what is left in the refined grain is the endosperm that's composed primarily of starch and protein. Since starch is a refined complex carbohydrate that is made up of sugar molecules attached together, just like sugar, it doesn't provide adequate nutrients needed for energy metabolism. Nutrients that were meant to be used in the starch's metabolism were removed during processing.

Nutrients Removed* When Wheat and Other Grains Are Refined

Biotin
Boron
Calcium
Chlorine
Choline
Chromium
Cobalt
Copper
Fiber
Fluorine
Folic acid
Inositol
Iodine
Iron

Lecithin
Linoleic acid
Linolenic acid
Magnesium
Manganese
Molybdenum
Niacin
Pantothenic acid
Para-aminobenzoic acid
Phenolic acids
Phosphorus
Phytochemicals yet to be
   recognized
Plant sterols

Potassium
Protein
Pyridoxine
Riboflavin
Selenium
Silicon
Sodium
Sulfur
Thiamine
Vanadium
Vitamin E
Vitamin K
Zinc

Either partially or almost totally

Don't think that enrichment of refined grains adds all or most of the important nutrients back. This is not so. Enrichment only adds five nutrients and not in as great a quantity as was originally there.

Nutrients Added During Enrichment

Thiamine	Riboflavin	Niacin	Iron	Folic acid

Our bodies need the nutrients that are provided by whole grains as well as other unrefined complex carbohydrate foods. Although I won't go into great detail, I'll briefly list some of the functions and deficiency symptoms of selected nutrients that are partially or almost totally removed in processing and not added back during enrichment. This will give you an idea of the importance of these nutrients to health. If you are interested in knowing about the other nutrients, please refer to nutrition books for information.

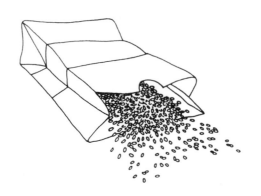

Some Nutrients Removed When Whole Grains Are Refined

Nutrient	Functions	Deficiency Signs
Pantothenic acid	Involved in carbohydrate, protein, and fat metabolism, cortisone plus other adrenal hormone production, and immunity. An anti-stress factor.	Fatigue, gastrointestinal disturbances, depression, irritability, decreased resistance to infection.
Vitamin B-6	Involved in carbohydrate, protein, and fat metabolism; red blood cell and antibody formation; and sodium-potassium balance.	Sore mouth, lips, and tongue, dermatitis, anemia, weakness, depression, nervousness, kidney stones.
Vitamin E	Involved in maintaining circulatory system and healing. Antioxidant and anticoagulant.	Heart disease, reproductive and muscular disorders.
Chromium	Involved in carbohydrate metabolism. Increases effectiveness of insulin. Helps normalize blood cholesterol and triglycerides.	Glucose intolerance, food cravings, atherosclerosis.
Magnesium	Involved in carbohydrate, protein, and fat metabolism, transmission of nerve impulses and muscle contractions, bone growth.	Kidney stones, nervousness, depression, confusion, muscle cramps, and tremors.
Zinc	Involved in many enzymes and insulin; wound healing and skin health; and bone formation. Needed for gastrointestinal tract, nervous, immune and reproductive systems.	Retarded growth, frequent infections, poor appetite and sense of smell and taste; fatigue.

Refined grains, although not totally devoid of nutrients, contribute to the same problems as sugar. Refined grains encourage blood sugar fluctuations, overeating and subsequent overweight, constipation, colon cancer, elevated blood cholesterol, *Candida* yeast overgrowth, plus much more.

Eliminating refined complex carbohydrates from your diet is a second way to improve your health. This book will show you how.

There are many terms used on ingredient lists indicating that a complex carbohydrate food has been refined. I have listed many of these terms on the following page. Become familiar with them so you'll know what to eliminate while you are on the *Perfect Whole Foods* diet. If you like, make a copy of these terms and carry them with you when you shop. There are other less common terms included in the **Quick Reference for Foods** and **Quick Reference for Additives** (see the **Appendix G** on page 348). You can check these references for any term about which you are uncertain.

Typical Terms and Sources for Refined Complex Carbohydrates

Refined corn
Bolted cornmeal
Corn (may be refined)
Corn flour
Corn pasta
Cornstarch
Degerminated corn
Enriched corn
Grits
Hominy
Hominy grits
Masa corn flour
Masa harina
Milled corn (may be refined)
Processed cornmeal
Stone ground corn (may be)
Unbolted (may be)
Whole hominy
Refined Barley
Pearled barley
Pot barley
Scotch barley
Refined Oats
Instant oatmeal
Oat flour
   (if bran is removed)
Refined rice
Converted rice
Enriched rice
Granulated rice
Instant rice
Long grain rice
Medium grain rice
Parboiled rice
Partially milled brown rice
Partially polished brown rice
Polished rice
Rice
Rice flour
White basmati rice
White rice

White rice flour
Wild rice blend
   (if it includes white rice)
Refined Rye
Light rye flour
Medium rye flour
Rye
Rye flour
Rye meal
Sifted rye flour
Sifted whole rye flour
Stone ground rye flour
White rye flour
Refined spelt
White spelt flour
Refined wheat
All-purpose flour
Bleached flour
Bleached wheat flour
Cake flour
Communion bread or wafers
Couscous
Durum
Durum flour
Durum pasta
Enriched flour
Enriched macaroni
Enriched pasta
Farina
Flour
Gluten
Gluten flour
High-gluten flour
Instantized flour
Macaroni
Noodles
Orzo
Pasta
Pastry flour
Patent flour
Pearled wheat

Seitan
Self-rising flour
Semolina
Semolina flour
Semolina pasta
Sifted flour
Sifted whole wheat flour
Spaghetti
Stone ground wheat flour
Unbleached flour
Vermicelli
Wheat
Wheat farina
Wheat flour
Wheat grits
White flour
Other Refined Complex Carbohydrates
Arrowroot
Arrowroot flour
Arrowroot starch
Baking powder
Dried potatoes
Glue on stamps and envelops
Hydrolyzed cereal solids
Kudzu
Kuzu
Maltodextrin
Mashed potatoes (if peeled)
Modified food starch
Peeled potatoes
Poi
Potato chips
Potato flour
Potato starch
Starch
Tapioca
Tapioca grits
Taro root
Vegetable food starch

*These terms, when listed on an ingredient list, denote that the grain has been refined. Grains like rice, barley, rye, and wheat are refined when the ingredient list doesn't list them as brown rice, whole or hulled barley, whole rye, and whole wheat. There are many additional, less commonly used terms for refined grains. Please check the **Quick Reference for Foods** in the **Appendix G** (p. 348) for terms about which you are uncertain.*

Why Should I Eliminate Alcohol?

Because it is more socially acceptable than taking other drugs, alcohol consumption is the most common form of drug abuse. Even if alcohol never interferes with your work or personal life, regular drinking can do great harm to your health.

If you are trying to improve your health or prevent disease, alcohol should be eliminated from your diet because it acts just like a refined carbohydrate in the body. Alcohol doesn't contain the nutrients that are needed for its metabolism. It is considered, like sugar, to be an empty calorie food, depleting the body of important nutrients. It is quickly absorbed and can be extremely addictive. Alcohol is harmful to the body in a number of other ways.

Alcohol:

* Is a depressant, affecting every organ of the body.

* Affects the brain and nervous system causing behavior problems, poor judgment, and accidents; destroying brain cells which are not replaceable; and impairing memory.

* Has a devastating effect on the lives of those addicted as well as their families.

* Interacts with other drugs, amplifying some and impairing others.

* Irritates the gastrointestinal system, causing problems with the esophagus, stomach, and intestines. These problems can include poor absorption of nutrients and food, including lactose intolerance.

* Damages the liver and pancreas and depresses the immune system.

* Is associated with high blood pressure, increased pulse rate, increased blood triglycerides, and heart disease.

* Contributes to the *Candida*-related complex by encouraging the growth of yeast in the body.

* Contributes to osteoporosis because of its diuretic effects which increase urine production and mineral and vitamin depletion.

* Is linked with an increased risk of developing cancer.

* Causes fetal alcohol syndrome during pregnancy which can cause a baby to be mentally retarded or have various physical defects.

Alcohol-Containing Products

All alcoholic beverages including beer, liquor, liqueurs, wine, and wine-coolers
Many vanilla and other flavoring extracts
Non-stick cooking sprays
Tamari soy sauce with alcohol added
Shoyu soy sauce with alcohol added
Mouthwashes

---

*Studies have shown that cooking does not evaporate all alcohol in food. Therefore, all products listed above should be totally eliminated on the **Perfect Whole Foods** diet.*

If you want to improve your health, totally eliminate alcohol while on the ***Perfect Whole Foods*** diet. *Note*: If you have a physical addiction to alcohol, please seek help from a qualified health professional.

Why Should I Eliminate Caffeine?

Many people resist when they learn they must stop drinking coffee on the perfect diet. Caffeine, the drug (yes, drug) present in coffee, is very habit-forming or addictive in that it causes both psychological and physical dependence. The body gets used to having it and develops uncomfortable symptoms when it isn't available. Headaches are the most frequent symptom of caffeine withdrawal.

When you drink coffee, tea, or colas to get a lift, you may be actually getting more than you bargained for. The lift comes from adrenalin and other stress hormones which cause the release of glycogen (sugar) stored in the liver. This glycogen then causes the pancreas to produce insulin. The resulting insulin, in some people, makes the blood sugar drop to levels lower than it was originally, and you, therefore, become tired and in need of another lift. Another cup of coffee or coke then makes you feel better—again temporarily.

Caffeine is a stimulant that affects many parts of the body. Caffeine influences the heart and the central nervous system, digestive, endocrine, reproductive, and respiratory systems. Here are several other specific ways in which caffeine affects the body:

• Headaches are caused both by the caffeine itself and by withdrawal when addicted. The central nervous system may also be affected by feelings of anxiety, panic attacks, sleeping problems, nervousness, muscle twitching, lack of balance, poor memory, and tremor.

• Caffeine increases the secretion of stomach acid which contributes to heartburn and digestive upset and can aggravate ulcers. It also causes a decreased absorption of iron.

• Caffeine belongs to a class of compounds called methylxanthines (also theophylline in tea and theobromide in chocolate). These compounds have been linked to fibrocystic breast disease in women and prostate problems in men. Caffeine affects hormonal balance in women, contributing to menstrual cramps, premenstrual water retention, PMS, and, in some cases, infertility. Caffeine affects a baby before birth and, after birth, through mother's milk.

• Caffeine, other methylxanthines, and chemicals called purines present in some other foods are converted into uric acid in the body. Uric acid causes gout which is a form of painful arthritis. Caffeine also interferes with the laboratory testing of uric acid so that gout is not properly diagnosed.

• Because of its diuretic effects, caffeine increases urine production, depleting the body of water, B-vitamins, vitamin C, and certain minerals (calcium, zinc, magnesium, potassium, and iron). Because they act as diuretics, coffee, tea, and colas do not quench thirst, but actually remove more water than was originally in the tissues. A loss of calcium and other minerals is a contributing factor in osteoporosis.

• Caffeine's impact on the cardiovascular system includes influences on the heart rate, heart rhythm, blood vessel diameter, blood cholesterol, and blood pressure. Some people have heart palpitations as a result of caffeine.

• Behavior problems in children can be caused by even small amounts of caffeine. It has been calculated that the caffeine in one soft drink for a young child is equal to four cups of coffee for an adult. Most parents wouldn't consider giving a child four cups of coffee, yet they think nothing of giving him or her a soft drink with caffeine (plus sugar and phosphates).

Eliminating caffeine from your diet is another step to better health. Withdrawal symptoms may occur, especially if you have been consuming caffeine regularly and in moderate to large amounts. Symptoms can include headaches, fatigue, depression, irritability, fuzzy thinking, nausea, vomiting, and runny nose, and they often last three or four days. If you do experience withdrawal symptoms, realize that they are indicators that caffeine has been adversely affecting your body and its health.

Caffeine-Containing Products

Coffee, regular and decaffeinated
Tea, black and green (regular and decaffeinated) including Assam, Darjeeling, Keemun, Lapsong Souchong, Formosa, Earl Grey, English Breakfast, Orange Pekoe, and Oolong tea
Herb teas that contain caffeine including Guarana, Yopo, Morning Thunder, New Brazilian Breakfast, Mate (or yerba mate or Paraguay tea), and Cassina (or yaupon, Christmas berry tree, or North American tea plant)
Macrobiotic bancha, kukicha, and twig teas
Many soft drinks
Chocolate/cocoa and white chocolate
Kola or kola nut (not gotu kola)
Over-the-counter drugs like Dristan, Anacin, and Excedrin

*Even decaffeinated coffee and tea contain a very small amount of caffeine and should be eliminated on the **Perfect Whole Foods** diet.*

Why Should I *Totally* Eliminate Refined Carbohydrates, Alcohol, and Caffeine?

Dr. Stoll, in his medical practice, has found that patients who are *perfect* in their total elimination of refined carbohydrates, alcohol, and caffeine make quick and dramatic health improvements. He says that problems not responding to the diet become much easier to treat medically. Those who are not *perfect* with the diet improve their health but progress is much slower.

To Make Quick and Dramatic Health Improvements

Totally Eliminate	**Avoid**
All sugars	Excessive fat
All refined complex carbohydrates	Hydrogenated fats including margarine
All alcohol	Refined oils
All dried fruit	Dry cereals
All fruit juices*	Most additives
All caffeine	Tap water
Most canned foods	

*Freshly squeezed vegetable juices are okay (limit carrot juice to 1 serving per day of 1 cup); canned tomato juice and V-8 juice are okay to use in cooking, not as beverages.

Totally Eliminate means just that. Become almost fanatic about these foods while you're on the perfect diet. Do not eat any food that you are asked to totally eliminate. When I speak about being *perfect* with the diet, the *Totally Eliminate* list of foods are the ones to which I'm referring.

Avoid means to try to refrain from these. Although for one reason or another these foods are not health-promoting, their occasional inclusion in your diet will not stop progress of the ***Perfect Whole Foods*** diet.

The *Perfect Whole Foods* diet stabilizes your blood sugar. That's why it's so helpful if you have diabetes or hypoglycemia or are overweight, suffer from fatigue, or other symptoms of unstable blood sugar. If your health needs improving, if you'd like to feel better and have more energy, then try the diet. It can definitely help!

An Important Note

If you are diabetic or if you have been eating a typical American diet consisting of excessive amounts of sugar, white flour, caffeine, or alcohol, it is critical that you begin the *Perfect Whole Foods* diet only under the direction of a physician who can provide guidance and medical monitoring. Diabetics may have reduced insulin requirements. A sudden, total elimination of refined carbohydrates may result in withdrawal symptoms.

If you are making changes in your diet without a physician's supervision, I suggest that you move in the direction of the perfect diet by making gradual diet improvements. Do not eliminate refined carbohydrates, caffeine, and alcohol all at once because of the withdrawal symptoms you may experience. How long you take to make these diet improvements varies from person to person.

Why Should I Avoid Margarine?

TV and magazine commercials expounding how margarine is less saturated than butter have led us to believe that margarine is a healthier choice than butter; likewise, health and nutrition books encourage us to use margarine. Margarine *does* contain less saturated fat than butter, but consider the following reasons to avoid it (as well as shortening and commercially refined oils).

Margarine, Shortening, and Commercially Refined Oils Are

Sources of pesticide residues
Sources of chemical solvent residues (not present in expeller-pressed oils)
Sources of toxic trans-fatty acids* and other damaged or altered fat products
Sources of toxic free-radicals**
Lacking in health-promoting lecithin, vitamin E, chlorophyll, beta carotene, and minerals naturally present in the food source from which the product is made as a result of degumming, alkali refining, bleaching, deodorizing, and winterizing***
Sources of toxic forms of nickel if the product is hydrogenated or partially hydrogenated
Sources of unnatural antioxidants (BHT, BHA, TBHQ)
Sources of antifoaming agents

Trans-fatty acids are twisted fatty acids that do not function as their normal form. Trans-fats are formed during hydrogenation and are associated with heart disease and other diseases.

**Free radicals are highly unstable particles, produced or present in fats. They can initiate chain reactions at the cellular level that lead to abnormal biochemical functions, toxicity, and ultimately aging, cancer, heart disease, and other diseases.*

***Degumming, alkali refining, bleaching, deodorizing, and winterizing are complex steps that refined oils go through, taking 3 to 4 hours and involving temperatures over 500° F.*

Margarine, shortening, and commercially refined oils are equivalent to white flour and sugar in that they provide none of the co-factors (vitamins, minerals, and sulfur-containing amino acids) needed for their own metabolism and therefore rob the body of essential nutrients. The major difference between commercially refined oils (available from grocery stores) and expeller-pressed oils (available in natural foods stores and co-ops) is that the expeller-pressed oils are mechanically pressed and, therefore, do not have the chemical solvent residues. Both oils are refined, lacking in essential nutrients, and are sources of free radicals, trans-fatty acids, and other altered fats.

Terms for Hydrogenated Fat or Oil

Hydrogenated oil	Pure vegetable shortening
Margarine	Shortening
Partially-hydrogenated oil	Vegetable shortening

Sometimes a label boasts cholesterol-free *to get your attention and make you think that it's a good product. Always consider the* type *and* amount *of fat in a product, not simply whether or not it contains cholesterol. (Remember, only animal products contain cholesterol.) Try to avoid products with any of the ingredients listed above.*

What Can I Eat?

You may have the idea by now that there's not much to eat on this diet. That absolutely isn't so. There are hundreds of foods to eat and enjoy. Up to now, I have stressed the negative to impress upon you the importance of eliminating refined carbohydrates, alcohol, and caffeine. It's now time to move on to the positive. To give you some idea of what you can eat, I will list some typical foods. You might want to use this list to help you get started. I'll tell you how to prepare these foods, as well as many others, throughout the book.

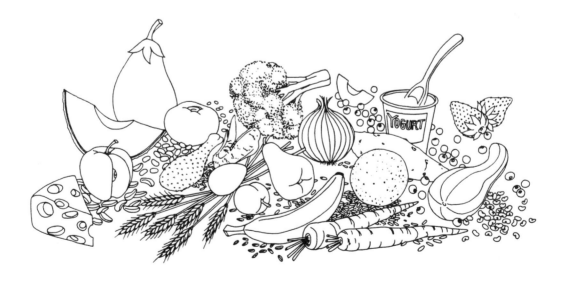

Typical Foods to Eat on the *Perfect Whole Foods* Diet

Vegetables: all kinds if fresh or frozen, raw or cooked; includes broccoli, carrots, celery, corn, mushrooms, parsley, spinach, tomatoes, lettuce, cauliflower, kale, onions, garlic, squash, peas, beets, and potatoes including the skin; organically grown when possible

Whole grains: includes brown rice, rolled oats (oatmeal), oat bran, millet, hulled barley, popcorn, whole corn grits, whole cornmeal, whole wheat flour, and unsweetened 100% whole grain bread and crackers; organically grown when possible

Beans: includes dried beans and peas (like pintos, navy beans, split peas, lentils, and black beans), tofu, and tempeh; organically grown when possible

Nuts and seeds: fresh, never rancid; includes natural peanut butter, almond butter, cashew butter, tahini, raw or plain roasted nuts and seeds like almonds, walnuts, pecans, pumpkin seeds, sesame seeds, and sunflower seeds; organically grown when available

Beverages: spring water, peppermint tea, camomile tea, ginger tea

Meat, fish, poultry: includes unbreaded fish, canned tuna in spring water, unbreaded and skinned chicken, fresh turkey, and lean beef; organically raised when available

Dairy products: plain, nonfat or low fat yogurt; skim milk or low fat milk; natural cheeses (like Colby, cheddar, and Mozzarella); and nonfat dry milk; organic when possible

Fruit: all whole fruit if fresh or frozen without sugar; organically grown when possible; avoid during *Candida* treatment

Eggs: farm eggs; organic when possible

Fats: unrefined oils and butter; organic when possible

Condiments and seasonings: fresh and dried herbs and spices, apple cider vinegar, mineral salt, unsweetened canned tomato products, carob powder, and baking yeast and baking soda for leavening; all organically grown when available

---

How Long Do I Stay on the *Perfect Whole Foods* Diet?

Most people see significant improvement in their health when they follow the perfect diet. They are amazed when symptoms that have been around for years disappear. They feel more energetic and have an increasing sense of well-being. Most people are, however, eager to liberalize their diet. It is important that you stay on the **Perfect Whole Foods** diet as long as you continue to notice an improvement in how you feel (usually 3 to 6 months). Then, with your doctor's approval, try the following test.

Test to Determine If You Are Ready to Liberalize Your Diet

Eat one bite of something containing just a little refined carbohydrate—for example, whole wheat bread sweetened with honey or molasses—just one bite! If you have a return of a previous symptom or simply don't feel well after the test, you know that you're not ready to liberalize. If you mistakenly eat something containing a refined carbohydrate and are not ready to liberalize, you will get the same reaction.

*Don't try this test until you have been on the **Perfect Whole Foods** diet at least three months (6 months if you are being treated for* Candida*) since it will slow progress if you're not ready to liberalize.*

In most cases, your body becomes super-sensitive to refined foods when you first totally eliminate them from your diet—so sensitive that if you do eat a small amount of sugar, refined complex carbohydrate, alcohol, or caffeine, you are likely to have a return of one or more of your symptoms. After you have been on the perfect diet for 3 to 6 months, the sensitivity will disappear. Your health will have improved so that you're able to eat refined foods occasionally without provoking symptoms. Since re-contact with refined foods during the sensitivity period slows progress, it's important to be patient and remain on the perfect diet long enough.

What If I Don't Feel Better on the Perfect Diet?

The *Perfect Whole Foods* diet is meant to help you get immediate results. Within a week to ten days of starting the diet (after withdrawal symptoms subside), most people notice a dramatic improvement in how they feel. If you do not experience this improvement, one or more of these may be possible:

- You have not *totally* eliminated refined carbohydrates. Check your diet carefully to determine if this is the case.

- You should also eliminate several sources of carbohydrates to which you could be reacting, including all fruit, bee pollen, bee propolis, commercially canned products that include distilled vinegar (like sugar-free mayonnaise and pickles), products made with koji starter (like miso and tempeh), naturally fermented products that could have trace amounts of alcohol (all tamari and shoyu, not just those with alcohol added), alcohol-free vanilla which could have trace amounts of alcohol, as well as any other food sources of glycerin as listed on the ingredient list.

- You may be allergic or sensitive to one or more foods you are eating or to chemicals in your environment. This is more difficult to determine and resolve. Read about **If You Have Food Allergies** (p. 317) and **If You Have Food Sensitivities** (p. 323) and check with your doctor about possible allergy testing. You may also have *Candidiasis* and need treatment for that (see **If You Have Candidiasis** in the **Appendix A** for a diet during treatment).

- You may have a medical problem that requires additional treatment. Please talk to your doctor.

How Do I Liberalize?

By liberalizing your diet, I'm not suggesting that you go for a banana split or a piece of chocolate cake or return to white bread and jelly. Liberalizing your diet means that you don't have to be 100 percent perfect with your diet. You don't have to read the fine print on *all* labels. Most of your food, however, should continue to be whole, natural, and unrefined.

When you begin liberalizing, it's easy to gradually drift from your whole foods diet: a switch to whole grain bread with honey...then to part whole wheat—part white flour bread...dressings with sweeteners...cereal with a little sugar in it...a cup of coffee here and there...just one ice cream cone...fast food hamburger, french fries, and catsup...canned vegetables tonight...a donut...Aunt Mary's birthday cake...your birthday cake...Fourth of July celebration...vacation splurge...Labor Day picnic...Thanksgiving feast...Christmas parties...New Year's Eve party...that special wedding reception...then...*I really don't know why I'm not feeling as well as I have been.*

If you suddenly or gradually return to your former eating habits, you will gradually lose all the health benefits you had gained while on the **Perfect Whole Foods** diet. Poor health or simply not feeling well is often a motivating factor to make lifestyle changes. Once that feeling of well-being returns, sometimes it's easy to forget what helped you feel better. That's human nature. If you return to your former lifestyle, to the same things that contributed to the illness in the first place, your health will suffer. Be on guard against this.

If you stray too far from the diet and begin to have symptoms, return to the perfect diet for a while and learn from your experience. Don't drift far from whole foods in the future.

I have found that by being on the perfect diet almost totally at home but not when I go out to eat, I'm not tempted to stray too far from whole foods. This won't work, however, if you go out to eat daily or even several times a week. I've also found, from working with patients on the diet, that because of individual differences, some can liberalize a little more than others. You must find out what's right for you.

Those who maintain a healthy lifestyle (including regular exercise and some kind of stress management technique), further improve their health. Those people are usually better able to liberalize their diet and maintain that super-healthy feeling.

GETTING STARTED

I've found that many people who need to make improvements in their diet have few kitchen skills. Use this portion of the book as a reference for practical information about kitchen equipment, food storage, label reading, menu planning, saving time, and avoiding toxic chemicals around the house.

An Encouraging Word

This section is written for you if you are starting the *Perfect Whole Foods* diet. If you've read the book up to this point, you may be discouraged. The diet may seem difficult, perhaps even impossible, to follow.

In the beginning, it does seem to be overwhelming, especially if you eat a poor diet, eat out a lot, really don't know how to cook, and don't feel very well either.

Whenever you make a change in your lifestyle, it is stressful until you know what you're doing. That's the case here. If you read this book thoroughly, relax, and maintain a positive attitude, you'll do fine. In a couple of weeks, you'll wonder why you were so concerned.

Let me mention one problem you may have and let you know that it's common. Other people, including friends and relatives, may try to influence you. Some will not understand why you're being so strict—even if you explain it to them. They might not intentionally try to get you off your diet, but they won't feel it's that important. Others will try to get you to go off—or to go to your limits. Be firm with them, but polite, about your diet. It is your choice to follow the diet and improve your health, and you have ultimate control over what you choose to eat.

Don't force your family or friends into following the perfect diet. You might encourage them to sample some of your food, but don't insist. A person must be ready to make diet changes or any lifestyle change. Unfortunately, that readiness often hinges on an illness. Some people will silently observe your progress and want to know more. Those who are curious will ask you questions. Forcing the issue on those not ready will turn them off.

It might be comforting to know that you won't be on the *Perfect Whole Foods* diet forever. The length of time is an individual matter. Stress management, regular exercise, and nutritional supplements, all based on your needs, will help you improve your health more quickly. Also, the better you adhere to the perfect diet or the more nearly perfect you are, the sooner you should be able to liberalize. Just knowing that you'll be able to add some foods to your diet later should make it easier to keep a positive outlook.

Don't, however, make the mistake of going back to your former poor eating habits when you are ready to liberalize. If you do, the benefits you accomplish will gradually vanish and your health will suffer. I have known a number of people who have returned to their old habits; their original symptoms returned. The liberal diet is meant to be a whole foods diet without the strict elimination of all traces of refined foods. How much you will be able to liberalize varies from person to person.

Equipping the Kitchen

The whole foods kitchen may be equipped simply with a few basic pans, an iron or *SilverStone* skillet, a steaming basket, a couple of good sharp knives, pot holders, some measuring cups and spoons, and a tempered glass cutting board (not plastic or wooden). Or, it may be more elaborate and also include such things as a food processor, slow cooker, hot-air popcorn popper, electric mixer, bread machine, pressure cooker, blender, wok, and grain grinder.

When Equipping the Whole Foods Kitchen, Remember These Principles

• Avoid equipment which may be harmful to you or the food you are going to eat.
• Select as many time-saving devices as your budget will allow and you will use.

Following the first principle, you should avoid pans made of toxic metals. Many people use aluminum pans because of their relatively inexpensive cost. Aluminum is, however, a toxic metal that can leach into your food, especially when cooking an acid ingredient like tomato sauce. Copper pans, too, should be avoided if food will touch the copper.

So, if aluminum and copper pans are to be avoided, what kind of pans should be used? Stainless steel, which doesn't react with food, is a good material for pans. Since it is a poor conductor of heat, better stainless steel pans have some other metal sandwiched or clad to the bottom, outside of the pan. These metals, often copper or aluminum, are fine used this way since they don't come into contact with food.

Cast iron is another good material. Although it does react with acid foods, the reaction is beneficial since iron salts are formed that the body can use. Cast iron skillets are generally less expensive than other good cookware. When buying cast iron, make certain a plastic coating has not been applied to the surface. Although the coating will keep the skillet from rusting, you'll be getting plastic in your food.

New cast iron cookware must be seasoned before using. To do this, generously oil the inside and bake it in the oven at a low temperature for several hours. Remove excess oil with a paper towel before using. Do not scour cast iron with a soap pad or you will need to season it again. Also don't use soap or detergent on it. To prevent rusting, dry cast iron thoroughly after washing by placing it either on a heated burner for a few seconds or in a warm oven for a few minutes.

SilverStone is a another good choice for cooking, especially for low-fat cooking. It must be handled properly to keep it safe and in good condition. Do not leave an empty pan on a hot stove since potentially dangerous fumes may be given off when *SilverStone* is heated to very high temperatures. The coating is nonreactive in the body, but to protect your *SilverStone* pans, use plastic spatulas and spoons for stirring since *SilverStone* is easily scratched with metal. *Pyrex* and *Corning Ware* are other good selections for cookware.

The question of microwave oven safety often comes up when whole foods are being discussed. The dangers of microwave emissions are recognized by scientists, some of whom believe that our government's standard for safe emissions is too lenient. The former Soviet Union standard is 1000 times stricter than ours. There is also the belief that microwave ovens may harm the food. Although studies have shown that the nutritional quality of food is not affected by microwaves, long-term testing of the effects of eating microwaved food has not been adequately carried out. Since the perfect diet encourages only health-promoting foods and cooking techniques, microwaved foods should used very little until more testing has been done.

If you like the convenience of reheating foods in the microwave, try instead heating stews and grains in the top of a double boiler. Although it is not as fast as a microwave oven, if you allow time while you are preparing your vegetables, the stew or grain will be ready when you are. Food will not stick to the pan if you oil it first with a little *Oil-Lecithin Combination* (p. 205).

The second principle in equipping a whole foods kitchen concerns time-saving devices. Select and buy them gradually as your budget allows. Such equipment as a slow cooker, food processor, or hand blender makes an excellent birthday or holiday gift. Because they are rather expensive and take extra space in the kitchen, be selective. An unused slow cooker will only take up space, and it won't save you time.

Smaller, less expensive gadgets and equipment that you may want to consider buying include a cheese cutter, hand-held grater, garlic press, tongs, a pancake turner, heat-resistant plastic stirring spoons, soup ladle, a colander, mixing bowls, cookie sheets, bread pans, and muffin tins.

Equipment Facts

Blender: Of all the kitchen equipment I own, I use my blender least of all. I don't recommend that you buy one, but if you already have a blender, you can use it to purée soups, make dressings and mayonnaise, and prepare *Overnight Blender Pancakes* batter (p. 232). Don't try using it to prepare thick dishes that call for a food processor unless the recipe also recommends a blender. Heavy dips like *Creamy Spinach Dip* (p. 260) and *Mexican Bean Dip* (p. 114) can overheat the motor of a blender. Read about the more versatile food processor in this section.

Bread Machine: A machine that will prepare bread dough, allow it to rise, and bake, all in one pan. These are excellent for those on the ***Perfect Whole Foods*** diet who don't have access to commercially baked unsweetened 100% whole grain bread. Before buying such a machine, make certain it can handle the heaviness of all whole grain flour by checking in the recipe booklet that accompanies the machine or by calling the company. (See recipe for *Whole Wheat Machine Bread (Unsweetened, 100% Whole Grain)* on page 210).

Champion Juicer: A vegetable/fruit juicer that will not only extract juice but will also, with proper attachments, make nut butters and frozen desserts. Fresh vegetable juices are used on the *Perfect Whole Foods* diet, but fruit juices should be eliminated. For a delicious frozen dessert made from bananas with a *Champion Juicer*, see the recipe for *Banana Ice Cream* on page 277.

Double Boiler: A set of two pans, one fitting inside the other. The contents of the upper pan is cooked or heated by boiling water in the lower pan. The water in the lower pan should not touch the upper pan. A double boiler is often used to cook *Whole Grain Corn Grits* (p. 131). It is also useful for heating leftovers that are thick and would stick if heated in a regular pan.

Foley Food Mill: A utensil with which you can manually puree cooked foods.

Food Processor: An appliance I couldn't be without. I use it often for shredding carrots for salads, chopping cabbage and other vegetables for slaw, shredding cheese, puréeing soups, making bread or cracker crumbs, and making pecan butter.

Hand Blender: A portable blender for puréeing cream soups and making salad dressings.

Hand-Cranked Grain Flaker: Another favorite appliance, although difficult to find in stores. I flake whole grains as needed and either cook them like oatmeal or soak them briefly for nutritious, delicious, and economical breakfasts. Call *HealthWays Nutrition* at (800) 870-5378 or (606) 223-2270 for information on ordering this unique appliance.

Seed and Nut Grinder: Since tiny seeds like flax are hard to chew and are, therefore, usually swallowed whole, they mostly pass through the intestinal tract without being digested. Grinding a large amount at a time in a blender or food processor is not recommended since the oil gets rancid quickly. A seed and nut grinder allows you to grind small amounts of flax and other seeds or nuts so the body can utilize their essential fatty acids.

Steaming Basket: An adjustable basket made of stainless steel that is used for cooking vegetables over boiling water rather than in water. Steaming baskets are also used for warming cooked foods like brown rice that would stick if heated in a pan.

Vita Mix: An appliance that will grind wheat berries and make bread dough for one loaf of bread, all in a few minutes. The bread is then shaped by hand, allowed to rise, and baked in an oven. Although it is expensive, if you don't have access to fresh, unsweetened whole grain breads, you might want to consider getting a *Vita Mix* or a bread machine. See recipe for *Whole Wheat Vita Mix Bread (Unsweetened, 100% Whole Grain)* on page 211. Don't buy a *Vita Mix* for the purpose of making fresh juice since this appliance makes vegetable purée rather than juice. Most recipes call for a liquid base like apple juice, orange juice, or fresh tomatoes for adding a small amount of vegetables such as carrots and celery. With fruit juice not used on the perfect diet and good fresh tomatoes available only in the summer, the purée would be usable only in the summer. (Canned tomatoes should not be used in quantity on the perfect diet.)

Water Purifier: A reverse osmosis water purifier is recommended if you want to purify your water rather than buy spring water.

Suggested Grocery List for the Beginner

Grains
Brown rice (long grain)
Rolled oats (oatmeal)
Hulled barley (for *Vegetable Barley Soup* on page 186)
Whole wheat spaghetti (or spelt or brown rice)
Whole wheat flour (pastry and hard varieties)
Whole cornmeal

Dried Beans
Pinto
Navy
Lentils

Beverages
Spring water
Camomile tea bags
Peppermint tea bags

Flavorings
Mineral salt or sea salt (not if iodized)
Lemon oil
Alcohol-free vanilla flavoring
Salsa (check ingredient list to eliminate sugar)
Raw apple cider vinegar
Tamari or shoyu sauce (make certain it doesn't have alcohol as an ingredient)

Nut Butters
Natural peanut butter
Natural almond or cashew butter

Oils
Extra virgin olive oil
Unrefined sesame oil

Dairy
Skim milk for cooking
Plain, nonfat yogurt (check ingredient list to eliminate those with whey, tapioca, sugar, or other refined carbohydrates)

If you're just going on the **Perfect Whole Foods** *diet and haven't had a chance to study this book, then use the list above to help you get started. Pay close attention to ingredient lists when selecting processed foods. Also buy a good variety of fresh fruit (unless you are being treated for* Candida*), fresh vegetables, and, if desired, some lean meat, poultry, and fish.*

Shopping for Groceries

If you've looked through the recipes, you may be wondering where you are going to find some of the unusual sounding foods like unrefined or expeller-pressed oils, mineral salt, tamari or shoyu, dulse, spelt, quinoa, and amaranth.

A natural foods co-op or grocery is the best place to do most of your grocery shopping. Health food stores and health food sections of grocery stores are also fine if they have a good supply of unprocessed foods. Wherever you shop, make certain that the turnover of products is fast so the food will be fresh and, therefore, more nutritious.

If you don't know where the nearest food co-op, natural foods grocery, or health food store is, check the yellow pages of your phone book or the phone book of a near-by larger city if you live in a small town. Look under *health food*. If you can't find a listing in the phone book, then call a local chiropractor or massage therapist for help. The larger the store you find, the greater the variety of foods from which you'll have to choose.

Those who live in the Central Kentucky area are fortunate to be able to shop at Good Foods Co-op in Lexington. The staff is always willing to help you. If you can find a friendly store like this one, you'll soon feel at home. Having a good place to shop can help make your whole foods experience a positive one from the start.

Other places to do some of your shopping include grocery stores, whole grain bakeries, produce stands, farmers' markets, and local farmers.

Reading Labels

Whether or not you are following the **Perfect Whole Foods** diet, it's important to get into the habit of reading food labels. To make wise food choices, you must know what you are buying. Keep in mind these facts about label reading:

• The list of ingredients on a label is given in the descending order by weight. In other words, the product contains more of the first ingredient than the second, and so on.

• Sometimes several similar ingredients are used in a product. If they were combined as one ingredient, they would be listed first or second. For example, when corn syrup, sugar, and honey are used in a cereal, the individual sugars are listed toward the end of the ingredient list. Manufacturers sometimes deliberately do this so the consumer won't realize how much sugar is in a product.

- Some foods do not have their ingredients listed on the label because they have a *standard of identity* set by the FDA. The manufacturer may list some of the ingredients, but not necessarily *all* of the ingredients. Foods that have the standard of identity include dairy products, frozen desserts, bread, flour, macaroni, cocoa, salad dressings, canned fruit, and canned vegetables.

- Beware of such words as *natural* and *pure* on labels. Sugar and white flour are considered natural and pure by manufacturers. Many times *no sugar added* products have honey or sorbitol in them. Pay close attention to ingredient lists.

- Words such as *enriched* or *fortified* are guarantees that a grain product is refined. These terms refer to the few nutrients added to a grain after the germ and bran have been removed. Enrichment adds nutrients, usually just four, that were originally in the food, but not necessarily in as great a quantity. Fortification adds vitamins and minerals which were not originally in the food or were present in much lower amounts.

- If a grain used in a product is *whole* rather than refined, the ingredient list must specify *whole* wheat, *whole* rye, *brown* rice, or *whole* or *hulled* barley rather than simply wheat, rye, rice, or barley or pearled barley. An exception to this rule concerns corn. Read specifically about corn under **Whole Grain and Cereal Facts** on page 123.

- Do not let the name of the product influence your purchase. Read the ingredient list for the facts. For example, breads and crackers may include *whole rye* or *whole wheat* in the name yet include some refined flour.

- *Lite* and *light* products are not necessarily better than regular products. Canned tuna in spring water, for example, is much lower in fat than the *lite* tuna which has less oil than tuna in oil, but does contain added oil. Don't reach for a *light* product without reading the labels carefully. Some *lite* dressings have sugar added where there is none in the regular dressing.

- Read the ingredient lists on labels in health food stores and food co-ops as well as in grocery stores. Don't assume a product is without refined flour or sugar just because it's found at a health food store. I've noticed that many of the candies at health food stores have sugar as their first ingredient. Yet people often buy it, thinking they're getting something better than grocery store candy.

- Read the ingredient lists on all products even if you do not think it would have sugar in it. Products that often have sugar include frozen turkeys and turkey breasts, roast beef and turkey from the deli, sausage, bacon, hot dogs, and ham.

- Read ingredient lists on familiar products. Products change. Don't assume that just because a product is acceptable today it won't have an objectionable ingredient in the future. Examples of products which have changed recently include *Ragu* Homestyle Spaghetti Sauce and *Louis Rich* Breakfast Turkey Sausage. These two products were originally okay for the *Perfect Whole Foods* diet—until sugar was added.

Selecting and Using Fats and Oils

If you are just beginning the **Perfect Whole Foods** diet and have been eating fats like margarine, shortening, fried foods, and vegetable oil, you might, for now, want to switch from margarine to *butter* and buy some *unrefined sesame oil* and *unrefined safflower oil* to use in place of the shortening and vegetable oils you're currently using. Study this section thoroughly when you are comfortable with your new diet. Although the material presented here is important in making health improvements, I don't want to overwhelm you with too much new information. On the perfect diet, it's not necessary to be absolutely perfect all of the time in choosing the best fats and oils as it is in eliminating refined sugars, refined complex carbohydrates, alcohol, and caffeine.

Even though I just advised you to use butter instead of margarine, I want to clarify that advice. Although butter is a natural product that's been used for thousands of years, nutritionally it has its faults. Butter is a food that's high in calories, total fat, and saturated fat; it lacks the essential fatty acids (read on for the discussion of essential fatty acids). Butter should, therefore, be used in small amounts only. If you need to follow the **Very Low Fat Diet** (p. 342) or restrict saturated fats, then there's definitely no room for butter in your diet.

Don't buy vegetables oils sold in supermarkets (oils like *Mazola, Puritan,* and *Crisco*) if you are on the **Perfect Whole Foods** diet. When possible, also avoid oils labeled as *expeller-pressed.* The only difference between oils sold in supermarkets and expeller-pressed (previously called cold-pressed) oils from natural food stores is that the supermarket oil is chemically expressed while the expeller-pressed oil is mechanically pressed. Both are further processed or *refined.* Refining removes health-promoting lecithin, vitamin E, chlorophyll, beta carotene, and minerals naturally present in the food source from which the product is made, adds undesirable chemicals, and uses very high temperatures. Refined oils, whether they are chemically or mechanically extracted, are undesirable. Try to avoid commercial products made with either of the two types of refined oils. (There are a few products like sugar-free mayonnaise and dressings that you can use occasionally, but don't get in the habit of using them often since they are high in total fat and are not made of the best oils.) Use *unrefined oils* for most of your cooking.

In an attempt to lose weight, lower blood cholesterol, and improve health, don't become obsessed with avoiding all fats unless you are temporarily on the **Very Low Fat Diet.** While it's true that we should eliminate much fat, our body needs some to be healthy. It's especially important that you not severely restrict the fat intake of infants and children under two years old since they need a variety of fats for proper growth and development. Low fat and nonfat milk products are not appropriate for young children. Neither are fried foods and margarine which provide too much highly processed fat.

Good fats provide *essential fatty acids.* These fatty acids are necessary because the body cannot make them; they must be provided in food (or supplements) to maintain good health. Unfortunately, the bad fats are much more plentiful in the typical American diet: rancid or old fats, most commercially-processed fat products, and saturated animal fats. These fats should be avoided or limited (see the two lists that follow).

Avoid These Fats

Margarine (contains partially-hydrogenated oil)
Shortening (contains hydrogenated oils)
Partially hydrogenated oils
Refined vegetable oils (are highly refined, chemically-extracted oils that lack health-promoting lecithin, vitamin E, chlorophyll, beta carotene, and minerals naturally present in the food source from which the product is made)*
Fried foods (high temperature frying causes destruction of the oil)
Saturated tropical oils (palm, palm kernel, and coconut oils)
Old nuts, seeds, oils, grains, or other fatty foods (contain rancid oil)
Shelled nuts, seeds, oils, grains, or other high fat foods stored improperly (should be stored in the refrigerator and away from oxygen)
Poultry fat and skin (contain highly saturated fats)

Although the perfect diet permits occasional refined oils in a few convenience products, less is better!

The fats in the preceding list (other than poultry fat and skin which are saturated animal fats) have undergone chemical changes so that, even if their original sources provided essential fatty acids, they no longer do. In fact, eating these fats (as well as sugar, refined complex carbohydrates, caffeine, and alcohol) interferes with the ability of essential fatty acids to function properly in the body.

Limit These Fats

Saturated Animal Fats
Beef, pork, and lamb (buy the leanest cuts)
Dairy fat: butter, sour cream, whole milk, cheese (buy certain nonfat and low fat dairy products)
Chicken and turkey products with 15% or more fat by weight (this includes most commercial turkey sausage, ground turkey, turkey and chicken hot dogs—select leaner products)

*Eliminate most or all of these saturated animal fats if you are on the **Very Low Fat Diet** (p. 342) or if you choose a vegetarian diet.*

The two essential fatty acids are *linolenic acid* (an Omega-3 fat) and *linoleic acid* (an Omega-6 fat). To avoid confusion since these two words are so similar, I'll refer to them with their Omega number. Note that there are other forms of Omega-3 and Omega-6 fats, but I won't be discussing them. Although neither of these two fatty acids can be produced in the body, our food supply typically provides more linoleic acid (Omega-6) than linolenic (Omega-3). You'll see why when you read the list of sources on page 47. Medical scientists recognize that these essential fats are vital to good health. Be certain to include sources of each in your diet every day.

Insufficient essential fatty acids in the diet create a variety of problems. Your body needs essential fatty acids for maintaining the membranes of every cell and for making hormone-like substances called prostaglandins. A lack can contribute to heart and skin disorders (from easy bruising, flaking skin and dandruff to sun sensitivity), arthritis, allergies, obesity, behavior problems (from moodiness and anxiety to depression and hallucinations), digestive and immune system disorders, premenstrual syndrome, toxemia of pregnancy, plus many other problems. Several factors determine exactly how much we need, including age, weight, genetic background, and present diet. The typical high fat American diet composed of white flour, white sugar, beef, and hydrogenated fats (margarine, shortening, and oils) contains almost no essential fatty acids. Their shortage contributes to the many medical problems common today.

Our typical food supply provides a shortage of essential fatty acids for a variety of reasons. A major reason is that food manufacturers process vegetable oils so they won't become rancid so easily. (The hydrogenation process began its large-scale use in the 1930's and was developed to provide a less expensive alternative to butter and lard.) Refining and hydrogenating oils do indeed extend the shelf life of these products but they also destroy the essential fatty acids naturally present in the food source of the oil. A second reason for our lack of essential fatty acids is that when whole grains are refined, essential fatty acids as well as many other nutrients are removed. Note that refined grains (with the germ and bran removed) produce products with a longer shelf life than products made of whole grains since it's the essential fatty acids in whole grains that turn rancid. And finally, commercially grown beef, poultry, eggs, and dairy products do not provide the essential fatty acids that free-range products do. These free-range products are now the exception rather than the norm as was once the case.

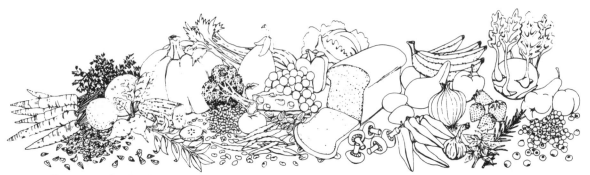

Let go of all anxiety and concern. Be at peace. God is touching, healing, loving, providing for each need in ways that surpass your greatest expectations.   ***Bridget Meehan, SSC, D.Min.***

Foods That Provide Essential Fatty Acids

Linolenic Acid (Omega-3)
Best Sources:
Flaxseed oil or flax oil (when fresh, mechanically-pressed, organic, unrefined, sold in opaque bottles, and refrigerated)
Fish (dark, cold-water, fatty fish especially mackerel, sardines, tuna, trout, cold-water salmon, not farm-raised varieties)

Lesser amounts:
Northern beans such as kidney, navy, pinto, red, soybeans, yankee beans (other beans and peas are nutritious, but not important sources of Omega-3 fatty acids)
Northern nuts such as walnuts, beechnuts, and chestnuts
Raw flax and pumpkin seeds
Whole grains, especially the fresh wheat germ from wheat
Unrefined canola oil*
Farm eggs (if the hens were fed natural grains, seeds, and greens)
Free-range grown beef, turkeys, and chickens (includes grass-fed beef rather than grain-fed)
Full-fat soy products like tofu, tempeh, and soy milk (don't count on soy oil as a source of linolenic acid because the refining process destroys it and unrefined soy oil is not available)
Breast milk (this is just one reason it's better to nurse babies rather than give them formula)

Linoleic Acid (Omega-6)
Whole grains, especially corn
Unrefined corn oil*
Sunflower seeds and unrefined sunflower oil (not the high-oleic variety of oil)
Sesame seeds and unrefined sesame oil*
Soybeans and full-fat soybean products like tofu, tempeh and soy milk (Don't count on refined soy oil as a source of linoleic acid because the processing destroys it. Unrefined soy oil is not available.)
Unrefined canola oil*
Unrefined safflower oil (not the high-oleic variety of oil)*

Because the essential fatty acids are polyunsaturated, they are unstable, become rancid easily, and are therefore easily destroyed, both in storage and in the body. Since Omega-3 is more polyunsaturated than Omega-6, it is more easily destroyed in processing and storage. Proper storage before they are consumed, proper use in cooking, and sufficient antioxidants in the body (like vitamins E and C, beta-carotene, and selenium) are necessary to protect the essential fatty acids. A well-planned whole foods diet (many health professionals also recommend supplements) will provide antioxidants.

*Unfortunately, these oils are not yet available as fresh and unrefined, so select the next best, the kind labelled unrefined.

Characteristics of The Best Oils

Fresh
Unrefined
Mechanically pressed at temperature below 118° F.
Processed in the absence of light
Processed in the absence of oxygen
Organically grown food source
Stored in sealed, dark, nonmetal containers
Refrigerated after sealed container is opened due to the presence of oxygen

---

Fresh flaxseed oil, an excellent source of the essential fatty acids, is currently available processed and sold with these specifications.

If you can't find fresh flaxseed oil processed to the preceding specifications, then ask your co-op or natural foods store buyer about ordering it. If it's not available, then other unrefined oils are considered to be the next best choice and are usually available.

Extra virgin olive oil conforms to many of the specifications of a good oil since it is mechanically pressed, unrefined, and is readily available. Many health and nutrition books encourage us to use it when we use oil. Olive oil is said to be one of the better oils since it helps reduce our blood LDL (low density lipoproteins), the "bad" component that deposits cholesterol in arteries. Olive oil is also good in the sense that it is more stable than most oils (since it is monounsaturated). Olive oil, however, is *not* a good source of the essential fatty acids. Therefore, we should not rely on it as our only source of oil.

Other fat sources that I've not yet discussed include almonds, cashews, pecans, filberts, nut butters, avocados and olives. As with olive oil, these do not provide essential fatty acids. Occasional use of these high fat foods should be fine unless you need to severely lower your fat intake as with the *Very Low Fat Diet* (p. 342).

To keep all fats and oils fresh, it's important to store them properly and use them fairly quickly since any fat can partially decompose or become rancid with time, particularly the polyunsaturated oils. Rancid foods taste and smell bad and are harmful to eat. Some people who have been accustomed to eating rancid foods do not recognize the bad taste.

Store All Foods Rich in Fat

Away from heat (refrigerate)
Away from light (opaque container)
Away from oxygen (airtight container)
Away from metal (nonmetal container)

Use these guidelines to store oils, nuts, seeds, nut butters, and other foods rich in fat. Monounsaturated oils like olive oil will harden in the refrigerator. To use them in their liquid state, simply remove them to room temperature briefly before using.

It's very important to use each kind of oil properly. For example, using flaxseed oil to stir-fry or sauté is not a good idea. Because heat destroys the unstable essential fatty acids, flaxseed oil should only be used raw. Select a monounsaturated or saturated fat for stir-frying and sautéing since these fats are more stable and can withstand moderate heat.

Use These Oils and Fats in Stir-frying and Sautéing

Monounsaturated Oils
Olive oil
Expeller-pressed safflower oil (high-oleic)*
Expeller-pressed sunflower oil (high-oleic)*
Unrefined sesame oil

Saturated Fats
Butter
Ghee

Fats and oils should never be used for high temperature frying or deep-frying since high temperatures create toxic trans-fatty acids.

*These two are the least desirable to use since they have been refined. The high-oleic variety of safflower and sunflower oils are monounsaturated while the regular varieties are polyunsaturated.

Use These Oils in Salad Dressings

Polyunsaturated oils
Unrefined fresh flaxseed oil*
Unrefined safflower oil (regular, not high-oleic)
Unrefined sunflower oil (regular, not high-oleic)

Monounsaturated oils
Unrefined canola oil
Extra virgin olive oil

*Never cook fresh flaxseed oil since cooking destroys fragile linolenic acid (Omega-3).

It's good to use a polyunsaturated oil daily, especially fresh flaxseed oil since it is an excellent source of the harder-to-get essential fatty acid, linolenic acid (Omega 3). When you use flaxseed oil or any polyunsaturated oil, it's very important to have adequate antioxidants like vitamins E and C, beta carotene, and selenium in your whole foods diet or supplements. These antioxidants prevent the fat from becoming rancid in the body. One simple way to help preserve the oil before you use it is to add your own preservative—about 200 units of vitamin E oil to each pint. Vitamin E is available in dropper bottles or in capsules that you can prick with a needle and squeeze into the oil. (Store vitamin E in the refrigerator as you do other oils.)

Uses for Fresh Flaxseed Oils

In salad dressings (see *Dressing a Salad*, p. 187)
On popcorn (p. 131)
Over cooked vegetables (after they are cooked)
On baked potato as a topping
On bread as a spread
In *Sunshine Butter* (p. 258)
With yogurt or cottage cheese

Never cook fresh flaxseed oil.

Use These Oils in Baking

Polyunsaturated Oils
Unrefined safflower oil (regular)
Unrefined sunflower oil (regular)

Monounsaturated
Extra virgin olive oil
Unrefined canola oil
Expeller-pressed safflower oil (high-oleic)*
Expeller-pressed sunflower oil (high-oleic)*

You may use polyunsaturated oils in baking muffins, breads, and cakes since baking raises the internal temperature of a product to only 212° F. Use a monounsaturated oil for baking foods that become crunchy—like Baked Fries (p. 172) and cookies since their surface temperatures are elevated to high temperatures.
*These two are the least desirable to use since they have been refined. The high-oleic variety of safflower and sunflower oils are monounsaturated while the regular varieties are polyunsaturated.

The bottom line, when it comes to oils, is to select the correct oil for what you plan to do with it, store all oils properly, include sources of the essential fatty acids in your diet daily, protect the essential fatty acids with antioxidants, and, as with all high fat foods, use oils in small amounts.

Storing Whole Foods

To keep natural, whole foods fresh and good-tasting, as well as to preserve their nutrients and protect them from becoming rancid, they must be stored properly. Beans, nuts, seeds, dried fruit, grains, and flours should be stored in glass or rigid plastic, airtight containers to keep bugs out. Avoid metal since it may react with the food, speeding rancidity of the natural oils. Plastic and paper bags are okay for storage if you're going to use the food within a day or so, but they will not protect the food from insects for long-term storage. Also, paper absorbs oil from the food and moisture from the air.

In storing foods at room temperature, keep foods away from light and in a dry, cool place, not exceeding 65 or 70 degrees. For safe cold storage, make certain that the temperature in your refrigerator is between 34 and 40 degrees. Your home freezer should be 0 degrees or lower. It's imperative that your refrigerator and freezer containers are air-tight, moisture-proof, and vaporproof in order to maintain good food quality during storage.

If you are like most shoppers and occasionally buy foods that you don't use immediately, keep track of their age. Date the container when you transfer food from bag to jar, using either pen and tape or a china marker. Ideally, foods should be eaten soon after they are harvested. Flour should be used soon after the grain is ground. But since that's not always possible, use the chart on the next page as a guide to food storage.

Keep This in Mind

If in doubt, throw it out!

If there's any question about a food being contaminated, moldy, or rancid, don't eat it.

Please Note: In the chart that follows, when a range of storage time is given, the shorter time is preferred; the longer is maximum. Less is always better since the food will be fresher and provide more nutrients. Foods that don't store well should be purchased in small amounts. Although freezing food prevents its fat from becoming rancid, it also destroys the vitamin E. Nuts and whole grain flours that have been frozen will have less vitamin E than those not frozen. (Storage of fruits and vegetables are discussed separately at the bottom of page 53.)

A merry heart doeth good like a medicine.   *Proverbs 17:22*

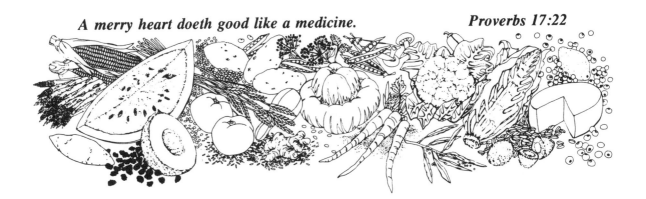

Maximum Storage Times for Whole Foods

FOOD	ROOM TEMPERATURE	REFRIGERATOR	FREEZER
Alfalfa seeds	3-4 months	Longer	
Sprouts	No	4 days	No
Baking powder	1 year		
Baking soda	2 years+		
Barley, hulled	6-12 months	Longer	
Barley malt syrup	1 year	Longer	
Beans, dried	1 year+		
Cooked	No	5 days	2-6 months
Bee pollen	Few weeks	Longer	
Bread	3-5 days	2-3 weeks	3-6 months
Brown rice	2-4 weeks	Longer	
Buckwheat flour	No	Yes	Yes
Groats	Weeks	Months	
Bulgur	1 month	Longer	Longer
Butter	No	Few weeks	6-8 months
Canned goods:			
Unopened	1 year		No
Opened	No	3 days	Yes
Tomato-based	No	5 days	Yes
Carob powder	Months		
Cheese, hard	No	2-4 weeks	4-6 months
Cottage	No	7-10 days	
Chicken, raw	No	1-2 days	6 months
Cooked	No	3-4 days	6 months
Cornmeal	No	Yes	Yes
Eggs, fresh	No	Weeks	If shelled
Eggwhite powder	Several months	Year	
Fish, raw	No	1 day	1-2 months
Cooked	No	1-2 days	Longer
Flour, most whole grain	2-4 weeks	4 months	6-8 months
Fruit, dried	Weeks	Longer	
Gluten flour	3-6 months	Longer	
Grains, raw	Vary	Vary	
Cooked	1 day	5 days	Longer
Herbs, dried	6-12 months	No	
Fresh	While growing	1 week	Longer
Honey	1 year+	No	No
Jam, opened	No	Months	
Lecithin granules	Weeks	Months	
Liquid	Weeks	Months	
Maple syrup	No	Months	
Meat, raw Ground	No	1-2 days	4-6 months
Steaks, roasts	No	3-5 days	9-12 months
Cooked	No	3-4 days	3 months
Cured	No	3-5 days	1-3 months
Milk, fresh	No	1 week	1-4 months
Nonfat dried	6 months	Longer	
Miso		1 year+	
Mustard	Weeks	6-8 months	
Nut butters	Not if opened	8-10 weeks	
Nuts, in shell	1 year+		
Shelled	No	2-4 months	Longer
Oat bran	2-4 weeks	1-2 months	Longer
Oat flour	2-4 weeks	1-2 months	Longer
Oats, rolled	2-4 weeks	1-2 months	Longer

FOOD	ROOM TEMPERATURE	REFRIGERATOR	FREEZER
Oils, fresh flax Walnut/soy/pumpkin Safflower, sunflower, sesame Olive	No 6 mo. (unopened) 9-12 mo (") 2 years (")	6 weeks after opening 1-2 months 2-3 months 6-9 months	Yes No No No
Pasta, whole grain	2-4 weeks	Longer	
Salad dressing	1 yr. (unopened)	2-3 months	No
Salsa, catsup	Not if opened	6 months, opened	
Sea vegetables	1-2 years		
Seeds, unhulled Hulled	1 year No	 2-4 months	
Soy flour Milk powder	No No	Yes Yes	
Spices, most	6-12 months	Cayenne, paprika are best refrigerated.	
Tamari soy sauce	Weeks	Months	
Tempeh	No	2 wks. unopened 4-5 days opened	Months
Tofu, fresh/bulk Shrink-wrap Mori-Nu Silken	No No Yes, check date	10 days Yes, check date	Months Months
Turkey, raw Cooked Deli sliced	No No No	To defrost 3-4 days 3 days	12 months 6 months
TVP	Year+		
Vegetables, dried Fresh	4 months Varies	Varies	6-8 months
Vinegar	2 years+		
Wheat berries Bran Germ, raw Germ, toasted Flour, whole	Year+ Weeks No No 2-4 weeks	Yes Months Use immediately 2 months 2 months	Yes Year+ 2-6 months Longer
Yeast, baking Nutritional	No Year+	4 Months	Year+

Store most vegetables in the refrigerator as quickly as possible after harvesting. More nutrients will be retained if they are prepared and eaten soon after harvest. Store potatoes, sweet potatoes, onions, garlic, winter squash, eggplant, rutabagas, and turnips in a cool, not cold, dark place. Potatoes stored in light will turn green due to the toxic alkaloid *solanine*. Do not eat the green portion of potatoes. Also, do not store potatoes and onions together; doing so will make the potatoes soften.

Vegetables purchased frozen should be put back into the home freezer as quickly as possible after shopping. If vegetables are defrosted, nutrients will be destroyed. Food value also decreases with time. The longer the vegetable is frozen, the more nutrients are destroyed.

Store fruits in the refrigerator when they are ripe. To slow the ripening process of bananas, store them in an opaque plastic bag in the refrigerator. Remove all of the air and close the bag with a twist tie before refrigerating it.

Menu Planning

When making changes in your diet, it helps to have some practical ideas to guide you. Simply knowing what you can eat and what you can't is usually not enough. Since you'll probably be eating foods that are new to you, keep in mind that what seems different and perhaps awkward to you now will soon become an everyday food. Maintaining a positive attitude about your new diet will help you accept it better.

The most important thing I can stress to you in menu planning is to plan ahead. Learn to be organized. It takes longer to cook whole foods than it does instant or processed foods that you may be using now. Whole foods don't usually need your constant attention, but they do need time for soaking, rising, sprouting, and cooking. Therefore, you must plan ahead in order to have food prepared when you need it.

Don't think that you are going to be in the kitchen all of the time. By planning and organizing, meals will become easy to prepare. First of all, in planning meals for the next few days, you need to consider not only the foods you have available in the cupboard and refrigerator, but also the time you have available. For example, if you know that you're going to be home all day on Monday but will be gone most of Tuesday through Thursday, why not prepare a few things ahead on Monday? Bake some bread and prepare a big pot of pinto beans to serve Monday night plain. And with the left-overs, prepare the *Mexican Bean Dip* (p. 114) for a sandwich spread for lunches. You could also start some alfalfa sprouts. They only take a few minutes to get started.

If you work outside your home all day, begin your next evening's meal the night before. Measure staple ingredients, look over grains for stones, and even cook grains, quick breads or a pot of soup ahead of time. You will want to prepare your vegetables fresh at each meal to preserve the nutrients. Avoid coming home from work not knowing what you are going to fix. Plan ahead! It makes life easier.

Plan around leftovers. Cook extra brown rice so you can prepare *Gooey Brown Rice* (p. 138) for a side dish. A good meal based on leftovers is to serve cooked kidney or pinto beans over brown rice and top them with *Pace* Picante Sauce or sauteed mushrooms, onions, and garlic. Also, serve a fresh vegetable salad and whole grain bread. This meal is simple to prepare, and it doesn't look like leftovers.

You can also make soup from leftovers! I recently had some left-over *New Orleans Red Beans and Brown Rice* (p. 88) as well as *Kasha* (p. 130). I combined these in a pan, added some leftover homemade pasta sauce and water. I had an instant soup which received more compliments from my family than the original dishes. Leftover steamed vegetables can be added, too. Be creative with your leftovers and they will look like a freshly cooked meal.

Breakfast is an often-neglected meal. It is important to allow time in your schedule to prepare and eat a good breakfast. If you're in a hurry at breakfast-time, select the recipes for wholesome grains that are pre-cooked, soaked ahead of time, or will cook in 15 minutes or less.

Use time-saving appliances to help you. Slow cookers are good for cooking foods all day and having them ready when it's time to eat. Soups, stews, beans, grains, and even baked potatoes can be cooked in them. If you have a slow cooker, you'll want to try *Chicken in a Crock Pot* (p. 104). Check the recipe booklet that came with your appliance for recipes you can adjust to include all whole foods.

The food processor is also an excellent time-saving appliance. It's great for chopping and shredding vegetables, shredding cheese, pureeing soups, and chopping nuts.

Use other members of the family to help in food preparation! If your husband, wife, or teenager gets home before you do, have him or her start preparing foods that take longer to cook. Have a certain spot in the kitchen where you can leave instructions. Just a few minutes of their time can help tremendously.

When you make your grocery list, plan in terms of meals and dishes. Don't just buy bulgur and then a couple of days later wish you had other ingredients to make *Tabouli* (p. 146). Take the time to make a complete grocery list and then go shopping when you are not too rushed.

Whole foods cooking can either be a rewarding or a frustrating experience. As I said at the beginning of this section and I'll repeat, *organization is the secret*. As with any worthwhile project, good planning is one of the keys to success.

Several people have asked me for a menu guide. Use the guide that follows to help you plan menus, but keep in mind that we're all different, and, therefore, our dietary requirements vary somewhat. One person may be overweight and need to restrict quantity, while the underweight person needs to try to eat more. Some people have food allergies and sensitivities. One person may be lactose intolerant and unable to use milk; another person may be sensitive to gluten and, therefore, unable to eat wheat, rye, triticale, oats, and barley. Some must restrict fat and salt because of other problems. A few absolutely cannot stand to eat certain foods. Of course, not all people fit into these categories. There are many who can eat and will eat anything and everything.

Whole Foods Menu Guide

The number of servings and serving sizes of the food categories listed here and on the following pages depend on your age and energy requirements. Make certain you eat a variety of foods. Don't eat the same foods day after day.

• Plan each lunch and dinner around a main dish—legumes, poultry, fish, and occasionally cheese, eggs, and red meats.

• Plan breakfast around whole grain cereals with milk, yogurt, soymilk, or nut milk, occasionally having an egg, whole grain pancakes, or even leftovers from dinner.

• Include cooked whole grains 2 to 3 times per day unless you have an allergy to grains. Serve cooked brown rice, rolled oats, hulled barley, millet, buckwheat, quinoa, spelt, and others.

- Include some raw food at each meal. Select from raw fruit, vegetable salads, carrot sticks, fresh vegetable juice, and uncooked nuts.

- Include at least three (preferably more) servings of vegetables each day, raw, cooked, and juiced. Select a variety of colors of vegetables—dark green leafy, yellow or orange, green, red, and white.

- Include whole grain breads or crackers daily—quantity depends upon energy requirements.

- Include good sources of vitamin C daily. These include citrus fruits, strawberries, cabbage, green peppers, and tomatoes.

- Include good calcium sources daily. These include, in addition to dairy products, greens (turnip, collard, mustard, and kale), sea vegetables, sardines and salmon with bones, and almonds. Less calcium-packed but still good sources are broccoli, soy products, carob powder, sesame and sunflower seeds, and most beans.

- Use all pure fats (butter and unrefined or expeller-pressed oils), nuts, and seeds in limited amounts. Avoid fried foods, margarine, refined oils (from the grocery store) and fatty meats. Include sources of the essential fatty acids daily such as fresh flax oil, cold-water fish (mackerel, sardines, tuna, trout, and cold-water salmon), certain nuts and seeds (walnuts, hazelnuts, beechnuts, chestnuts, and pumpkin seeds), and certain beans and bean products (soybeans, tofu, tempeh, kidney, navy, pinto, red, and yankee beans).

- Use salt and salty foods in limited amounts.

- When you use a recipe with more than 30% calories from fat, compensate for the fat by serving other dishes lower in fat.

- Help yourself with weight loss goals by selecting most foods and recipes with a low percent calories from fat, 20% or less.

Over the years, I have had numerous requests for sample menus. I hesitate to provide these as each person's needs and preferences are different. However, I am including a **Sample Meal Plan** as well as **Sample Menus** for the *Perfect Whole Foods* diet with the explanation that these are, just as the name states, *samples*. You can and should vary your meals.

Sample Meal Plan

Breakfast
Fresh fruit
Whole grain cereal
Nonfat dairy product
100% whole grain bread
Fat*
Beverage

Lunch
Main dish
100% whole grain bread
Raw vegetable or fresh vegetable juice
Fat*
Fresh fruit
Beverage

Dinner
Main dish
Whole grain
Cooked vegetable
Raw vegetable
100% whole grain bread
Fat*
Beverage

Optional Evening Snack
Varies

Used in cooking or added to food at table.

A Sample Menu for the Perfect Whole Foods Diet

Breakfast
Fresh Grapefruit
Oatmeal (p. 134)
Skim Milk
Whole Grain Toast (Unsweetened)
Almond Butter
Peppermint Tea

Lunch
Tofu Salad in Pita Bread (p. 118)
Fresh Apple
Spring Water

Dinner
Grilled Chicken (p. 104)
Country Garden Rice (p. 139)
Fresh Steamed Broccoli (p. 166)
Fresh Vegetable Salad
Homemade Dressing
Whole Wheat Yeast Biscuits (p. 212)
Butter
Ginger Tea

Optional Evening Snack
Plain Yogurt with sprinkle of
  Pecan Meal

Saving Time

Most people, even those who like to cook, have other responsibilities and don't want to be in the kitchen any longer than necessary. Those who hold a full-time job outside the home, have young children at home, or have older children always on the go must find ways to save time. Whole foods cooking does take longer than cooking convenience foods. However, by developing a few habits, time in the kitchen can be kept to a minimum.

Here are some ways to work at full efficiency:

• Clean up small messes in the kitchen as you cook. For example, clean up vegetable scraps and wash the food processor while your soup is coming to a boil. The clean-up after your meal will be quicker and easier.

• Soak pans for a little while to make clean-up go faster. Pans that have had grains cooked in them (or any starchy food) should be soaked in cold water, while greasy or oily pans and skillets should be soaked in hot water to help dissolve the fat.

• Have your cupboards organized so that you know where everything belongs. Think of how much time you waste when you have to look for something. Keep grains together on one shelf and dried legumes on another. Organize your herbs and spices so you can find them immediately and put them back where they belong when you are finished. I store my herbs and spices in small, clear, labeled jars lined up in a drawer. Baby food jars fit in my drawer perfectly. I've labeled the rows according to:

Powders (for chili powder, granulated garlic, granulated onion, etc.)
Leaves (basil, oregano, thyme, etc.)
Seeds (celery, dill, poppy, etc.)
Sea Vegetables (dulse flakes, kelp, etc.)
Sweet Spices (cinnamon, nutmeg, etc.)

The jars in each row are arranged alphabetically. Until I organized them this way, I wasted so much time looking through all of the jars. Now, I can find them immediately.

• To avoid being caught without a staple ingredient and to save time in planning your grocery list, don't throw an empty box of food away or wash an empty jar that stored bulk food until you've added that food to your grocery list.

• Make use of convenience appliances such as the slow cooker and the food processor. If you don't have these, consider putting them on your "want list" for holiday or birthday gifts.

• If your oven has an automatic timer, use it in time-saving ways. Pre-set it to come on and cook your grain or potatoes you have placed in the oven earlier in the day. (See the recipe for *Baked Brown Rice* on page 137.)

• Freeze leftovers in single-size portions so you can eat them when the rest of the family has something you can't eat. Nobody likes to prepare two separate meals at one mealtime, and this will save you from that drudgery.

• Ask family members to help you in the kitchen. Not only does it save your time, but it helps others learn to cook. Everyone should be able to cook and not totally depend upon someone else to do it for them.

Eating Out

If you're on the *Perfect Whole Foods* diet, it's next to impossible to drop in at a fast-food restaurant for a bite to eat and still adhere to the diet. About the only way to do it is to order the salad bar and then be *very* careful about what you select. If you plan ahead, you can take your own salad dressing; otherwise, you'd better skip theirs unless you can find separate bottles of oil and vinegar. The oil won't be expeller-pressed or unrefined, but, at least, it won't have sugar added. If you must have a dressing, then you'd better plan on taking your own since many salad bars do not offer plain oil and plain vinegar.

When selecting from the salad bar, of course avoid foods that are obvious sources of sugar or refined starch—like croutons, crackers, salad dressings, slaw, macaroni salad, and bacon bits or fake bacon bits. Stick with the plain, fresh vegetables—lettuce, cucumbers, green peppers, onions, radishes, etc. The sunflower seeds are often rancid, so you'd better sample one before sprinkling them on your salad.

Such items as garbanzo beans are probably canned and might have sugar added; pickles may be sweetened; ranch-style fried potatoes could be sugared since some chain restaurants dip potatoes in a sugar solution to make them brown better.

Sometimes when I go to fast-food restaurants that serve prepared salads, I carry with me a 3-ounce can of water-packed tuna and use that to top the salad. It not only adds protein to the salad but also takes the place of a dressing.

If you want more to eat than salad, sometimes it helps to call ahead and see what a restaurant has to offer. First of all, make certain the person to whom you speak is qualified to give accurate information. You should probably ask for the manager. The more times restaurant managers are questioned about how food is prepared and what is available, the sooner fresh, sugar-free, low fat, whole grain foods will be widely available. Here are some questions you might ask when calling.

Questions to Ask Managers of Restaurants While You're on the Perfect Diet

Beef
- Is your hamburger 100% ground beef?
- Is the meat injected with, marinated in, or basted with anything to tenderize it or make it juicier?
- Is your roast beef self-basting? (If it is, the basting solution injected into it probably has sugar, salt, and fat.)
- Is roast beef kept warm in gravy?

Turkey
- What is the source of your turkey? Fresh, frozen, turkey roll, precooked slices, precooked turkey? Probably all except a fresh turkey will have sugar added.

Chicken
• Do you have baked or broiled chicken without breading?
• Is it marinated before cooking or is a basting sauce added?

Fish
• Do you serve fish baked, broiled, or grilled without breading?
• Is it cooked in butter, margarine, or oil?
• Can it be prepared with no fat added?

Vegetables
• Is a plain baked potato available without fat?
• Are your cooked vegetables fresh, frozen, or canned?
• How are cooked vegetables seasoned? Butter or margarine?
• Is corn on the cob available? (If so, ask that margarine not be spread on it.)
• Is a salad bar or plain fresh vegetable salad available?

Grains
• Is brown rice available? (If wild rice is available, it is probably blended with white rice.)
• Do you have 100% whole grain bread? (For the *Perfect Whole Foods* diet, it is best to assume the bread is sweetened, but asking will let the manager know there's a demand for it.)

Condiments
• Are plain oil and vinegar available for salad?
• Is butter or margarine served?

Fruit
• Is fresh fruit available?
• If fresh fruit compote is available, does it have sweetener added? Is canned fruit added to the fruit compote?

Beverages
• Is herb tea available? (If so, make certain it isn't blended with a caffeine-containing tea.)
• Is hot water available for your own herbal teabags?

General questions
• Do all restaurants in this chain prepare foods the same way?
• Do you use a microwave in cooking?
• If yes, then to cook what foods?

Select questions according to the type of restaurant.

Avoiding Toxic Household Chemicals

Although complete books are written on this subject, use the following hints to become aware of toxic household products. Even though we don't ingest them like food, the fumes of many products are dangerous, the products may burn the eyes and skin or cause a rash, and they may be environmental pollutants.

Some people are more sensitive to chemicals than others. For all of us, they are an unnecessary stress to our bodies. If we're being so careful about what we eat, then we also need to be cautious about what we breathe and touch. The following are suggestions for avoiding a few commonly-used products:

Anti-Perspirants: These contain aluminum, a toxic metal. By selecting *deodorants* instead of *anti-perspirants*, you will avoid the possible absorption of aluminum into your body. Or, by powdering your underarms with dry baking soda, you can avoid commercial deodorant altogether. Deodorant stones have become popular recently, but it is my understanding that, although they do not contain aluminum chlorhydrate, they do contain other forms of aluminum.

Cleansers: By using dry baking soda in place of toxic cleansers, you'll not only avoid the chemicals but will also not add scratches to your porcelain tubs and basins.

Fabric Softeners: Add ¼ cup distilled vinegar or baking soda to the first rinse cycle.

Mildew Remover: Wipe with distilled vinegar.

Window Cleaner: Add 1 tablespoon distilled vinegar to 1 quart water. Store in squirt bottle, apply, and wipe with paper towels.

For more information about avoiding toxic household chemicals, read *Nontoxic and Natural, a Guide for Consumers* by Debra Lynn Dadd (Los Angeles: Jeremy P. Tarcher, Inc., 1984). Note that not all products recommended in this book are nontoxic.

Explaining the Recipes

Use the information below to help with the recipes that follow:

Measuring cups and spoons should be filled and leveled with a flat knife or spatula when measuring dry ingredients. Do not tap cup to pack more ingredients into it. For more accurate measure, have both types of measuring cups specifically made for liquid and dry ingredients (use nested measuring cups for dry measure and clear, usually glass, cups with various measures marked on side for liquids).

Not all recipes included in the book are appropriate for the perfect diet; some are meant to be used later. If you are on **Perfect Whole Foods**, check before preparing any recipe, to see if you can have it now. Look toward the end of the recipe, just before the *Percent Calories From Fat*. If the perfect diet should eliminate a particular recipe or make specific changes, information will be found here. If there is no mention of the perfect diet, the recipe is okay.

Most recipes (except for breakfast cereals) are for family-size quantities. Some recipes that reheat well will serve more. If you live alone or will be the only one eating the food, you can prepare only a half portion of many recipes.

Some people have a greater desire for salt, herbs, and spices than others. In many recipes in this book, the amount of salt is given as a range. If you prefer little salt, use the lesser amount. You might also want to adjust the spices and herbs after you try a recipe once. If you find recipes you don't like soon after you begin eating whole foods, try them again in a month or so. Because your taste for whole foods will change when you stop eating refined ones, you might like the whole foods recipe later.

When I refer to a recipe in the text, I have italicized the titles and listed their page numbers so you can find them easily.

Use These Measurement Conversions to Help You Increase or Decrease a Recipe

3 teaspoons = 1 tablespoon
1 cup = 8 ounces = 16 tablespoons
½ cup = 4 ounces = 8 tablespoons
⅓ cup = 5 tablespoons + 1 teaspoon
¼ cup = 2 ounces = 4 tablespoons
⅛ cup = 1 ounce = 2 tablespoons
2 cups = 1 pint
4 cups = 2 pints = 1 quart
4 quarts = 1 gallon
1 pound = 16 ounces = approximately 2 cups

Nutrition Calculations

• Calculations are based on each recipe without optional ingredients.
• Variations are not calculated.
• When a recipe calls for a range of amounts of an ingredient, the lesser amount is calculated.
• When a recipe suggests ingredients but not amounts, calculations are not made since they would vary according to quantities used.
• When a recipe calls for whole grain flour, whole wheat is used in the calculation.
• When an unspecified kind of cheese is called for, low-fat cheddar is used in the calculations.
• Fat in *Oil-Lecithin Combination* (p. 205) used to oil pans is not calculated. Use as little as possible.
• Calculations are made using:
  Dine Right Software, Dine Systems, Inc., Amherst, N.Y., 1992.
  Pennington and Church's *Food Values of Portions Commonly Used*, 14th and 15th Editions.
  Robertson, Flinders, and Ruppenthal's *The New Laurel's Kitchen*, 1986.
  Data from individual manufacturers.

MAIN DISHES

Most people plan their menus around a main dish. This is usually a meat, poultry, fish, dried beans, eggs, or cheese dish. The recipes in this section include all of these; some are traditional-type recipes: *Grilled Chicken*, *Baked Fish*, and *Navy Bean Soup*. Others include more unusual ingredients like TVP (textured vegetable protein), tofu, and tempeh: *Vegetarian Sloppy Joes*, *Grecian Tofu Balls*, and *Tempeh Stew*. If you're ready to try foods that are unfamiliar, you'll discover a whole new world of foods.

Some main dish recipes in this book are higher in fat than others. Those especially high in fat should be used infrequently. If you need to restrict fat because of a medical problem, you shouldn't use the higher fat main dishes at all. If you need to restrict calories, eliminate these recipes also.

If you have been eating meat, poultry, fish, eggs, or cheese one, two, or even three times a day, substituting legumes (dried beans, peas and lentils) for some of these is a tasty and economical way of increasing unrefined complex carbohydrates and decreasing fat in your diet. When you eat whole grains and legumes, you will be receiving what is called *complementary protein*—together the grains and the legumes will provide complete protein that's just as adequate as animal protein. This is the basis of the vegetarian diet. There are several combinations of incomplete protein foods which eaten together supply complete protein. The following chart summarizes these combinations.

You Don't Have to Eat Animal Products for Complete Protein

Complement whole grains with
Legumes (dried beans, peas, and lentils) *or*

Complement legumes with
Whole grains (brown rice, whole wheat, millet, and oats,) *or*
Nuts and seeds *or*
Wheat germ

Complement nuts and seeds with
Legumes *or*
Wheat germ

Supplement whole grains, legumes, and nuts and seeds with
Milk products *or*
Eggs

Although it was at one time believed that these food combinations should be included at the same meal, it is no longer thought to be necessary.

Eating legumes or beans with grains is the most typical vegetarian combination. Unless you are already familiar with the vegetarian concept, you may not realize that two common food combinations provide complete protein—a peanut butter sandwich (peanuts are a legume and bread is a grain) and dried beans with cornbread. Other typical combinations are dried beans with brown rice, dried beans with whole grain pasta, and tofu (soy) served with whole grain bread.

Although the **Perfect Whole Foods** diet is not a vegetarian diet, those who eat meat will benefit nutritionally by incorporating more plant-based foods into their meals. Also, most vegetarians will benefit from the perfect diet.

Some Reasons Vegetarian Diets Are Nutritionally Beneficial

Well-chosen vegetarian diets generally provide
- Less total fat than meat-containing diets
- Less saturated fat than meat-containing diets
- Less cholesterol than meat-containing diets because plant foods contain no cholesterol (only foods of animal sources contain cholesterol)
- Less protein than meat-containing diets (an advantage in preventing osteoporosis)
- Fewer pesticide residues than meat-containing diets since most farm animals are regularly fed pesticide-containing plant foods and pesticide residues accumulate in flesh and fat
- More fiber than non-vegetarian diets since animal products contain no fiber
- A greater amount of essential fatty acids than meat-containing diets
- Fewer calories than non-vegetarian diets

A well-chosen lacto-ovo-vegetarian diet contains a limited amount of eggs and high-fat dairy products. Vegan diets contain no eggs or dairy products.

Legumes

Before you cook legumes (dried beans, peas, and lentils), sort or remove any stones, dirt, and shriveled beans. If you don't do this, you could break a tooth since little stones are sometimes found among the beans. After you sort the dried beans, wash them in running water and drain.

When Legumes (Dried Beans) Are Cooked

They double or triple in volume.
One cup (approximately ½ pound) will yield 2 to 3 cups of cooked beans.

Most legumes should be soaked before cooking. Lentils, split peas, and black-eyed peas are exceptions since they cook quickly. There are two soaking methods, overnight soaking and quick soaking. Legumes can be soaked overnight (or for 4 to 8 hours) in 3 to 4 times their volume of room temperature water. Because soy beans ferment easily, they should be soaked in the refrigerator. The quick method of soaking is to bring the legumes to a brisk boil, turn off the heat, cover, and let them sit for an hour. Since beans absorb water during the soaking period, the cooking time is considerably shorter than if you cook beans that have not been soaked.

Legumes should be cooked slowly. Rapid boiling often results in their skins breaking open. Use plenty of water to keep the beans covered and cover the pot with a lid. Do not salt legumes (except lentils and split peas) until after they are cooked since salt draws moisture out of the bean, increasing their cooking time. Recipes in some books say to add baking soda to beans to decrease their cooking time. Although soda *will* shorten the time, it *also* destroys thiamine, a B-vitamin. Therefore, do not use baking soda in cooking beans or any vegetable.

Digestibility

Many people complain that beans are hard to digest and are gas-forming. Beans contain two indigestible starches called stachyose and raffinose that are split by intestinal bacteria into carbon dioxide and hydrogen (main constituents of intestinal gas). Several steps can be taken to overcome this problem. Experiment to determine the techniques that help you.

Techniques to Improve the Digestibility of Dried Beans

- Soak beans in plenty of water overnight or longer—up to 36 hours. Refrigerate if you soak longer than overnight. After soaking, pour off the excess water and add fresh. Some nutrients will be poured off, but so will the indigestible starches.

- Cook beans until they are *very* tender.

- The legumes least likely to cause intestinal problems are adzuki, split peas, lentils, mung beans, and lima beans. Enjoy these while eating others in small amounts and gradually increase their serving sizes as your body starts digesting them better.

- Certain herbs and vegetables make beans more digestible when they are cooked together. They include anise seed, cloves, cinnamon, coriander, cumin, dill seed, garlic, ginger, parsley, rosemary, sage, savory, and tumeric. Or try adding a 3 or 4-inch strip of kombu, a sea vegetable, to each cup of dried legumes while they are cooking to make them easier to digest.

- Add up to ¼ cup of apple cider vinegar per cup of dried beans (measured before soaking and cooking) during their last half hour of cooking to improve digestibility.

- Eat beans earlier in the day (at lunch or even at breakfast) rather than for supper or dinner. Your digestion is likely to be better while you are more active.

- After soaking, sprout the beans for 2 days and then cook until tender. This technique often works when the others fail.

- Use the liquid product, *Beano*, to provide the enzymes necessary for digesting beans. Simply add a few drops (check the label for the exact instructions) of *Beano* to the beans on your plate. Do not add the product to beans while they are cooking; cooking destroys the enzymes.

Cooking Time

The length of time beans should be cooked depends upon what beans you are cooking, the method of cooking, as well as the age of the beans. Older beans require longer cooking since they become drier with age. The following chart summarizes the approximate cooking times for various legumes.

Cooking Times for Dried Beans and Peas

Bean/Peas	Cooking Time After Soaking (hours)
Anasazi	1½ - 2
Aduki	1 - 2
Black-eyed peas	1 - 2 (no soaking)
Black turtle	1½ - 2
Garbanzo (chickpeas)	3 - 4
Great northern	1½ - 2
Kidney	1 - 2
Lentils, green	½ - ¾ (no soaking)
Lentils, red	½
Lima, baby	1 - 1½
Lima, large	1½ - 2
Mung	1 - 1½
Navy	2 - 3
Pinto	1½ - 2½
Red Mexican	2 - 3
Split peas, green or yellow	1 - 2 (no soaking)
Soy	3 - 3½

Slow cookers or crock pots are useful for cooking beans since they can be turned on the low setting and almost forgotten. Because slow cookers vary in heating capacity, the length of time for cooking legumes varies greatly. You will need to experiment to determine how long beans need to cook in your particular pot. On low, soaked beans may take as long as 16 to 20 hours or as short as 8 hours. On high, you should watch the beans (or any food) carefully and add hot water as it evaporates. Beans must be covered with water at all times to cook properly. If you don't want to cook the beans for 16 to 20 hours in your slow cooker, try cooking them 2 or 3 hours on high and then 6 to 8 hours on low, making certain there's plenty of liquid to keep them covered.

Most legumes can be cooked in a pressure cooker. Follow the manufacturer's manual for instructions. Certain beans and peas are not recommended to be cooked by this method since they might foam and clog the vent. Check your manual concerning the specific beans to avoid.

If you're on a liberal whole foods diet, you may find plain canned beans (with no sweeteners added) handy to have on hand for when you don't have time to cook beans from scratch. Although the canning process destroys nutrients, there are fewer nutrients lost in canned legumes than there are in other canned vegetables like green beans, greens, and carrots. If you're on the perfect diet, you should prepare dried beans and peas at home.

Cheese

Many people substitute cheese for meat when they decide to cut down on red meat in an attempt to decrease fat. Unfortunately, cheese often contains as much fat, sometimes more, than meat. Unless you must follow an extremely low-fat diet (10% fat), eating cheese occasionally, especially low-fat varieties, should be okay. If you're on the *Perfect Whole Foods* diet and fat is not your main concern right now, don't get into the habit of having cheese often. It's easy to acquire such a habit since cheese is convenient and good-tasting. If you don't have cooking skills to prepare a variety of other foods, take the time to develop them by studying this book and practicing what you learn.

Low-fat cheeses have become available at most stores. Part-skim milk cheeses have approximately 5 grams of fat per ounce. Since five grams here and there add up quickly, don't overeat low-fat cheese. Avoid processed cheeses such as American cheese and cheese foods as they contain additives like phosphates that are not health-promoting. Most of the extremely low-fat or fat-free cheeses contain starches which are totally eliminated on the *Perfect Whole Foods* diet. Check the ingredient lists of labels carefully.

If low-fat cheese is not available, then try using a sharp cheese such as sharp cheddar. With more flavor than other cheeses, these sharp cheeses let you use less, and, therefore, control your fat intake. Compare popular cheeses in the following chart with some low-fat varieties.

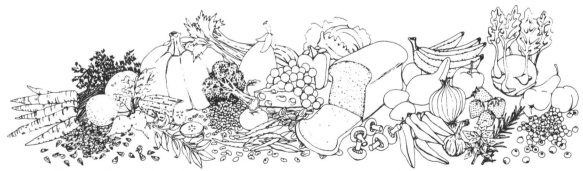

If you always do what you've always done, you'll always get what you've always gotten.   *Unknown*

A Comparison of Various Cheeses

Cheese	Fat Grams	Percent Calories from Fat
Cream cheese, 2 tablespoons	9.5	87
Neufchatel, 2 tablespoons	6.5	80
Cream cheese, light, 2 tablespoons	5.0	68
Nonfat yogurt cheese, 2 tablespoons	0.0	0
Cheddar	9.5	74
Colby	9.0	73
Muenster	8.5	73
Monterey	8.5	73
Swiss	8.0	66
Blue	8.0	74
Provolone	7.5	68
Low-fat cheddar	5.0	60
Whole milk mozzarella	6.0	69
Part-skim milk mozzarella	4.5	56
Parmesan, 2 tablespoons	2.5	60
Cottage, 4% fat by weight, 2 tablespoons	9.5	38
Cottage, 2% fat by weight, 2 tablespoons	0.5	20
Cottage, 1% fat by weight, 2 tablespoons	0.3	13
Cottage, dry curd, 2 tablespoons	0.1	4

Grams of fat are given for one ounce of cheese. One ounce is equal to 1/4 cup shredded (not packed), two 1-inch cubes of hard cheese, or 2 tablespoons of soft cheese like cream and cottage cheeses.

When slicing or shredding cheese, be careful not to touch with your bare fingers the cheese that you will be storing in the refrigerator. Once cheese is touched, even with *clean* hands, mold begins to grow on the surface fairly quickly. How many times have you opened a partially-used package of cheese only to find mold on it? Although mold will grow on untouched cheese, it occurs sooner when the cheese as been contaminated.

Read the ingredient list on the label carefully when buying cottage cheese. I have noticed more and more brands with modified food starch, lactose, and whey added. These and other refined carbohydrates should be eliminated while on the **Perfect Whole Foods** diet. Low-fat cottage cheeses (1% and 2% fat) are better than regular cottage cheese (4% fat) because of the reduced fat; they are, however, more likely to have starch added.

Eggs

Eggs are used as main dishes since they are a good source of protein. Fresh farm eggs or free-range eggs, as they are often called, should be eaten rather than commercial or battery eggs. Although farm eggs are sometimes more expensive than commercial ones, they are worth the additional cost since they provide essential fatty acids (linoleic and linolenic acids). These essential fatty acids come from the farm hen's natural diet. Free-running, uncaged farm hens eat natural grains, seeds, greens, and occasional insects. Commercial hens, however, are given processed feed that is rich in oleic acid (a non-essential fatty acid). This fatty acid is more stable than the essential ones, thus making the commercial feed more suitable for large-scale transport and storage. Commercial feed is also often medicated with antibiotics, hormones, and growth stimulators. Because hens raised on small local farms are healthier than commercially raised hens, their eggs are much less likely to contain salmonella bacteria that can cause intestinal illnesses or, in some cases, death.

The Advantages Of Farm Eggs

- Farm eggs provide both linoleic and linolenic fatty acids (the body can't make these essential fatty acids), while commercial eggs provide monounsaturated oleic fatty acids (not essential).
- Farm hens are not medicated with antibiotics, hormones, and growth stimulators.
- Farm eggs are much less likely to contain salmonella bacteria than commercial eggs.

Some people have the mistaken notion that brown-shelled eggs are more nutritious than white eggs. Actually, brown eggs are from a different variety of hens. Although farm eggs are often brown, the color alone does not indicate whether they are farm or commercial eggs. How the hens are fed and treated determines that. Before you buy farm eggs, make certain that's what you're getting by finding out how the hens are fed.

Watch for and avoid synthetic hard cooked eggs which are used at some salad bars and on some prepared fast food restaurant salads. If you are not certain if eggs are real or synthetic, ask. Even if you recognize that they are synthetic, it's good to voice your opinion. Tell the manager of the restaurant that you prefer the real thing.

Fat in Eggs

Percent Calories from Fat		Total Grams Of Fat	
1 whole large egg	64	1 whole large egg	6
1 egg yolk	80	1 egg yolk	6
1 egg white	0	1 egg white	0

If you are restricting fat or cholesterol, egg whites can be used in place of whole eggs in many recipes. Substitute two whites for one whole egg. Recipes throughout this book suggest using egg whites where appropriate. To avoid buying whole eggs and discarding the yolks, egg white powder (from *Now* Natural Foods) is available and can be reconstituted by mixing with water.

Reconstituting Egg White Powder

For 1 egg white
Mix 2 teaspoons egg white powder with 2 tablespoons water in a small jar. Let it sit for a few minutes and shake to remove lumps. If necessary, let sit a few minutes longer and shake again.

Do not use dehydrated egg whites that are meant for making confections. These egg whites include sugar and starches. Now Eggwhite Powder contains only dried egg whites.

Various egg replacers are available in grocery stores and natural food stores. Before you buy any of these, read the ingredient list carefully. Most contain starches that should be eliminated on the *Perfect Whole Foods* diet.

Poultry

Many people are eating more poultry in an attempt to reduce fat in their diets. Baked or stewed without the skin, the light meat of most poultry is, indeed, lower in fat than many flesh foods. The dark meat contains about twice as much fat as the light. (That's why it's more moist and flavorful than the light meat.) Add the skin and you'll add about half again as much fat. If you fry the dark meat of the chicken with the skin, you'll have about the same amount of fat as you would in a similar amount of hamburger. In order to reduce your fat intake, you must be selective.

When shopping for the perfect diet, carefully read the ingredient lists on labels of frozen hens, turkeys, turkey breasts, turkey roasts as well as pre-cooked turkey breast and deli turkey. Most of these have sugar or fat injected into the muscle. The fat added is usually hydrogenated (a process that makes the fat saturated). Fresh turkeys and turkey parts are available throughout the year in large grocery stores. If they are not available, then they are usually plentiful at holiday times. You might buy and freeze them for later use if fresh turkeys are not available all year round. A frozen turkey can be stored in a home freezer for as long as a year.

The best choice is organically grown fresh or frozen poultry. It's often available from food co-ops and natural food stores.

Whole chickens, turkeys, ducks, and geese can all be roasted using a roasting pan and traditional directions (about 20 to 30 minutes per pound weight at 325° and until the internal temperature reaches 180° on a meat thermometer).

If you need to keep the fat content of your poultry as low as possible, remove the skin and fat from the bird before cooking it and do not add additional fat. Since a bird roasted this way will be dry, add some water to the bottom of the pan so the meat will be steamed rather than roasted. When using the broth from cooked poultry (beef, too), chill it first and remove the solidified fat to make the broth free of fat. Avoid domestic ducks and geese since over half of their calories come from fat. An easy way to cook a turkey breast half or portion is to use a slow cooker. See the recipe for *Turkey Breast in Slow Cooker* (p. 107).

Ground turkey has become a popular main dish item. It is used like ground beef. Because the flavor is so mild, make certain you add adequate seasonings. Several brands of ground turkey are available. I have seen ground turkey with 15, 10, and 7 percent fat by weight. The lean ground turkey with 7 percent fat is preferable since fat and skin has not been ground with the lean meat. The other two have these sources of fat added.

Turkey sausage, ham, bologna, hot dogs, and even bacon are available but they almost always contain sugar as do similar pork products. For years a brand name breakfast turkey sausage was sold which had no added sugar. Then some time ago, I picked up a package from the grocery store freezer and noticed that the label stated the product was *improved!* Suspiciously, I read the fine print and found that sugar, indeed, had been added! That incident has prompted my advice that you should routinely read labels if on the perfect diet. I have since developed a recipe for *Homemade Turkey Sausage* (p. 108).

Food co-ops and natural food stores usually have turkey hot dogs, bologna, and sausage without sugar and other undesirable additives like nitrates and phosphates. They usually contain more fat (and sodium as well) than is desirable, so don't eat them too often. I discovered that one chicken hot dog (a popular natural foods brand) contains 9 grams of fat whereas a typical hot dog from the grocery store contains 13 grams of fat. With such a large amount of fat in a small hot dog, it apparently includes the skin of the chicken.

When cooking raw poultry as well as any flesh food, certain precautions should be taken to avoid contamination with salmonella, a bacteria that can cause intestinal illnesses and even, in some cases, death. Poultry is sometimes infected with bacteria during the processing.

Psalm 50:15
And call upon me in the day of trouble: I will deliver thee, and thou shalt glorify me.

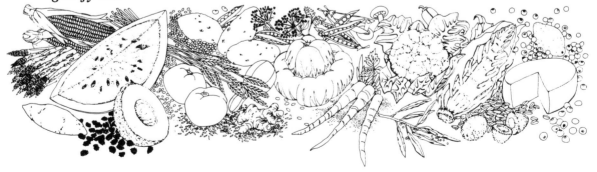

Precautions to Prevent Salmonella Poisoning When Handling Poultry

- Keep poultry cold until ready for use. If you plan to keep it longer than a couple of days after purchase, freeze it. When it's time to use the poultry, defrost it in the refrigerator.

- Before cooking poultry, rinse it carefully with cold water.

- Cook poultry thoroughly. There should be no pink color left after cooking. A meat thermometer inserted into the thickest part of the bird should read 180° to insure thorough cooking.

- Wash carefully with hot soapy water anything that has come into contact with the raw poultry (utensils, counter surfaces, cutting boards, as well as your hands and under your nails). Don't forget about the dish cloth. After the clean-up, put it with the laundry and get a fresh one.

- Avoid using a wooden cutting board since bacteria can lodge in the pores of the wood. Plastic cutting boards can be cleaned more thoroughly.

An Important Reminder for Those on the Perfect Diet

Read very carefully the ingredient lists of these and all poultry products:

Cooked turkey and chicken luncheon meat	Turkey bologna
Deli turkey and chicken	Turkey ham
Frozen chicken pieces	Turkey and chicken hot dogs
Frozen whole turkeys	Turkey roasts
Frozen turkey breasts	Turkey rolls
Frozen hens	Turkey sausage
Turkey bacon	

Fish

The oil naturally present in fish is the only animal fat that is actually beneficial to the human body. Fish oil is one of the major sources of the essential Omega-3 fatty acids.

Fish can be a delicious as well as nutritious food, yet many people don't cook it properly. Because it is so easily overcooked, fish is often served tough, dry, and rubbery. No wonder many people don't like it! Cooking fish is simple if you know how. (I share some of my favorite techniques with you on page 73.)

Hints For Cooking Fish

- Buy only truly fresh fish or else buy it frozen. Not-so-fresh fresh fish will have a strong flavor.

- Allow approximately ⅓ pound of fillets or steaks per person.

- Cook fish 10 minutes per inch thickness. This time can be used whether the fish is baked, broiled, sauteed, poached, or steamed; the fish can be fillets, steaks, or whole. If the fish is frozen, double the cooking time to 20 minutes per inch thickness. The 10 minute rule of thumb is not applicable to shellfish or crustaceans.

- A test for doneness of fish is to check it with a fork. When done, the fish will flake. Also, it should turn from translucent to opaque.

Whatever method you choose to cook fish, incorporate these hints for moist, tender fish.

Methods of Cooking Fish

Baking: Heat oven to 425 to 450°.
When a lid or paper is used to cover fish, add about 5 minutes to time for heat to reach fish.

Broiling: Preheat oven.
If 1-inch thick, cook 4 inches from the heat.
If less than 1-inch, cook up to 6 inches from the heat.
Turn over halfway through cooking.
If fish is very thin, you may want to it broil without turning.
If desired, brush with a small amount of butter or oil to prevent fish from drying out.

Sautéing: Use a small amount of hot oil, but don't allow the oil to smoke; or use a *Silverstone* skillet or griddle without oil.

Poaching: Put fish into boiling water, begin timing when water starts simmering again.

Steaming: Water under the fish should be boiling.

Beef

Although beef is usually implicated as being high in fat, certain cuts are actually much lower than many cheeses. Some of the leanest cuts of beef include rump, round, tenderloin, and flank. With all visible fat trimmed from these cuts, they have less than 3 grams of fat per ounce of lean meat or less than 10 percent fat by weight. Don't let this 10 percent figure or any listing of percent fat by weight confuse or fool you. It is not the same as percent calories from fat. Based on calories and grams of fat, these lean cuts of beef have at least 30 percent calories from fat. However, this is still lower than most cheeses.

Cuts of beef with a high percentage of fat should definitely be restricted or, better yet, eliminated from a health-promoting diet. The percent of fat listed on some packages of lean ground beef is often 20 or 30. They are listed as percentage fat by weight, not calories as I give you in this book. Ground beef that is 20 percent fat by weight (sometimes expressed as 80 percent lean) has about 68 percent of its calories from fat. Beef that is 30 percent fat by weight has about 78 percent calories from fat! Even worse, a marbled T-bone steak, broiled, has over 80 percent of its calories from fat!

Whatever cut of beef you do select, to lessen your intake of fat, choose meats that have little or no marbling (visible streaks of fat within the lean) and cut all visible fat from the meat before cooking it. Some stores sell meat with visible fat already removed from the edges. Look for terms such as 100 percent lean trim, total trim, and 0-inch trim. Although sometimes difficult to find, the best beef is raised without the use of steroids, antibiotics, or other additives.

Pork

Pork is generally a high fat meat, often having more fat than beef. Popular items such as cooked pork sausages and bacon range from 75 to 95 percent calories from fat. Also, pork products like bacon, ham, luncheon meats, and hot dogs are usually cured with the chemicals sodium or potassium nitrate or nitrite which are suspected of causing cancer. (Cured beef and turkey products are also prepared with these chemicals.) If you choose to eat pork, have small portions only occasionally and select lean cuts with all visible fat trimmed before cooking.

Sandwiches

Many people have the idea that sandwiches are not healthy. But they easily can be if you prepare them on 100 percent whole grain bread, include plenty of fresh vegetables on them, and don't use high fat ingredients. Sandwiches make a quick main dish when you don't have the time to cook. They often require some pre-preparation or you'll end up with a cheese or peanut butter sandwich. Try the sandwich recipes included in this book and create original ones. Some of the recipes simply list the ingredients to use. I may suggest a specific kind of bread, but vary that according to your own preferences, whether you are on the perfect or liberal diet, and what breads are available to you.

Several burger recipes given in this book (tempeh, tuna, and taco) are panfried in oil. Very little oil is needed. Use an oil that does not break down easily at high temperatures—like expeller-pressed high oleic-monounsaturated safflower oil. Oil is not needed to prevent sticking if you use a *SilverStone* griddle or skillet. However, a little oil is desirable for these burgers since they will brown better and have a slightly better flavor. Omit the oil on an extremely low-fat diet (10 percent calories from fat).

Check your local co-op or natural food store for grainburger and instant refried beans mixes that are available. They're handy when time is short; many can be included on the *Perfect Whole Foods* diet. As always, pay attention to the ingredient lists on all labels.

Main Dish Facts

Avidin: A protein component in egg whites that, when eaten raw, blocks the absorption of the vitamin biotin (present in the yolk). Cooking inactivates avidin. Raw eggs should not be eaten regularly (because of the problem with avidin as well as the possibility of eggs being infected with salmonella bacteria). Read below about **Eggs, Raw**.

Boil: To cook in a liquid with bubbles rising and breaking on the surface.

Cheese: A high-fat dairy product that should be eaten only in limited amounts. Don't touch cheese that will not be eaten immediately since it will mold more quickly. While cutting cheese, keep the portion that you will be holding and touching covered with plastic wrap.
¼ pound = 4 ounces = 1 cup shredded.
1 ounce = ¼ cup shredded or two 1-inch cubes.

Cheese, Cottage: While you're on the perfect diet, select cottage cheeses without added starches such as tapioca or added whey. Store brands often include these refined carbohydrates.

Chicken: 3½ pound raw chicken = approximately 3 cups cooked, diced chicken.

Egg Replacers: Be cautious about using egg replacers on the perfect diet since they usually have starch as an ingredient. Read the ingredient list carefully.

Eggs, Raw: Because raw and undercooked commercial eggs have been linked to salmonella poisoning (a serious and potentially fatal food poisoning), extreme caution must be taken if using recipes in which the eggs are not cooked or are undercooked! All raw eggs as well as foods containing raw eggs should be kept refrigerated at *all* times (below 45°). Farm eggs are less likely to be contaminated with salmonella bacteria than commercial eggs.

Garbanzo Beans: Are also known as chickpeas. They are popular in Middle Eastern dishes.

Grilling, Charcoal or Gas: Avoid or use very occasionally since the smoke formed when meat is grilled contains potential cancer-causing substances which contaminate the food. The combination of amino acids and creatinine in meat and the presence of high temperatures cooking create the conditions for the cancer-causing substances to be formed. Since soy products do not contain creatinine, charcoal or gas grilling these products do not form cancer-causing substances.

Legumes: Dried beans and peas. Legumes, along with a whole grain dish, make a nutritious main dish that will substitute for meat.
1 pound legumes = 2¼ to 2½ cups uncooked dried beans or peas.
1 cup uncooked dried beans or peas = 2 to 3 cups cooked.

Lentils: A small flat legume that cooks quickly and does not need soaking. Lentils are excellent in soups and stews. Cooked and drained lentils can often be substituted for cooked ground beef in casseroles and other mixed dishes. When you make this replacement, you'll drastically reduce the fat content of the dish, eliminate cholesterol, and include beneficial fiber.

Nitrates/Nitrites: Curing agents in meat products such as ham, bacon, hot dogs, and luncheon meats. These preservatives have been associated with cancer and should be avoided.

Okara: Soy pulp, a by-product of making tofu. You may find okara in commercially prepared products. It can be used on **Perfect Whole Foods** if other ingredients are okay.

Peanut Butter, Natural: Select pure peanut butter without added sugar or hydrogenated oils. Since peanuts are a legume, serving peanut butter on whole grain bread is a way of providing complementary protein.
Percent Calories From Fat: 77
Fat Grams In 1 Tablespoon: 8

Simmer: To cook a liquid slightly below the boiling point with bubbles forming slowly and collapsing below the surface.

Soy Milk: Unsweetened commercial soynilk products include vaccuum-packed *WestSoy Westbrae* Natural Unsweetened Non-Dairy Beverage and powdered *EnerG* Pure SoyQuik. See page 206 for instructions on preparing soy milk from soy or soya milk powder. Soy milk can also be made at home from soy beans. You can find a good recipe for making soy milk in the cookbook *The New Laurel's Kitchen* by Robertson, Flinders, and Ruppenthal (Ten Speed Press, 1986).

Tempeh: (TEM-pay) Is a cultured food with meat-like texture made from whole soy beans, a bacteria culture, and sometimes whole grains. The beans and grains stick together and form a *cake*. Tempeh should not be eaten raw. Cook it at least 10 to 20 minutes before eating.
Percent Calories From Fat: 40
Fat Grams In 2 ounces: 4

Tofu: (TOE-fu) Is a non-fermented soy product made into a soft, cheese-like product. It is sometimes called bean curd. Because it is bland, seasonings should be added to dishes prepared with tofu. The tofu absorbs the flavors of the seasonings. Tofu is a popular food to prepare as a meat substitute. It is usually available as *soft* and *firm*. Soft tofu has more water than firm and is used for dips or foods in which the tofu is blended. Firm tofu is used for recipes in which the tofu should hold its shape. Tofu that comes packed in water or tofu leftover from vacuum-sealed packages should be stored submerged in cold water in the refrigerator. The water should be changed daily. Fresh tofu should have a delicate, not sour, scent to it. Try freezing tofu (drain it first) and then thawing it (at room temperature or by pouring boiling water over it) for a meat-like texture. 1 pound tofu = approximately 2 cups mashed.
Percent Calories From Fat: 53
Fat Grams In 4 ounces: 5

Tuna: Always buy fresh or canned tuna packed in water. If you are sensitive to MSG, select brands that have only tuna, water, and salt. Those brands with *vegetable broth* or *hydrolyzed vegetable protein* will have MSG present in these ingredients. Don't make the mistake of reaching for the *lite* canned tuna since it has oil added, although less oil than the tuna packed in oil. Canned tuna is extremely high in sodium unless especially canned with less or no salt.
Percent Calories From Fat: 8 (water-packed or fresh)
Fat Grams In 2 ounces: 1

TVP: Textured vegetable protein is a very low-fat meat substitute made from soy beans. It is generally harder to digest than beans. To reconstitute TVP, mix 1 cup water with 2 cups TVP, stir, and let it sit for 5 to 10 minutes. Reconstitution is not necessary in soups and stews if you allow enough liquid in the dish to be absorbed by the TVP.
Percent Calories From Fat: 6
Fat Grams In ½ Cup Dry TVP: 1

Vegan Diet: A very strict vegetarian diet that excludes all animal products. No dairy products or eggs are eaten. Since the vegan diet contains no source of vitamin B-12, vegans must make certain they have a reliable source from either fortified foods or a vitamin supplement. A deficiency of vitamin B-12 can result after B-12 reserves in the body are used up, usually several years after eliminating all animal products from the diet. A vitamin B-12 deficiency can cause serious neurological problems that are not reversible. Vegan diets also are often excessively high in carbohydrates (refined carbohydrates in many cases) and, unless really well planned, will not provide adequate protein, minerals, or essential fatty acids. Also, it can be difficult for young children on a vegan diet to get adequate calories as well as the nutrients just listed.

Vegetarian Sloppy Joe Mix: A combination of 1½ cups TVP, ¼ cup dried onion flakes, and ¼ cup dried mixed vegetables, used in **Bean Supreme** (p. 84) and **Vegetarian Sloppy Joes** (p. 117).

Please Read These Important Notes:

If you have strictly followed the *Perfect Whole Foods* diet for at least two weeks, but you are not feeling dramatically better, see page 35 for additional steps that may be necessary.

If you are allergic to wheat, do not substitute spelt or kamut without first determining that you can tolerate them.

If you are being treated for *Candida*, please see specific guidelines on page 315, Appendix A: If You Have Candidiasis.

Main Dish Recipes

Black Bean Soup

1½ cup dried black beans, sorted, rinsed, and drained
½ cup millet
2 bay leaves
1 teaspoon dried oregano leaves
1 onion, chopped
3 garlic cloves, minced
2 carrots, chopped
2 celery ribs, chopped
5 or 6 drops *Tabasco* Sauce, or more to taste
2 tablespoons cider vinegar
¼ to ½ teaspoon salt, optional

Place beans in a large pot with 8 cups of water and bay leaves. Bring to a boil, turn off heat, cover, and let sit for 1 hour. Add remaining ingredients except vinegar and salt. Bring to a boil, cover, reduce heat, and simmer until beans are almost tender. Add vinegar and cook about 30 minutes longer. Total cooking time will be about 2 hours. Remove bay leaves and add optional salt. Remove 4 or 5 cups of soup and purée in food processor or blender. Stir into remaining soup, dilute with some water if you prefer a thinner soup, heat, and serve. This is good as a main dish served with a large fresh vegetable salad, steamed vegetable, and whole grain bread. Makes about 9 cups.

Black Bean Soup Using a Slow Cooker: Soak beans overnight in slow cooker; in the morning, heat beans and water on high while preparing and adding other ingredients. In about 1 hour, reduce heat to low and cook at least 12 hours. To decrease the cooking time, cook longer on high, adding water if necessary.

Percent Calories From Fat: 6
Total Fat Grams In Recipe: 10

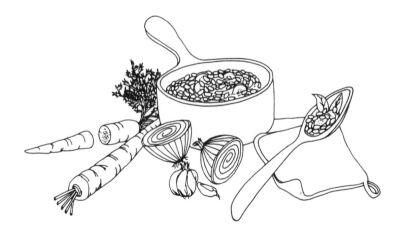

Lentil Soup

If you've never had lentils, try this recipe or the one for Lentil Stew *(p. 82). Lentils are small, flat legumes which do not need soaking and take an hour or less to cook.*

1½ cups dried lentils, sorted, rinsed, and drained
1 large onion, chopped
1 green pepper, chopped
1 teaspoon oil
2 tablespoons whole grain flour
1 cup tomato purée
½ cup long grain brown rice, sorted and rinsed
4 carrots, sliced
3 ribs celery, sliced
½ teaspoon each of dried marjoram, thyme, and parsley
2 bay leaves
9 cups water
¼ to ½ teaspoon salt, optional

Using a large pot, cook the onion and green pepper in oil for a couple of minutes. Add flour and stir briefly. Add remaining ingredients, stir until soup comes to a boil, reduce heat, cover, and simmer for about an hour, stirring occasionally. Remove bay leaves and add optional salt. Makes about 12 cups.

Percent Calories From Fat: 5
Total Fat Grams In Recipe: 9

Red Lentil Soup

If you have children in the family, try this recipe. It's a simple and soothing soup.

1 large onion, chopped
1 teaspoon butter
2 teaspoons olive oil
2 or 3 garlic cloves, minced
1½ cups red lentils, sorted, rinsed, and drained
¼ teaspoon salt
Juice from 1 lemon
Black pepper, optional

Sauté the onion slowly in the butter and oil for about 10 minutes or until the onion is soft but not browned. Add the garlic, lentils, and 6 cups of water. Bring to a boil, cover, reduce heat, and simmer for 20 to 30 minutes. Cool slightly and purée with a food processor, blender, or hand blender. Add salt, lemon juice, and pepper. Heat and serve. Makes about 8 cups.

Perfect Whole Foods: *Substitute 1 drop of lemon oil for the lemon juice.*
Percent Calories From Fat: 13
Total Fat Grams In Recipe: 14

Split Pea Soup

Prepare Split Pea Soup early in the morning in the slow cooker and it will be ready by dinner time. Serve with a cooked whole grain or whole grain bread to complement the protein of the peas.

2 cups dried split peas (green or yellow), sorted, rinsed, and drained
1 onion, chopped
2 celery ribs, chopped
2 carrots, chopped
¾ cup chopped cabbage
2 garlic cloves, minced
1 bay leaf
½ to ¾ teaspoon salt
6 whole peppercorns

Place peas in a slow cooker or pan along with 5 cups of water. Chop vegetables in food processor or by hand. Add vegetables, minced garlic, bay leaf, and peppercorns to crockpot or pan. Cook until everything is very tender and peas have become smooth and thick. A slow cooker will take about 10 to 12 hours on low or 8 hours starting on high and turning to low when hot. Simmering in a pan will take about 2 hours. Before serving, remove peppercorns and bay leaf and add salt. Makes about 8 cups.

Percent Calories From Fat: 3
Total Fat Grams In Recipe: 2

Navy Bean Soup

2 cups dried navy beans, sorted, rinsed, and drained
2 or 3 carrots, sliced
2 garlic cloves, halved
1 potato, scrubbed and sliced
1 large onion, sliced
1 or 2 celery ribs, sliced
½ to ¾ teaspoon salt, optional
Black pepper to taste, optional

Place beans and 6 cups of water in soup pot. Bring to a boil, turn off heat, cover, and allow to sit for 1 hour. Bring to a boil again, reduce heat, and simmer until beans are very tender or 2 to 3 hours. While beans are cooking, place 1 cup of water in another pan along with the vegetables. Cook until tender and then purée the vegetables and liquid in a food processor or with a hand blender until smooth. Add to cooked beans with salt and pepper, if desired. Stir, heat, and serve. Makes about 8 cups.

Percent Calories From Fat: 2
Total Fat Grams In Recipe: 5

Smokey Mountain Bean Soup

This soup is traditionally made with bacon that's high in saturated fat and contains nitrates. I use a soy bacon called Fakin'Bacon *made by Tempehworks, Inc. It has bacon flavor without the undesirables. Next time you cook kidney or pinto beans, add about 1 cup extra uncooked beans to the bean pot so you can prepare this soup using 2 or 3 cups of leftover beans.*

1 cup dried kidney or pinto beans, cooked until tender and drained
½ cup long grain brown rice, sorted, rinsed, drained, and cooked in 1 cup water (or 1½ cups cooked)
1 onion, chopped
2 garlic cloves, minced
1 teaspoon olive oil
½ of a 6-ounce package *Fakin'Bacon*
2 large tomatoes, diced
½ teaspoon paprika
¼ teaspoon black pepper
½ teaspoon salt, optional
4½ cups water

In a soup pot, sauté the onion and garlic in the oil for 3 or 4 minutes. Coarsely chop the *Fakin'Bacon* while sautéing the vegetables. Add beans, cooked rice, tomatoes, seasonings, bacon, and 4½ cups of water to the soup pot. Cover and simmer soup for 1 hour. Soup is delicious at this point, but even better the next day! Makes about 10 cups.

Variation: If good fresh tomatoes are not available, use a 16-ounce can of whole tomatoes in juice, coarsely chopping the tomatoes.

Perfect Whole Foods: No since Fakin'Bacon *has honey in it.*
Percent Calories From Fat: 7
Total Fat Grams In Recipe: 7

Quick-N-Easy Chili

If you cook the kidney beans ahead of time, you can have a delicious pot of chili in just 10 or 15 minutes.

1½ cups dried kidney beans, cooked until tender and drained (or 3 to 4 cups cooked)
½ cup TVP (textured vegetable protein) flakes
½ cup water
16-ounce jar *McIlhenny's Tabasco* 7 Spice Chili Recipe (Regular or Spicy)

Combine ingredients and simmer for 10 to 15 minutes. Makes 4 cups.

Perfect Whole Foods: Check ingredient list of McIlhenny's to make certain sugar and starch are not added.
Percent Calories From Fat: 3
Total Fat Grams In Recipe: 3

Lentil Stew

This Middle Eastern dish is easy to prepare. It's one of my many favorites. The salad and dressing are traditionally served on top of the lentils and brown rice. Children and some adults may prefer their salads served separately.

1 large onion, chopped
2 or 3 garlic cloves, minced
2 or 3 carrots, sliced
2 or 3 celery ribs, sliced
1 teaspoon olive oil
¾ cup lentils, sorted, rinsed, and drained
1 cup long grain brown rice, sorted, rinsed, and drained
¼ to ½ teaspoon salt, optional

Sauté vegetables in oil for 1 or 2 minutes.   Add lentils and rice, sautéing for few minutes longer. Add 4 cups of water, bring to a boil, reduce heat, cover, and simmer for 40 to 45 minutes or until all water is absorbed. Add optional salt. Makes about 7 cups.

To serve: Prepare salad using your choice of dark salad greens, tomatoes, onions, cucumbers, radishes, green peppers, and celery. Serve salad on top of the stew and drizzle the dressing (recipe below) over the salad.

Lentil Stew Dressing
2 tablespoons olive oil
2 tablespoons lemon juice (or raw cider vinegar)
½ teaspoon paprika
¼ teaspoon dry mustard
1 clove garlic, minced
Salt to taste, optional

Combine ingredients in a jar, add lid, and shake briefly.

Perfect Whole Foods: Use raw cider vinegar rather than lemon juice.
Percent Calories From Fat: 6, 89, or 22 (Stew only, dressing only, or stew, dressing, and salad together)
Total Fat Grams In Recipe: 8, 26, or 35 (Stew only, dressing only, or stew, dressing, and salad together)

Split Pea Stew: Use yellow split peas in place of the lentils. Serve salad of your choice separately.

Quick Lentil Soup: Dilute leftover *Lentil Stew* with water and sugar-free homemade or commercial spaghetti sauce to make a quick soup.

Baked Potato Bar

This is a quick-serve meal if you have your beans already cooked and take just a few minutes in the morning for preparation. Scrub potatoes, prick them with a fork, place in cold oven, and set timer to come on so the potatoes will be ready when you come in from work or are ready to eat. Just before dinner, prepare the toppings that you and your family prefer. Since children often don't like their foods mixed, let them have their ingredients separate while you make a good baked potato even better with toppings.

Toppings you may want to prepare:
Cooked pinto, kidney, or black beans
Raw sunflower seeds
Sliced mushrooms, sautéed
Celery slices, sautéed
Raw or sautéed chopped onions
Shredded low-fat cheese
Chopped fresh tomatoes
Avocado chunks
Plain, nonfat yogurt

Perfect Whole Foods*: Select a small potato and eat it all, including the skin.*

Beans and Brown Rice

Here's a simple recipe that's quick to prepare if you have leftover cooked brown rice and beans.

Cooked long grain brown rice (I like basmati brown rice)
Cooked beans (my favorites are pintos and black beans)
Picante sauce (*Pace* is a good brand—however, read the ingredient list)
Fresh lime wedges

On each person's plate, top brown rice with cooked beans. Add picante sauce to taste and a couple of lime wedges as a garnish. Squeeze lime juice over the beans and rice before eating.

Perfect Whole Foods*: Omit the lime or use the pulp of the lime as well as the juice.*

Bean Supreme

*This recipe was created by Dr. Walt Stoll who wrote the **Introduction** to this book. He uses several techniques to make the dried beans more digestible. Bean Supreme is delicious served:*

- *hot, over cooked brown rice or whole grain pasta*
- *cold, spread on rice cakes (blended or as is)*
- *hot, as a soup or stew (depending on consistency)*
- *cold, as condiment (sprinkle with cheese as desired)*
- *as substitute for refried beans in Mexican dishes.*

The recipe below is for 1 cup of beans. Double the recipe if you like. The seasonings, as called for, make a very tasty and spicy product. If you prefer a mild flavor, reduce the amount of spices.

1 cup dried beans, sorted, rinsed, and drained (any kind—the more different kinds used together,
    the better—it's also great with pintos!)
1 large green pepper, chopped fine
2 medium onions, chopped fine
2 large garlic cloves, sliced thin
¼ recipe *Sloppy Joe Mix* (p. 117)
1 cup spaghetti sauce (commercial or homemade)
2 tablespoons butter or unrefined sesame oil
2 teaspoons tamari or shoyu soy sauce (alcohol-free)
¼ cup apple cider vinegar
¾ teaspoon salt

Mix these spices together:
1 tablespoon chili powder
2 tablespoons dried parsley
½ teaspoon each of dried savory, rosemary, cumin, tumeric, coriander, and sage
⅛ teaspoon black pepper (freshly ground)

Soak beans overnight in 3 cups of filtered or spring water (longer—up to 36 hours—may be helpful to reduce gas-forming tendencies). Bring to a boil, reduce heat, cover, and simmer for about 4 hours or until all beans are soft. Turn off beans and add vinegar. Allow to soak while preparing the sautéed portion—at least ½ hour. This greatly reduces gas and adds to the flavor.

Place butter or sesame oil in skillet. Sauté the garlic, adding the onions and peppers after a couple of minutes. Sprinkle the spices over the mixture and sauté until spices are brown. Turn the beans back on, simmer while sautéing, and add in this order:
Sloppy Joe Mix, spaghetti sauce, tamari or shoyu soy sauce (alcohol-free), and sautéed ingredients. Simmer until desired thickness—the longer, the tastier (20 minutes minimum). Sometime during this process, add the salt. Tastes better the longer it stands after preparation. Makes about 5 cups.

Perfect Whole Foods: Use a sugar-free spaghetti sauce.
Percent Calories From Fat: 27
Total Fat Grams In Recipe: 29

Pinto Bean Salad

This makes a delicious main dish for summer. It's quick and easy if you have leftover beans.

2 tablespoons oil
2 tablespoons raw cider vinegar
2 tablespoons water
½ teaspoon chili powder
1 small onion, chopped
½ teaspoon dried oregano leaves
4 cups leaf lettuce, torn into bite-size pieces
15 to 20 sliced red radishes
1½ cups cooked pinto beans, drained

Mix oil, vinegar, water, onion, and seasonings to make dressing. Let sit for 30 minutes or longer before mixing with other ingredients. Mix vegetables and beans, add dressing and mix again. Makes about 6 cups.

Percent Calories From Fat: 37
Total Fat Grams In Recipe: 30

Creole Limas

1 cup dried baby limas, sorted, rinsed, and drained
2 garlic cloves, minced
1 large onion, chopped
1 bay leaf
1½ teaspoon dried thyme
½ teaspoon crushed red pepper
1 large or 2 medium-sized fresh tomatoes or a 16-ounce can of tomatoes, coarsely chopped
1 green pepper, coarsely chopped
¼ to ½ teaspoon salt, optional
1 cup long grain brown rice, sorted, rinsed, drained, and cooked in 2 cups water

Bring beans to a boil in 3¼ cups of water, cover, turn heat off, and let stand for 1 hour. Add remaining ingredients except tomatoes, green pepper, and rice. Bring to a boil again, reduce heat, and simmer while covered until almost tender, about 30 minutes to 1 hour. Drain about half of the juice from the tomatoes if they are canned. Add chopped tomatoes and pepper, cooking until beans are very tender, about 30 minutes longer. Season with salt, if desired. Serve in a bowl over the cooked brown rice. Makes 5 to 6 cups (without rice).

Percent Calories From Fat: 5
Total Fat Grams In Recipe: 8

Brazilian Black Beans and Brown Rice

Serve this vegetarian dish with cornbread and a tossed salad for a traditional South American meal. To let flavors blend, prepare the beans ahead of time and reheat when time to serve.

1½ cups black beans, sorted, rinsed, and drained
1 onion, peeled and studded with 4 whole cloves
3 garlic cloves, 2 whole and 1 minced
¾ teaspoon dried thyme
¾ teaspoon dried oregano
1 large onion, chopped
1 green pepper, diced
2 teaspoons oil
2 tomatoes, chopped
¼ to ½ teaspoon salt, optional
2 cups long grain brown rice, sorted, rinsed, drained, and cooked in 4 cups water
Salsa or Picante Sauce
Garnishes: Fresh orange slices and plain, nonfat yogurt

Bring beans to a boil in 4 cups of water, turn off heat, cover, and let sit for 1 hour. Add clove-studded onion, whole garlic, thyme, and oregano and simmer for about 1½ hours or until beans are tender. Sauté chopped onion, pepper, and minced garlic in oil for about 5 minutes. Add to beans along with tomatoes. Cook for 15 to 20 minutes. Remove 2 cups of the bean mixture and mash or purée in food processor. Return to beans and continue cooking while stirring for a few minutes longer. Add optional salt. To serve, remove whole onion and garlic. Dish brown rice onto serving platter or individual plates. Top with bean mixture and salsa. Garnish with orange slices and yogurt. Makes about 7 cups of beans, excluding the rice.

Perfect Whole Foods: Eat the pulp of the orange as well as the juice. Make certain Salsa or Picante Sauce contains no sugar.
Percent Calories From Fat: 10 (without garnish)
Total Fat Grams In Recipe: 19

Variation: If you like a bacon-like flavor and are not on the **Perfect Whole Foods** diet, add ¼ package of coarsely chopped *Fakin' Bacon* to the beans while they are cooking.

Mexican Fiesta Salad

Layer or sprinkle the ingredients (in the order listed) in the center of a large platter, starting with bean dip on the bottom. Leave room for baked whole grain corn chips around the edge. Have guests dip the chips into the salad for a fun and flavorful dish.

Baked whole grain corn chips
Mexican Bean Dip (p. 114)
Low-fat sour cream
Shredded lettuce

Cherry tomatoes, halved
Green onions, sliced
Black olives, sliced
Low-fat cheese, shredded

Perfect Whole Foods Diet: Check the ingredient list of low-fat sour cream or use plain, nonfat yogurt.

Hoppin' John

The Staff of Good Foods Co-op where I work pitched in one afternoon and came up with this recipe after preparing another Hoppin' John recipe we found in a cookbook. This one is tastier and more attractive. Hoppin' John is traditionally served with cornbread or biscuits—whole grain, of course!

1 cups black-eyed peas, sorted, rinsed, and drained
¾ to 1½ teaspoons crushed red pepper
1 large onion, coarsely chopped
1 small green pepper, chopped
1 large fresh tomato, chopped
1 teaspoon or more *Parsley Patch* It's a Dilly Seasoning Blend
¼ to ½ teaspoon salt, optional
1½ cups long grain brown rice, sorted, rinsed, drained, and cooked in 3 cups water
1 cup shredded low-fat cheddar or colby cheese
Fresh tomato wedges for garnish
Louisiana Hot Sauce, to taste

Combine peas and 2 cups of water. Add crushed red pepper, bring to a boil, reduce heat, cover, and simmer for about 1 hour. Add onion, green pepper, tomato, *Parsley Patch* seasoning, and more water if necessary. Cook for about 45 minutes longer or until peas are tender. Add salt, if desired. Serve over the cooked rice, garnishing with shredded cheese and tomato wedges. Have the *Louisiana* Hot Sauce on the table for individual seasoning. Makes 4 to 5 cups of Hoppin' John, excluding the brown rice.

If good fresh tomatoes are not available, substitute a 16-ounce can of tomatoes, using the tomato juice in place of an equal amount of water.

Perfect Whole Foods: *Read the label of the seasoning blend to make certain it's okay.*
Percent Calories From Fat: 25 with cheese, 20 without (excluding the brown rice)
Total Fat Grams In Recipe: 25 with cheese, 3 without (excluding the brown rice)

Mexican Salad

Serve this main dish salad in place of tacos or taco salad. The usual crisp corn tacos, tortillas, and corn chips, besides being high in fat and salt, often have coconut oil or hydrogenated fat as an ingredient. Garnish this salad with whole grain baked corn chips if they are available.

Crisp lettuce, broken or shredded
Whole kernel corn, steamed
Cooked dried beans such as pinto or kidney
Chopped fresh tomatoes
Chopped onions, raw
Celery slices, raw
Green pepper, coarsely chopped
Shredded cheese
Avocado chunks
Salsa, Picante Sauce, or Guacamole
Plain, nonfat yogurt
Whole grain baked corn chips as a garnish

Serve these ingredients separately and let each person make his own salad.

Perfect Whole Foods: *Check ingredient lists carefully if you use commercial salsa or picante sauce.*

New Orleans Red Beans and Brown Rice

2 cups dried red Mexican beans, sorted, rinsed, and drained
1 bay leaf
2 teaspoons oil
3 celery ribs, chopped
2 garlic cloves, minced
1 large onion, chopped
2 to 3 teaspoons chili powder (or more)
1 tablespoon tamari or shoyu soy sauce (alcohol-free)
¾ cup tomato purée
1 cup long grain brown rice, cooked in 2 cups water

Bring beans to a boil in 6 cups of water, turn off heat, cover, and let sit for 1 hour. Add bay leaf and simmer for 1½ hours. While beans are cooking, sauté vegetables and chili powder in oil for about 10 minutes. Add to beans along with tamari or shoyu sauce and simmer for about 1 hour longer or until beans are soft. Stir in tomato purée and heat for a few minutes. Serve over cooked brown rice. Makes about 7 cups beans, excluding brown rice.

Percent Calories From Fat: 8 without rice, 7 with rice
Total Fat Grams In Recipe: 12 without rice, 14 with rice

Garbanzo Bean Stew

This stew is good served with a vegetable salad, whole grain bread, and fresh fruit in season.

1½ cups garbanzo beans (also called chickpeas), sorted, rinsed, and drained
2 bay leaves
2 teaspoons oil
1 large onion, chopped
3 or 4 carrots, sliced
3 or 4 celery ribs, sliced
3 garlic cloves, minced
2 potatoes, scrubbed and cut into 1-inch chunks
1½ teaspoons dried basil
2 tablespoons chopped fresh parsley
½ to ¾ teaspoon salt, optional
2 tablespoons nutritional yeast

Bring beans to a boil in 5 cups of water, turn off heat, cover, and sit for 1 hour. Add the bay leaves and simmer for 3 hours. While beans are cooking, sauté onion, carrots, celery, and garlic in oil for a couple of minutes. Add to partially cooked beans along with the potatoes, basil, and parsley. Cook until all are tender, about 20 minutes. Add yeast and salt. Makes 7 cups.

Percent Calories From Fat: 11
Total Fat Grams In Recipe: 20

Lima Bean Stew: Use lima beans in place of the garbanzo beans, cooking them about 1¼ hours.

Scrambled Tofu

Whether or not you eat eggs, you'll like this egg-like scramble. Serve it with Whole Grain Corn Grits *(p. 131), steamed broccoli, and fresh fruit in season.*

1-pound package soft or medium tofu, rinsed, drained, and mashed
2 teaspoons tamari or shoyu soy sauce (alcohol-free)
¼ teaspoon turmeric
1 tablespoon nutritional yeast
¼ teaspoon granulated garlic
1 teaspoon granulated onion

Oil skillet lightly. Mix ingredients in a bowl. Pour into skillet and cook on low to medium heat until hot throughout and flavors are blended or about 15 minutes, stirring occasionally. Makes 3 cups.

Percent Calories From Fat: 49
Total Fat Grams In Recipe: 20

Scrambled Tofu with Vegetables: Add sliced or chopped vegetables like mushrooms, green peppers, and green onions to mixture before cooking.

Tofu Curry

Serve this stuffed in Toasted Pitas *(p. 237) or over cooked whole grains such as brown rice or millet. Either way, it's delicious! Since leftovers of this recipe tend to become watery, make just half of it if you have only a couple of people to feed. Or, serve leftovers over cooked grains rather than in pita bread.*

1 large onion, chopped
6 medium mushrooms, sliced
2 or 3 carrots, thinly sliced
1 teaspoon oil
2 cups sliced cabbage
1-pound package medium or firm tofu, rinsed, drained, and crumbled
2 tablespoons whole grain flour
1 to 2 teaspoons curry powder or to taste
½ teaspoon salt
Cooked whole grain (millet or long grain brown rice) or *Toasted Pitas* (p. 237)

In a large skillet, sauté onions, mushrooms, and carrots in oil for a couple of minutes. Add cabbage and sauté for a couple of minutes more or until cabbage is somewhat wilted. Remove from heat. In a saucepan, combine water, flour, and seasonings, stirring until flour is dissolved and lumps are gone. Use 2 cups of water if you are serving the mixture over cooked whole grains and 1 cup if you are stuffing the pitas. Cook, while stirring, until liquid begins to boil and becomes slightly thickened. Add tofu. Finally, add tofu mixture to sautéed vegetables and heat only until hot. Serve immediately. Makes 7 cups, excluding the cooked whole grain.

Percent Calories from Fat: 35, excluding the grain or pitas
Total Fat Grams in Recipe: 25, excluding the grain or pitas

Tofu Swiss Steak

1-pound package firm tofu, frozen and thawed
3 tablespoons tamari or shoyu sauce (alcohol-free)
2 tablespoons apple cider vinegar
¼ teaspoon black pepper
½ teaspoon dried rubbed sage
Whole grain flour for dipping tofu
1 tablespoon oil
1 large onion, sliced
1 carrot, chopped
1 celery rib, chopped
½ green pepper, chopped
4 or 5 mushrooms, sliced
1 cup tomato purée

Gently squeeze the water from tofu and slice it into ⅜-inch slices. In the refrigerator, marinate tofu slices for several hours in a mixture of tamari, vinegar, black pepper, and poultry seasoning. Add oil to a large *SilverStone* skillet. Dip tofu in flour and brown it in oil, turning once and being careful not to break the pieces. Add vegetables, tomato purée mixed with ½ cup of water, and any remaining marinade, cover skillet, and cook over low heat for 1 hour. Makes about 16 pieces (each piece 2 x 3¼-inches). Serves 4 or 5.

Percent Calories From Fat: 40
Total Fat Grams In Recipe: 47

Grecian Tofu Balls

Serve these tofu balls plain at a party or with whole grain pasta and spaghetti sauce as a main dish.

1 cup short grain brown rice, sorted, rinsed, and drained
1-pound package medium tofu, rinsed, drained, and mashed
2 tablespoons tamari or shoyu soy sauce (alcohol-free)
1 cup pecan meal
1 cup fresh wheat germ
⅛ teaspoon black pepper
¼ teaspoon ground cinnamon
1 teaspoon granulated onion
½ teaspoon granulated garlic
1 teaspoon dried oregano leaves

Cook brown rice in 2 cups of water until almost all water is absorbed or about 35 minutes. Preheat oven to 350°. Oil 2 cookie sheets. Mix all ingredients together and form into 1-inch balls. Bake for 30 minutes on cookie sheets. Makes about 6 dozen.

Percent Calories From Fat: 45
Total Fat Grams In Recipe: 99 (less than 1.5 grams fat per tofu ball)

Szechuan Tofu Stir-Fry

My family's dentist, Michael H. Lerner, DMD, MSD, developed this colorful dish. Besides being an excellent dentist, Dr. Lerner is also a gourmet whole foods cook! (The Szechuan hot paste or sauce can be found in oriental food stores.)

1-pound package tofu, frozen, thawed, drained, and cut into ½-inch chunks
8 ounces whole wheat pasta (linguini or spaghetti), cooked and drained
2 tablespoons peanut oil, divided
3 tablespoons tamari soy sauce
2 tablespoons arrowroot or corn starch

Marinade:
4 garlic cloves, minced
1 to 2 teaspoons minced fresh ginger
4 green onions, diced
2 tablespoons low sodium tamari soy sauce
2 tablespoons fruit-sweetened apricot preserves (or Duck sauce)
2 tablespoons Szechuan hot paste or sauce (more or less to taste)
2 tablespoons sesame seeds
2 tablespoons wine

Vegetables:
½ zucchini
½ yellow squash
6 or 8 mushrooms
3 green onions
3 ribs celery
½ cup purple cabbage
2 cups bean sprouts
1 cup snow peas

Marinate tofu for 30 minutes. While marinating, cut vegetables into desired shapes. Drain tofu, reserving marinade. Stir-fry tofu in 1 tablespoon oil until tofu is brown. Set aside. Stir-fry vegetables in 1 tablespoon more oil until veggies are dark in color and still crisp. Combine tamari sauce and arrowroot with 1 cup water. Add to veggies, cook until thickened, then add tofu and leftover marinade. Stir in pasta and toss. Serve and enjoy! Makes about 12 cups.

Perfect Whole Foods: No
Percent Calories From Fat: 29
Total Fat Grams In Recipe: 60

Tofu Skillet Dinner

1 large onion, chopped
1 garlic clove, minced
2 ribs celery, sliced
1 cup mushrooms, sliced
½ green pepper, diced
2 teaspoons oil
1-pound package firm tofu, rinsed, drained, and cut in cubes
1 cup shredded cabbage
2 bay leaves
1 tablespoon tamari or shoyu soy sauce (alcohol-free)
½ cup frozen green peas, thawed
1 tablespoon arrowroot
1 cup raw long grain brown rice, cooked in 2 cups water

In a large skillet, sauté the onion, garlic, celery, mushrooms and green pepper in the oil for a couple of minutes. Add tofu, cabbage, bay leaves, 1 cup water and tamari. Bring to a boil, reduce heat, cover, and simmer for about 15 minutes. Add green peas. Mix arrowroot with ¼ cup additional water and stir into ingredients. Stir and cook until thickened. Do not allow the ingredients to boil after adding arrowroot. Serve over cooked brown rice. Makes about 6 cups of tofu and vegetables, excluding the brown rice.

Perfect Whole Foods: Omit arrowroot and stir 3 tablespoons whole wheat flour into the ¼ cup water; add to tofu-vegetable-tamari mixture and thicken by bringing it all to a boil while stirring constantly.
Percent Calories From Fat: 24
Total Fat Grams In Recipe: 34

Gingered Tofu

This is a simple yet tasty way to prepare tofu. It's good served with brown rice and Mushroom-Miso Soup (p.183). *Yoko Obata, a Japanese exchange student and friend of my daughter Heather, showed me how to prepare the tofu as well as wakame, a sea vegetable. She was all excited about having a Japanese meal in Kentucky. When it came time to eat and the wakame was passed to Yoko, she smiled and said, "No, thanks." She explained that in Japan, teenagers don't eat sea vegetables, only adults. Sounds like teenagers are similar from wherever they come!*

1 package (10.5 ounces) *Mori-Nu* Silken Soft Tofu, cold
2 teaspoons or more tamari or shoyu soy sauce (alcohol-free)
1 to 2 teaspoons grated fresh ginger
1 green onion, thinly sliced (use some of the green)

Drain, then slice the tofu into a serving bowl. Drizzle with soy sauce and top with the ginger and green onion. Serve cold. Serves 2 or 3.

Percent Calories From Fat: 36
Total Fat Grams In Recipe: 8

Tempeh (or Tofu) Stew

8-ounce package tempeh, defrosted and chopped fine (or ½ pound tofu, frozen, defrosted, drained, and cubed)
1 teaspoon oil
1 or 2 teaspoons tamari or shoyu soy sauce (alcohol-free)
¼ teaspoon dried sage
1 teaspoon dried basil
1 tablespoon dried parsley
½ teaspoon granulated garlic
½ teaspoon dried marjoram
3 to 5 carrots, sliced
3 to 5 celery ribs, sliced
1 onion, chopped
1 green pepper, chopped
10 to 12 fresh mushrooms, sliced
2 cups potatoes (scrubbed but not peeled), cut into chunks
¼ teaspoon salt, optional
½ cup shredded low-fat cheese, optional

Oil large skillet or dutch oven and cover cooking surface with tempeh or tofu. Sprinkle tamari and seasonings on top and stir to mix. Rearrange tempeh or tofu evenly over bottom of skillet. Add vegetables on top of the tempeh or tofu. Then pour 1 cup of water over the vegetables, and if desired, sprinkle salt and cheese on top. Cover, bring to a boil, reduce heat, and cook 30 to 45 minutes or until vegetables are tender. Do not stir while stew is cooking. Serve a fresh salad and whole grain bread with this stew to make a delicious meal. Makes about 8 cups.
Slow Cooker: 6 hours on low.

Percent Calories From Fat: 25 without cheese, 30 with cheese
Total Fat Grams In Recipe: 27 without cheese, 38 with cheese

Barbecued Tempeh

Since this recipe uses half of the Barbecue Sauce *recipe, use the other half by adding cooked turkey or chicken pieces for another appetizing main dish.*

8-ounce package tempeh, defrosted
1 teaspoon oil for panfrying (total)
½ recipe of *Barbecue Sauce* (p. 268)

Cut tempeh into 4 pieces and then slice each piece into 2 thin patties. Panfry in oil on both sides until crisp and brown. Add to already prepared and cooked *Barbecue Sauce*, simmering for at least 1 hour before serving. Or prepare everything ahead of time and marinate tempeh in cooked sauce in refrigerator instead of simmering. Cook 10 to 15 minutes and serve. Serves 3.

Percent Calories From Fat: 32
Total Fat Grams In Recipe: 26

Mexican Skillet Dinner

If you like Mexican food, you'll like this quick and simple dish.

6 soft whole grain corn or whole wheat tortillas, torn or cut into 2-inch pieces
1 onion, chopped
2 teaspoons oil
1 teaspoon or more chili powder
¼ teaspoon dried oregano
¾ cup low-fat (1%) cottage cheese
1 cup tomato sauce
¾ cup shredded low-fat cheese

Thinly coat a heavy skillet with *Oil-Lecithin Combination* (p. 205). (I like my iron skillet for this recipe.) Add the oil to the skillet and sauté onions until soft. Add chili powder, oregano, and tortilla pieces, stirring until pieces are lightly coated with oil and seasonings. Spoon cottage cheese over tortilla pieces. Pour sauce on top and then sprinkle with shredded cheese. Cover skillet and heat until cheese is melted and sauce is bubbly. Serve from skillet. Serves 3 or 4.

Perfect Whole Foods: If you can't find whole grain corn tortillas or are not certain whether or not they are whole grain, then use 100% whole wheat tortillas (with no baking powder added). Use cottage cheese and tomato sauce with no starches or sugars added.
Percent Calories From Fat: 31
Total Fat Grams In Recipe: 34

Variations:
• Substitute 1 package (10.5 ounces) *Mori-Nu* Silken Tofu (mashed) for cottage cheese.
• Substitute cooked, drained beans for cottage cheese.
• Add small can drained green chilies before sprinkling cheese.

Spaghetti Dinner

Serve this for a quick and easy yet delicious meal. It's an excellent main dish to try if you're wanting to reduce your meat intake.

Whole Grain Pasta, cooked and drained (p. 147)
Quick Pasta Sauce (p. 268) or commercial sauce with no sugar added
Your favorite vegetables such as pressed garlic, chopped onions, diced green peppers, and sliced
   mushrooms, zucchini, or yellow squash
Parmesan cheese

Cook vegetables in spaghetti sauce until just tender. Serve over cooked pasta and top with Parmesan cheese.

Wheat-Free Spaghetti Dinner: Try one of the several wheat-free, 100% whole grain pastas that are available–spelt, brown rice, or buckwheat. Or use baked spaghetti squash. Note that corn pasta, quinoa-corn pasta, and kamut pasta with corn are not 100% whole grain and should, therefore, not be used on the **Perfect Whole Foods** diet.

Vegetarian Lasagna

For many years of my journey with whole foods, I served this lasagna for special occasions with Whole Wheat French Bread *(p. 216) and a large fresh vegetable salad. Recently however, I've been using fewer animal products in my diet and have been preparing the* Dairy-Free or Vegan Lasagna *(p.96) recipe that follows this. Whichever you prefer, they are both good.*

1½ recipes of *Quick Pasta Sauce* (p. 268), previously prepared and refrigerated (or a sugar-free commercial spaghetti sauce)
2 cups low-fat (1%) cottage or ricotta cheese
2 eggs, beaten
¼ cup grated Parmesan cheese plus 1 or 2 tablespoons more Parmesan cheese
¼ cup fresh, chopped parsley or 2 tablespoons dried
8 ounces whole grain lasagna noodles, cooked and drained
½ pound shredded part-skim milk Mozzarella cheese

Preheat oven to 350 °. Combine cottage cheese with eggs, ¼ cup Parmesan cheese, and parsley. Set aside. Coat bottom of 9-inch x 13-inch baking dish with sauce. Don't use too much sauce each time you add it or lasagna will be soupy. You will not use all of the sauce—altogether, probably just a little more than one recipe. Layer half of the noodles, half of the Mozzarella, half of the cottage cheese mixture, and more sauce. Repeat. Sprinkle the top with 1 or 2 tablespoons Parmesan cheese before baking. Bake for 30 to 40 minutes. Let stand 10 to 15 minutes before serving. Serves 6 to 8.

Percent Calories From Fat: 24
Total Fat Grams In Recipe: 81

Vegetable-Vegetarian Lasagna: Partially cook sliced eggplant, zucchini, or spinach by steaming and add to casserole layers.

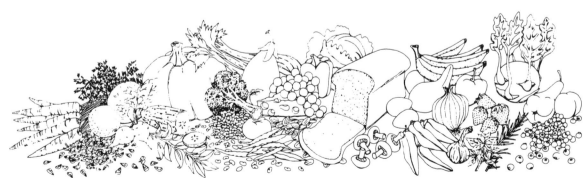

Health is truly a lot more than just being free of disease. Walt Stoll, M.D.

Dairy-Free or Vegan Lasagna

Whether you are allergic to dairy products, a vegan, or just want to avoid saturated animal fats, try this luscious lasagna.

8 ounces whole wheat lasagna noodles, cooked and drained
2 teaspoons olive oil
2 or 3 garlic cloves, minced
1 medium onion, chopped
10 or 12 mushrooms, sliced
1 green pepper, chopped
2 celery ribs, thinly sliced
2 teaspoons dried basil
1 teaspoon dried oregano leaves
½ teaspoon each dried marjoram and thyme
28 or 29-ounce can tomato purée
6-ounce can tomato paste
⅛ teaspoon black pepper
½ to ¾ teaspoon salt
1-pound package firm tofu, drained and mashed
2 tablespoons nutritional yeast

Preheat oven to 350°. In a large skillet, sauté fresh vegetables in oil for 5 minutes. Sprinkle herbs over vegetables and sauté a minute or so longer. Add tomato purée, tomato paste, salt, and pepper, stirring to mix. Bring to a boil, reduce heat and simmer sauce for about 10 minutes. Coat bottom of a 9-inch x 13-inch baking dish with about one-third of the sauce. Add a layer of cooked noodles, sprinkle with half of the tofu, and finally half of the nutritional yeast. Repeat the layers of sauce, noodles, tofu, and yeast, topping with the remaining sauce. Bake for 30 minutes. Serves 6 to 8.

Percent Calories From Fat: 24
Total Fat Grams In Recipe: 46

Dairy-Free Cheese

This recipe was given to me by a Co-op friend. It reminds me of processed American-type cheese and is good sliced on sandwiches or shredded on pizza. If you are allergic to dairy, beware of the soy cheeses that are available. They almost always are made with casein or caseinate which are dairy derivatives.

1 cup water at room temperature
⅓ cup + 1 rounded tablespoon unflavored gelatin*
1¼ cups boiling water
2 cups raw cashews
3 tablespoons nutritional yeast
2 teaspoons granulated onion
¼ teaspoon granulated garlic
2 to 3 tablespoons fresh lemon juice
2 teaspoons paprika
1½ teaspoons salt

Soak gelatin in room temperature water in blender. Pour boiling water over soaked gelatin and blend until gelatin is dissolved. Cool slightly. Add cashews and blend thoroughly. Add remaining ingredients, blend until mixture is consistency of creamy sauce. Pour into a bread pan, cover, and refrigerate overnight. Cheese may be frozen after it firms if desired. Makes about 3½ cups.

Perfect Whole Foods: Do not use because of lemon juice.
Percent Calories From Fat: 60
Total Fat Grams In Recipe: 131

* Vegan Cheese: To use agar in place of gelatin, use 3 tablespoons plus 1 teaspoon agar powder and follow these directions: Combine agar powder with 1½ cups water at room temperature. Bring to a boil, reduce heat, and simmer for 2 minutes. Slowly add ¾ cup more water. Pour into blender container, adding cashews and remaining ingredients. Blend until creamy and continue with instructions above.

Macaroni and Cheese

1½ cups uncooked whole grain macaroni
3 tablespoons whole wheat flour, hard or pastry
1½ cups skim milk
1½ cups shredded low-fat cheese
¾ teaspoon prepared mustard
½ teaspoon granulated onion
⅛ teaspoon black pepper, optional
⅛ teaspoon paprika

Cook macaroni in about 6 cups of boiling water until tender or about 10 to 12 minutes; drain. While macaroni is cooking, prepare sauce by whisking the flour into the milk until smooth and then cooking over medium heat and stirring constantly until sauce thickens. Stir in cheese, seasonings, and cooked macaroni. Heat until cheese melts. Sprinkle with more paprika if you like. Makes 4 cups.

Wheat-Free Macaroni and Cheese: Use spelt or brown rice macaroni and a whole grain flour other than wheat.

Percent Calories From Fat: 37
Total Fat Grams In Recipe: 59

Macaroni-O's

Children who like canned spaghetti products usually like this simple dish.

1½ cups uncooked whole wheat macaroni
15-ounce can tomato sauce
⅛ teaspoon granulated garlic
⅛ teaspoon granulated onion
⅛ teaspoon dried oregano leaves
⅛ teaspoon black pepper
1 cup shredded part-skim milk Mozzarella cheese

Cook macaroni in about 6 cups of boiling water until barely tender or about 10 minutes; drain. Mix in remaining ingredients and stir while heating over low heat until cheese is melted and blended in sauce. Makes 4 cups.

Wheat-Free Macaroni-O's: Use spelt or brown rice macaroni.

Perfect Whole Foods: Select a tomato sauce with no added sugar or starch.
Percent Calories From Fat: 17
Total Fat Grams In Recipe: 21

Light Pesto

Most pesto recipes are very high in fat, usually having ¼ to ½ cup of olive oil per recipe. My friend Debbie Graviss adapted a recipe to eliminate as much fat as possible and came up with this one. It's delicious!

1 tablespoon olive oil
1 large garlic clove, minced or crushed
4 cups loosely-packed fresh basil leaves, washed, drained, and dried with paper towels
1½ cups plain, nonfat yogurt
½ cup grated Parmesan cheese plus more for topping
½ teaspoon salt
¼ teaspoon black pepper

Combine oil and garlic in a small pan and cook over low heat for about 1 minute. Remove from heat and cool slightly. In food processor, purée all ingredients. Makes about 1¾ cups pesto. To serve, toss ¼ cup pesto (room temperature) with about 1 cup cooked whole grain pasta (about 2 ounces raw). Sprinkle with additional Parmesan cheese if you like.

Percent Calories From Fat: 38
Total Fat Grams In Recipe: 24

Instant Pita Pizza

Whole wheat pita bread (unsweetened)
Chopped or sliced raw vegetables such as mushrooms, green onions, and green peppers
Sliced black olives, optional
Granulated garlic
Granulated onion
Shredded part-skim milk Mozzarella cheese
Pizza sauce or spaghetti sauce (unsweetened)

Prepare pizza by spreading sauce on top of each pita, sprinkling vegetables and granulated garlic and onion over sauce, and topping vegetables with cheese. Broil in oven until cheese melts and becomes lightly browned.

Toasted Pizza: Substitute lightly toasted, 100% whole grain bread (unsweetened) for the pita bread.

English Muffin Pizza: Substitute split English muffins for the pita bread, lightly toasting the split muffins before preparing the pizza. If you are on the perfect diet, use homemade unsweetened English muffins. (You can use the recipe on page 217.)

Whole Grain Pizza

Prepare a scrumptious pizza using unsweetened, yeasted whole grain bread dough—wheat, spelt, or kamut! You can prepare the bread dough by hand, in a Vita Mix, *or in a bread machine. (See bread recipes beginning on page 208. Or, order ahead and buy the dough from a whole wheat bakery for an almost instant pizza. (Make certain the dough is unsweetened and 100% whole grain if you are on the perfect diet.)*

Bread dough containing 4 to 5 cups of whole grain flour
Sugar-free pizza sauce (commercial) or spaghetti sauce (homemade or commercial)
½ teaspoon oil
4 cups fresh vegetables (any or some of all: sliced mushrooms, chopped onions, coarsely chopped green pepper, sliced zucchini or yellow squash, or snow peas with ends removed)
Sliced black olives, optional
8-ounce package shredded part-skim milk mozzarella cheese
2 tablespoons Parmesan cheese
Granulated garlic
Granulated onion
Crushed red peppers, optional

Preheat oven to 500°. Oil two 14-inch pizza pans with *Oil-Lecithin Combination* (p. 205). In a skillet or pan, sauté vegetables in ½ teaspoon oil for about 5 minutes. Divide dough in half and, one half at a time, roll dough into a 10 to 12-inch circle on a counter that has been dusted with whole grain flour. Place dough on pan and, using fingers, stretch dough to cover pan. Spread sauce on dough, enough to lightly cover. Sprinkle half of vegetables on top of sauce. Arrange olives on vegetables, if you're using them. Sprinkle half of the mozzarella cheese and a little Parmesan cheese (optional) over the pizza. Next, sprinkle granulated garlic and onion plus a few crushed red peppers (optional) on top of the cheese. Bake immediately for 8 to 12 minutes or until dough is cooked and cheese is lightly browned.
Note: The *Whole Wheat Vita Mix Bread (Unsweetened, 100% Whole Wheat)* recipe on page 211 will make one pizza.

Dairy-Free Whole Grain Pizza: Use *Dairy-Free Cheese or Vegan Cheese* (p. 97) in place of mozzarella and Parmesan cheeses.

Percent Calories from Fat: 19
Total Fat Grams in Recipe: 51 (two 14-inch pizzas, without olives)

Mexicali Pizza

Soft whole grain corn tortillas or whole wheat tortillas or chapatis
Fresh tomatoes, thinly sliced
Mushrooms, thinly sliced
Green peppers, finely chopped
Onions, finely chopped
Part-skim milk mozzarella cheese, shredded

Preheat oven to 350°. Place tortillas or chapatis on a cookie sheet. Arrange tomatoes and mushrooms on top; sprinkle with green peppers, onions, and cheese. Bake until cheese melts.

Perfect Whole Foods: Make certain the flat bread is 100% whole grain and contains no baking powder.

Vegetable Quiche

Use Now *Eggwhite Powder in place of the two egg whites to avoid having to discard egg yolks. For two egg whites, mix 4 teaspoons powder with 4 tablespoons water, allow to sit for a few minutes, and mix again. Many dried egg white products are meant for candies and frostings and contain sugar and starch.*

Prepare 2 cups cleaned, coarsely chopped vegetables such as any of the following combinations:
• Spanish onions alone
• Onions, mushrooms, green peppers, and ½ teaspoon dried basil
• Broccoli and onions
• Cauliflower, carrots, onions, and green peppers
• Shredded zucchini, onions, and mushrooms

1 teaspoon butter
¾ cup skim milk
1 whole egg
2 egg whites (or another whole egg)
⅛ teaspoon black pepper
4 teaspoons whole grain flour
1 cup shredded low-fat cheese
Small amount grated Parmesan cheese
9-inch *Whole Grain Pie Crust* (p. 239), baked 10 minutes

Sauté vegetables in butter until tender but still crisp. Cool. If using juicy vegetables such as zucchini or mushrooms, drain off most of the liquid. Beat together the milk, eggs, and pepper. Preheat oven to 350°. Stir flour and shredded cheese into cooled vegetables, spoon vegetable mixture into pie crust, and then pour egg and milk mixture over the vegetabes, sprinkle with Parmesan cheese, and bake 35 or 40 minutes. Serves 5 or 6.

Wheat-Free Vegetable Quiche: Use spelt or triticale flour with the rolled oats in the crust. Check the *Whole Grain Pie Crust* recipe on page 239 for exact proportions.

Percent Calories From Fat: 37
Total Fat Grams In Recipe: 83

Cottage Cheese-Spinach Quiche

This crustless quiche is quickly made and is a great main dish when you're in a hurry. I use Now Eggwhite Powder in place of the two egg whites so I don't have to discard egg yolks. For two egg whites, mix 4 teaspoons powder with 4 tablespoons water and allow it to sit for several minutes and mix again. Be aware that many dried egg white products are meant for candies and frostings and contain sugar and starch.

10-ounce package frozen chopped spinach, steamed until tender
1 cup low-fat (1%) cottage cheese
1 whole egg
2 egg whites (or another whole egg)
⅛ teaspoon pepper
Pinch of nutmeg
¼ cup shredded low-fat cheddar cheese
1 tablespoon sunflower seeds or pinenuts

Preheat oven to 350°. Oil 8 or 9-inch pie pan with *Oil-Lecithin Combination* (p. 205). Beat egg and egg whites together with a fork. Drain spinach and place in mixing bowl. Add cottage cheese, eggs, pepper, and nutmeg. Pour into pie pan then sprinkle with cheese and nuts. Bake for 20 to 25 minutes. Serves 4.

Perfect Whole Foods: Read cottage cheese ingredient list carefully so you won't buy brands with added starch or whey.
Percent Calories From Fat: 31
Total Fat Grams In Recipe: 18

Hard Cooked Eggs

Until I learned this method, I had trouble peeling the shells from hard cooked eggs. Since fresh eggs are harder to peel than older ones (there's little air space between the shell and the whites of fresh eggs), use your older eggs when hard cooking them. If the yolks of hard cooked eggs turn green, they have been over-cooked.

Place eggs in cold water, cover, bring to a near boil, reduce heat, and simmer for about 15 to 20 minutes, time depending upon the size of the eggs. Remove from heat, add eggs to a bowl of ice water, reserving the hot water. Let eggs sit for about 2 minutes in the ice water. Place eggs back in hot water for 2 more minutes, then back into the ice water. When almost cool, crack the shells. Finish cooling in ice water and then remove shells.

Percent Calories From Fat: 64
Total Fat Grams In Recipe: 6 (1 large egg)

Frittatas

Frittata (pronounced frit-TA-ta) is the Italian word for omelet. Rather than being folded in half as are most omelets, frittatas are served open-faced, either hot or cold. The filling can include any variety of vegetables, cooked grains, as well as small pieces of cooked meat or poultry, if desired. Vegetables are sautéed in the skillet; grains and meats are added; then the beaten eggs are added and cooked until set. Frittatas make a quick main dish and can be varied according to preferences and food on hand. I find it an easy way to include vegetables in a Sunday brunch. Use the following tips to help prepare the frittata recipe I've included as well as your own original frittatas.

- A 10-inch *SilverStone* or iron skillet will accommodate a 4 to 8 egg frittata. Unless you're using the non-stick skillet, you'll need to use a thin layer of *Oil-Lecithin Combination* (p. 205) to prevent the frittata from sticking.
- Sauté the vegetables until they are almost tender before adding the egg mixture.
- Use low to medium heat once the eggs are added to avoid over-browning the bottom before the center sets.
- The total cooking time depends on the number of eggs you're using.
- To help cook the top of the frittata, broil it about 6 inches from the heat for a couple of minutes.
- A frittata can be served in several ways. Cut it into wedges and serve it from the skillet. Or slide the uncut frittata top-side up or inverted (browned-side-up) onto a platter and serve.

Basic Ingredients:
5 or 6 whole eggs
2 or 4 egg whites (or 1 or 2 more whole eggs but frittata will have more fat and cholesterol)
Oil-Lecithin Combination (p. 205), optional
½ teaspoon oil, optional
1 small onion, chopped
Fresh or dried herbs, to your taste
3 or 4 cups filling*: chopped, diced, or sliced vegetables; cooked grains; and meat
Shredded low-fat cheese, optional

*Here are two sample vegetable fillings you might enjoy.

Filling 1:
1 small zucchini, coarsely chopped
1 garlic clove, minced
½ small, firm eggplant chopped
1 cup sliced mushrooms
½ green pepper, diced
¼ teaspoon basil

Filling 2:
1 small zucchini, coarsely chopped
1 small yellow squash, coarsely chopped
1 small red pepper, diced
1 small green pepper, diced
Shredded Swiss cheese, optional

Prepare skillet with *Oil-Lecithin Combination* if you're not using a non-stick skillet. Sauté all vegetables in oil for a few minutes. Then add cooked grains, meat, and herbs, if used. Stir to mix ingredients and arrange them evenly in skillet. Beat eggs and egg whites together, then pour into skillet. Cook over low to medium heat until eggs are almost set. Add optional cheese and finish cooking the top by broiling in oven. Serve hot or cold. Serves 4 or 5.

Percent Calories From Fat: 47 (filled with vegetables, no cheese)
Total Fat Grams In Recipe: 25

Grilled Chicken

Here are several simple yet delicious ways to prepare grilled chicken. If you use a SilverStone skillet, there's no need to oil the pan before adding the chicken. It will not stick.

Boneless, skinless chicken breast halves
SilverStone skillet or griddle
Salt and pepper, optional

Cook chicken over medium heat, using a *SilverStone* skillet or griddle, until cooked throughout and browned on outside, turning the pieces over occasionally. Salt and pepper, as desired.

Lemon-Pepper Grilled Chicken: Sprinkle chicken with a seasoning like *Parsley Patch* Lemon Pepper Herb & Spice Blend. Grill as in recipe above. If you are on **Perfect Whole Foods**, make certain your seasoning does not contain sugar, lemon juice powder, lemon powder, or lemon flavor (sources of sugar). Lemon peel and lemon oil are okay.

Oriental Grilled Chicken: Begin cooking chicken according to recipe above and sprinkle pieces generously with granulated onion and granulated garlic while cooking. Next sprinkle with tamari or shoyu soy sauce. When you turn the chicken pieces over, repeat the seasonings. If you are on the perfect diet, make certain that soy sauce is free of sugar and alcohol.

Percent Calories From Fat: 17
Total Fat Grams In Recipe: 3 (1 breast half)

Chicken in a Crockpot

This is a favorite recipe at the Ballard Morgan home. Dr. Morgan and his wife Martha put these simple ingredients together in the slow cooker before going to work. They also prepare Baked Brown Rice (p. 137) by placing the ingredients in the oven and having the oven set to come on and cook later in the day. When they arrive home, all they have to fix is a fresh vegetable salad and a delicious dinner is ready! Dr. Morgan is a dentist in Lexington and Martha is his assistant.

5 carrots, sliced
1 or 2 onions, sliced or coarsely chopped
5 celery ribs, sliced
4 skinless chicken breast halves (with or without bones)
¼ teaspoon coarsely ground black pepper
½ teaspoon salt, optional

Place carrots, onions, and celery in the bottom of a slow cooker. Turn slow cooker on to begin heating. Rinse chicken under running water, place it in a saucepan, add 2 cups of water, salt, and pepper and heat to boiling. Transfer chicken and water to slow cooker. Cover and cook on low for 8 to 10 hours (or on high for 3 1/2 to 5 hours). Remove bones before serving. If desired, break chicken into small chunks. Makes about 8 cups.

Percent Calories From Fat: 16
Total Fat Grams In Recipe: 15

Snow on the Mountain

Serve this as a special company buffet. Have plenty of cooked brown rice and creamed turkey or chicken (use the Whole Grain Creamy Sauce *recipe on page 267). Guests select from the many toppings with coconut the final one, it being the "snow on the mountain." Vegetarians still have plenty from which to select when they omit the creamed turkey.*

Long grain brown rice, cooked
Cooked chicken or turkey chunks in *Whole Grain Creamy Sauce*

Toppings:

Chopped tomatoes
Chopped celery
Sautéed, sliced mushrooms
Pineapple chunks

Black or green olives
Chopped onions
Diced green pepper
Sliced almonds

Shredded low-fat cheese
Unsweetened shredded
coconut

Perfect Whole Foods: Omit pineapple chunks if they are canned and coconut if it is dried.

Chinese Chicken Salad

1½ cups cooked chicken chunks
5 cups fresh spinach, torn into pieces
8 medium-sized mushrooms, sliced
½ red onion, sliced and separated into rings
1 cup Chinese or green cabbage, thinly sliced
1 cup snow peas
2 tablespoons sesame seeds, toasted in a dry skillet
1 tablespoon oil
2 tablespoons raw wine vinegar
¼ cup tomato purée
¼ teaspoon tamari or shoyu soy sauce (alcohol-free)

Prepare dressing by combining oil, 2 tablespoons water, vinegar, tomato purée, and tamari. Pour dressing over chicken. Cover and refrigerate to chill. When ready to serve, gently toss the vegetables in a large bowl and arrange on 4 dinner plates. Top with chicken and dressing. Sprinkle with sesame seeds. Serves 4.

Percent Calories From Fat: 33
Total Fat Grams In Recipe: 42

Chicken and Dressing Casserole

This recipe takes a little longer than most in this book, but it's a family favorite! If you have leftover turkey with broth, save time by substituting it for the chicken.

4 chicken breast halves with skin removed
1 bay leaf
½ teaspoon celery seeds
5 carrots, sliced and steamed until tender-crisp
5 cups whole wheat bread cubes (bread that is starting to dry out is good)
1¼ teaspoon dried sage
½ teaspoon oil
1 onion, chopped
2 celery ribs, thinly sliced
¼ cup whole grain flour
1 cup shredded low-fat cheese

Early in the day, put chicken in pot with enough water to cover. Add bay leaf and celery seeds; simmer for an hour. Separate chicken and broth and cool both in the refrigerator; discard any hardened fat from the broth. Remove chicken from bones. Add enough water to the broth to make 3¼ cups total.

Prepare the dressing by tossing bread cubes with sage. Sauté onion and celery in oil for 5 to 7 minutes. Mix sautéed vegetables with bread cubes. Add 2 cups of the broth, mixing well and reserving remaining broth. Let sit while preparing sauce.

Oil a 10-inch square casserole dish with *Oil-Lecithin Combination* (p. 205). Preheat oven to 350°. Add the flour to 1¼ cups remaining broth, stirring until smooth. Cook, stirring constantly, until thickened and starting to boil. Add cheese and stir until melted; add chicken pieces and cooked carrots. Spread chicken mixture in casserole. Top with dressing. Cover and bake for 30 minutes. Makes about 6 servings.

Perfect Whole Foods: Use unsweetened, 100% whole grain bread.
Percent Calories From Fat: 25
Total Fat Grams In Recipe: 43

Broccoli-Turkey Bake

Here's another family favorite. This simple casserole can be prepared the night before and baked just before serving.

1 bunch broccoli
1½ cups turkey broth
5 tablespoons whole grain flour
1 small onion, chopped
3 cups sliced mushrooms (about 15 medium mushrooms or 8 ounces)
¼ to ½ teaspoon salt, optional
1½ cups cooked turkey, diced

Oil a 10-inch square casserole dish with *Oil-Lecithin Combination* (p. 205). Cut washed broccoli into bite-size pieces and steam until tender-crisp. While broccoli is cooking, combine broth and flour in medium size saucepan, stirring until free of lumps. Cook until thickened, stirring constantly. Add onion and mushrooms, stirring gently and cooking for 3 or 4 minutes. Add salt, if desired. Preheat oven to 375°. Place broccoli in casserole. Cover with diced turkey and then pour sauce over the turkey. Bake uncovered for 20 to 25 minutes. Makes about 6 servings.

Perfect Whole Foods: Make certain turkey and broth do not have sugar or starch added.
Percent Calories From Fat: 7 (using light meat of turkey with no skin)
Total Fat Grams In Recipe: 5

Turkey Breast in Slow Cooker

Remove skin from turkey breast half or portion, rinse the skinned turkey breast thoroughly under cold running water, and place it in pan. Add 1/2 cup water and bring water to a boil. Cook over medium heat until turkey is heated throughout. Transfer turkey and liquid to slow cooker container. If desired, add a whole onion and 2 or 3 whole garlic cloves. Turn cooker on low and cook for 8 hours. The internal temperature of the turkey should read 180 degrees on a meat thermometer when it's done.

Perfect Whole Foods: Most frozen turkey breasts have sugar and fats injected into them. Select fresh turkey or read ingredient list carefully to eliminate undesirable ingredients in frozen ones.
Percent Calories From Fat: 18
Fat Grams In 2 Ounces: 2

Crockpot Turkey Spoon Burger

Prepare this recipe for company, serving it on whole grain buns or over brown rice. Freeze extras in portions suitable for your family.

3 pounds lean ground turkey (7% fat), browned in skillet, chopped into small pieces, and drained
1 onion, chopped
1 or 2 garlic cloves, minced
3 or 4 ribs celery, chopped
1 green pepper, chopped
1 cup spaghetti sauce (sugar-free)
6-ounce can tomato paste
1 tablespoon tamari or shoyu sauce (alcohol-free)
2 tablespoons apple cider vinegar
1 teaspoon prepared mustard
½ teaspoon paprika
¼ teaspoon black pepper
½ to ¾ teaspoon salt

Place browned turkey in slow cooker. Mix remaining ingredients with 1¼ cups boiling water and stir it into the turkey. Cook for 6 hours on low or 3 to 4 hours on high, adding water as necessary if on high. Makes about 8 cups.

Perfect Whole Foods: Use buns or toast that are 100% whole grain and are unsweetened.
Percent Calories From Fat: 44
Total Fat Grams In Recipe: 101 (about 13 grams fat per cup)

Homemade Turkey Sausage

This breakfast turkey sausage is free of sugar and preservatives; it is also lower in salt and fat than commercial brands. Use lean ground turkey with less than the typical 85 percent lean by weight (or 15 percent fat) to avoid added turkey fat and skin.

1 pound lean ground turkey (7% fat by weight)
1½ teaspoons dried sage
1 teaspoon dried thyme
½ to ¾ teaspoon salt
½ to 1 teaspoon crushed red pepper, optional
½ teaspoon dried marjoram
¼ teaspoon granulated garlic
⅛ teaspoon black pepper

Using a food processor with blade attachment, combine all ingredients. Use immediately or freeze. Clean the equipment thoroughly with hot, soapy water. Makes 1 pound of sausage.

Percent Calories From Fat: 50
Total Fat Grams In Recipe: 32 (about 2 grams per ounce)

Sausage Quiche

½ pound *Homemade Turkey Sausage* (p. 108)
1 small onion, chopped
2 tablespoons diced green pepper
½ teaspoon dried basil
Dash of granulated garlic
¾ cup shredded low-fat cheese
2 egg whites
½ cup skim milk
9-inch unbaked *Whole Grain Pie Crust* (p. 239)

Preheat oven to 350°. Brown sausage in skillet and mix with onion, green pepper, basil, and garlic powder. Put mixture into pie crust. Sprinkle cheese on top. Beat egg whites and milk together and pour over sausage. Bake approximately 50 minutes or until egg and milk mixture is set and quiche is browned. Serves 5 or 6.

Percent Calories From Fat: 38
Total Fat Grams In Recipe: 83

Sausage-Cheese Balls

½ pound *Homemade Turkey Sausage* (p. 108)
1 cup shredded low-fat cheese
½ teaspoon granulated onion
1½ teaspoons poultry seasoning
⅛ to ¼ teaspoon crushed red pepper
¾ cup whole grain flour

Preheat oven to 350°. Combine seasonings with flour. Mix all ingredients together and shape into 1-inch balls. Bake on ungreased cookie sheet for 15 to 20 minutes. Makes 2 to 3 dozen.

Percent Calories From Fat: 36
Total Fat Grams In Recipe: 39

Baked Fish with Garlic Butter

1 pound fish fillets, such as haddock, perch, or cod
2 teaspoons butter or oil
1 garlic clove, finely minced

Preheat oven to 425°. Sauté garlic in butter until garlic is golden brown. Arrange fish in a single layer in a flat casserole with a lid and drizzle garlic butter over fish. Cover and bake until fish is opaque, about 10 minutes per inch thickness plus 5 minutes because of lid. Serves 3 or 4.

Percent Calories From Fat: 26 (using haddock)
Total Fat Grams In Recipe: 13

Fish Baked in Milk

Baking it in milk will help make strong-tasting fish have a milder flavor.

1 pound fish fillets, such as haddock, perch, or cod
Skim milk
Your choice of seasonings:

Salt	Parsley	Granulated garlic	Lime wedge
Pepper	Paprika	Granulated onion	Chives
Dill weed	Tarragon	Lemon wedge	

Preheat oven to 425°. Arrange fish in a single layer in flat baking dish and pour milk to half the depth of the fish. Bake until fish is opaque, approximately 10 minutes per inch thickness. Remove fish from baking dish and place on serving platter. Sprinkle with seasonings to taste. Serves 3 or 4.

Perfect Whole Foods: If you use lemon or lime, eat the pulp, not just the juice.
Percent Calories From Fat: 11
Total Fat Grams In Recipe: 5

Broiled Fish

1 pound fish fillets, such as haddock, perch, or cod
2 teaspoons oil
Salt, optional

Preheat broiler pan and brush with oil. Place fish on pan and broil 5 minutes per inch thickness, 4 to 6-inches from broiler. Brush with a little oil and turn fish over. Lightly brush other side with oil and broil 5 minutes longer or until fish flakes with a fork and has turned opaque. Do not overcook! Thin pieces may not require turning. Season with salt to taste. Serves 3 or 4.

Percent Calories From Fat: 28 (using haddock)
Total Fat Grams In Recipe: 14

Tom's Tuna

1 onion, chopped
1 or 2 carrots, sliced
½ teaspoon oil
6-ounce can water-packed tuna, drained
1 cup brown rice cooked in 2 cups water

In a skillet sauté onion and carrots in oil until carrots are tender-crisp. Add tuna and heat. Serve over cooked brown rice. Season with alcohol-free tamari or shoyu sauce. Serves 2 or 3.

Percent Calories From Fat: 8
Total Fat Grams In Recipe: 9

Seafood Creole

If you want to eat fish yet don't care for its taste, then try this recipe or the one on page 109 called Baked Fish with Garlic Butter.

1 pound fish fillets, such as haddock, perch, or cod
1 cup tomato purée
1 small onion, chopped
2 or 3 mushrooms, sliced
1 rib celery, sliced
¼ green pepper, diced
1 or 2 garlic cloves, minced

Preheat oven to 425°. Arrange fish in a single layer in baking dish with a lid. In small saucepan, cook vegetables in tomato purée for about 3 to 4 minutes. Pour over fish, cover, and bake until fish flakes when tested with a fork or about 10 minutes per inch thickness of fish. Serves 3 or 4.

Percent Calories From Fat: 11 (using haddock)
Total Fat Grams In Recipe: 6

Salmon Steaks in Lemon-Butter Sauce

Salmon is a very fatty fish that's rich in the beneficial Omega-3 fatty acids. These fatty acids are recognized for lowering blood cholesterol and promoting health in many other ways.

1 small salmon steak per person (approximately 1-inch thick)
½ teaspoon melted butter per steak
½ teaspoon lemon juice per steak
Dill weed

Preheat oven to 450°. Arrange salmon steaks in baking dish. Brush with butter mixed with lemon juice. Sprinkle with dill. Cover and bake for approximately 15 minutes.

Perfect Whole Foods: *Do not use the lemon juice.*
Percent Calories From Fat: 58
Total Fat Grams In Recipe: 23

Sautéed Scallops

Bay scallops are milder in flavor than sea scallops and are the smaller of the two. If you use the larger sea scallops, cook them longer, about 3 to 6 minutes altogether.

1 pound fresh bay scallops
4 teaspoons butter, total
Lemon wedges, optional

Rinse scallops and pat them dry with a paper towel. Melt 1 teaspoon butter in skillet. Sauté about one-fourth at a time, using moderate heat and cooking for 2 or 3 minutes. Add 1 teaspoon of butter each time you sauté more scallops. Serve with lemon wedges. Serves 3 or 4.

Perfect Whole Foods: Eat the pulp of the lemon as well as the juice.
Percent Calories From Fat: 24
Total Fat Grams In Recipe: 16

Sautéed Scallops and Mushrooms: Sauté 8-10 sliced fresh mushrooms and 2-3 sliced garlic cloves and set aside before sautéing the scallops. Mix with cooked scallops and serve with optional lemon juice.

Boiled Shrimp

1 pound fresh green shrimp
1 quart water
1 bay leaf
3 peppercorns
1 tablespoon apple cider vinegar
½ teaspoon salt, optional

Bring all ingredients except shrimp to a boil in a saucepan. Add shrimp, return water to a boil, reduce heat, cover, and simmer for 2 to 5 minutes or just until shrimp turn pink. Drain and cool shrimp in ice water. To remove shells, pull legs off with fingers and then peel back. Remove tail fins if shrimp will be used in a mixed dish or leave them on as a handle for dipping. Cut the back lengthwise with a paring knife just deep enough to remove the black vein with knife point or toothpick. Do this while rinsing under cold water. Refrigerate. Use in salads, stir-fries, or with hot sauce. Makes about ¾ pound.

Percent Calories From Fat: 10
Total Fat Grams In Recipe: 7

Tasty Tuna Salad

If you are sensitive to MSG, buy tuna that contains only tuna, water, and salt. Most canned tunas include hydrolyzed vegetable protein or vegetable broth which are likely to have naturally occurring MSG.

6-ounce can water-packed tuna, not drained
¼ cup raw rolled oats or oat bran
2 ribs celery, thinly sliced
1 tablespoon mayonnaise (unsweetened)
3 tablespoons or more plain, nonfat yogurt
½ teaspoon granulated onion

Combine all ingredients in a bowl and chill. Makes about 1¾ cups.

Percent Calories From Fat: 29
Total Fat Grams In Recipe: 15

Slow-Cooked Rump Roast

Rump roast, with all of the visible fat removed, is one of the leanest cuts of beef available.

2 to 3 pound rump roast, visible fat removed from surface
2 medium onions, cut in half
1 garlic cloves, minced
3 to 5 potatoes, scrubbed and halved, optional
2 to 4 carrots, cut into 2-inch pieces, optional

Heat roast in pan along with ½ cup of water until roast is warmed. Place garlic, onions, and optional vegetables in bottom of slow cooker. Add meat and water. Cook on low heat for 8 to 11 hours.

Reduced-Fat Slow-Cooked Rump Roast: To decrease the fat even more, cook overnight and refrigerate during the day, storing broth in a separate wide-mouth jar. Before using the broth, remove the solid fat from the top of the jar. This step is especially helpful if you cook a cut of meat that has more fat than the rump roast. Makes about 3 servings per pound of roast.

Rump Roast Cooked in Oven: Preheat oven to 325 to 350° and cook roast with vegetables in a dutch oven with a tight-fitting lid for 2 or 3 hours or until roast is tender and cooked throughout. Add more water during cooking if the liquid cooks away.

Percent Calories From Fat: 32
Fat Grams In 2 Ounces Cooked Rump Roast: 4

Mexican Bean Sandwich

2 slices 100% whole grain bread, lightly toasted if desired
¼ cup *Mexican Bean Dip* (see recipe below)
Toppings like tomato slices, green pepper rings, and onion slices broken into rings

Perfect Whole Foods: Use unsweetened whole grain bread.
Percent Calories From Fat: 15
Total Fat Grams In Recipe: 5

Mexican Bean Dip

This makes a lot of dip but it disappears fast, especially if there are teenagers around.

4 cups cooked pinto or kidney beans (2 cups dried beans makes about 5 cups cooked)
1 onion, cut into chunks or 1½ teaspoons granulated onion
¼ cup raw apple cider vinegar
¼ teaspoon black pepper
1 teaspoon dried oregano leaves
1 teaspoon granulated garlic
1 teaspoon chili powder

Drain beans (save some of bean liquid) and place in food processor (with blade attachment) along with remaining ingredients. Process until mixture is smooth, adding some bean liquid if necessary to thin. Serve warm or cold with raw vegetables or in tacos or use as a sandwich spread (see recipe above). Makes about 4½ cups.

Percent Calories From Fat: 4
Total Fat Grams In Recipe: 5

Chickpea Spread

2 cups cooked chickpeas, drained
2 ribs celery, thinly sliced
1 green onion, thinly sliced
1 tablespoon mayonnaise
2 tablespoons plain, nonfat yogurt
1 drop lemon oil
Salt and pepper, to taste

Chop chickpeas in food processor. Combine mayonnaise, yogurt, and lemon oil. Mix all ingredients together with a spoon and serve on whole grain bread with toppings like lettuce, sprouts, tomato slices, or cucumbers. Makes about 1½ cups.

Perfect Whole Foods Diet: Use mayonnaise that is sugar and starch-free.
Percent Calories From Fat: 29
Total Fat Grams In Recipe: 20

Black Bean Spread

Use this spread or the next, Navy Bean-Garlic Spread, to make satisfying lunch sandwiches for work or school. Add leaf lettuce or sprouts plus other toppings to suit your appetite.

1 cup black beans, sorted, rinsed and drained
½ teaspoon oil
1 onion, chopped
1 to 3 garlic cloves, minced
½ to 1 teaspoon crushed red peppers
½ teaspoon dried oregano
½ small can tomato paste
¼ teaspoon salt, optional

Bring beans to a boil in 3 cups water, turn off heat, cover, and let sit for 1 hour. Cook for 1½ to 2 hours or until beans are tender. While beans are cooking, sauté vegetables in oil until the onion is transparent. Drain beans, reserving the liquid. Using a food processor with blade attachment, purée beans, sautéed vegetables, tomato paste, and optional salt, adding some reserved liquid, if necessary, to made the right consistency for spreading. For a dip, add more liquid. Makes about 3 cups.

Percent Calories From Fat: 6
Total Fat Grams In Recipe: 5

Navy Bean-Garlic Spread

Don't be shocked at the amount of garlic in this recipe! Because it is slowly roasted whole, the garlic is mild in flavor.

1 cup navy or great northern beans, sorted, rinsed, and drained
1 or 2 medium-sized bulbs garlic (2 to 4 ounces), not peeled
1 to 2 teaspoons olive oil, optional
⅛ to ¼ teaspoon crushed red peppers
¼ teaspoon salt, optional

Bring beans to a boil in 3½ cups water, turn off heat, cover, and let sit for 1 hour. Cook for 2 to 3 hours or until beans are tender. While beans are cooking, turn oven to 300°. Remove only loose skin from garlic, place garlic bulbs in a small baking dish, and roast for 1½ to 2 hours or until garlic is very soft when pressed lightly. Cool 5 minutes. Peel garlic cloves and place in food processor with blade attachment. When beans are ready, drain, reserving liquid, and add to processor with remaining ingredients. Process until smooth, adding some reserved liquid, if necessary, to make the right consistency for spreading. For a dip, add more liquid. Makes about 2¼ cups.

Percent Calories From Fat: 7
Total Fat Grams In Recipe: 5

Taco Burgers

Children and teenagers love these burgers. Serve them on whole grain buns with salsa and watch them disappear.

3 cups cooked kidney beans, drained and coarsely mashed (not puréed)
1½ teaspoons onion powder
¾ teaspoon oregano
¼ teaspoon salt, optional
1 small can chopped green chilies
¼ cup parmesan cheese
Whole grain flour
Whole grain cornmeal
Small amount *Oil-Lecithin Combination* (p. 205)

Mix beans, seasonings, green chilies, and cheese. Shape into 6 to 8 patties. Dip each patty into a mixture of whole wheat flour and cornmeal. Rub a small amount of *Oil-Lecithin Combination* over a skillet or griddle, heat, and fry patties on both sides until browned. Makes 6 to 8 burgers.

Perfect Whole Foods: Use 100% whole grain buns without sweeteners added.
Percent Calories From Fat: 13
Total Fat Grams In Recipe: 12

Cottage Cheese Danish

Fix this for a quick low-fat breakfast.

1 piece 100% whole wheat bread, toasted
¼ cup low-fat (1%) cottage cheese
⅛ teaspoon alcohol-free vanilla extract, optional
Dash of cinnamon
Fruit of your choice, cut up (apple, banana, strawberries, peaches, apricot, pear, or whole
    blueberries)

Mix vanilla with cottage cheese and spread on toast. Sprinkle with cinnamon. Arrange fruit on top and put under broiler for 2 to 3 minutes or until cottage cheese just starts to brown.

Perfect Whole Foods: Use unsweetened 100% whole grain bread. Read the ingredient list of the cottage cheese carefully to make certain it has no starch or whey added.
Percent Calories From Fat: 6
Total Fat Grams In Recipe: 2

A Pocket Full of Veggies

1 large 100% whole wheat pita, slit in back for stuffing
1 cup shredded vegetables (cabbage, carrots, radishes, and green peppers)
1 tablespoon salsa
¼ cup shredded low-fat cheese

In bowl, combine vegetables, sauce, and cheese, stirring gently. Stuff pita with mixture and arrange on *SilverStone* griddle or skillet with slit on top. Heat until pita is browned and cheese inside is slightly melted, using a lid if desired. Serves 1 or 2.

Perfect Whole Foods: *Check to make certain the pita bread and salsa are not sweetened.*
Percent Calories From Fat: 31
Total Fat Grams In Recipe: 9

Vegetarian Sloppy Joes

This, surprisingly, has the taste and texture of sloppy joes made with ground beef. Prepare a Vegetarian Sloppy Joe Mix *(or several) by combining in a plastic bag or bags, ahead of time, the TVP, dried onion flakes, and dried mixed vegetables. Use this mix to prepare the recipe below or in* Bean Supreme *(see page 84).*

Mix these three ingredients together to make one *Sloppy Joe Mix*:
1½ cups TVP (textured vegetable protein)
¼ cup dried onion flakes
¼ cup dried mixed vegetables

Use these ingredients with the mix when preparing *Vegetarian Sloppy Joes*:
28 or 29-ounce can tomato purée
2 teaspoons tamari or shoyu soy sauce (alcohol-free)
1 tablespoon or more chili powder
1 teaspoon oil
2 teaspoons prepared mustard

To prepare a Sloppy Joe Mix, combine mix plus ingredients listed above in a large saucepan or skillet with 1 cup of water and simmer with lid on until vegetables are tender or about 20 minutes. Serve on whole grain buns or toast. Leftovers are good in tacos. Makes 5 cups.

Perfect Whole Foods: *Read the ingredient lists of mustard and bread carefully.*
Percent Calories From Fat: 11
Total Fat Grams In Recipe: 11

Almond Butter-Banana Sandwich

2 slices 100% whole grain bread, plain or toasted
1 tablespoon almond butter
1 sliced banana

Perfect Whole Foods: Use unsweetened 100% whole grain bread.
Percent Calories From Fat: 25
Total Fat Grams In Recipe: 11

Peanut Butter-Banana Sandwich: Substitute peanut butter for the almond butter.
Cashew Butter-Banana Sandwich: Substitute cashew butter for the almond butter.

Tofu Salad in Pita Pockets

This is one of my favorite ways to fix tofu. In addition to having a family dinner, I have enough salad for sandwiches for the next day's lunches.

1-pound package tofu, rinsed and drained (soft, firm, or medium tofu)
2 tablespoons mayonnaise
2 teaspoons tamari or shoyu soy sauce (alcohol-free)
2 teaspoons prepared mustard
½ teaspoon kelp powder, optional
¼ cup nutritional yeast
1 teaspoon paprika
1 teaspoon granulated onion
2 carrots, finely chopped
2 celery ribs, finely chopped
¼ cup finely chopped green pepper
¼ cup fresh parsley, snipped with scissors
2 tablespoons or more plain, nonfat yogurt

Mash tofu with a fork. Stir in other ingredients except yogurt, adding raw vegetables when other ingredients are well mixed. If mixture is dry, stir in some yogurt to moisten and help hold ingredients together. Makes 5 cups of *Tofu Salad*.

For sandwiches, prepare as follows:
3 or 4 whole wheat pita breads, each cut in half
Alfalfa sprouts
Tomato slices

Lightly toast pita bread halves in toaster. Open into pockets with knife or spatula. Let cool for 5 minutes. Stuff with tofu salad, sprouts, and tomato slices.

Perfect Whole Foods: Make certain mustard, mayonnaise, and 100% whole wheat pita bread have no sweeteners added. Mustard should have no wine or sweetener added.
Percent Calories From Fat: 52 (Tofu Salad only)
Total Fat Grams In Recipe: 43

Crispy Tofu Sandwich

If you've never tried tofu, here's a quick and easy recipe to prepare. With some imagination, it tastes like chicken. The good-tasting nutritional yeast can also be used to sprinkle over popcorn.

1-pound package firm tofu, rinsed and drained
¼ cup whole grain yellow cornmeal
¼ cup nutritional yeast
Pinch of cayenne pepper
Pinch salt, optional
⅛ teaspoon granulated garlic
⅛ teaspoon granulated onion
1 egg, beaten (or 2 egg whites)
1 tablespoon oil, total
Whole grain bread and toppings, as desired

Slice tofu into ⅜-inch thick pieces. Combine cornmeal, nutritional yeast, and seasonings in a flat bowl, stirring to mix well. Heat a little oil on griddle or skillet. Carefully dip tofu in egg and then into cornmeal mixture. Pan fry the tofu on both sides until crisp. Make into sandwiches with toasted whole grain bread, leaf lettuce, and tomato slices. Leftover tofu slices are good cold. Makes 5 or 6 slices (each 3 x 4-inches).

Percent Calories From Fat: 42 without bread and toppings
Total Fat Grams In Recipe: 40

Tempeh Burgers

Tempeh burgers are good cooked over a charcoal grill. If you are avoiding beef, take tempeh along when you go to a cook-out. (Grilling meat causes potential cancer-causing substances to be formed in the food, while grilling soy foods do not create these substances.) Use the following recipe as well for pan frying your tempeh burgers at home.

8-ounce package tempeh, defrosted
½ teaspoon oil
Whole wheat pita bread or buns
Your choice of toppings for burger: mayonnaise, mustard, sprouts or lettuce, sliced low-fat cheese, tomato slices, and mushroom slices

Cut tempeh in half, crosswise. Slice each piece into two thin patties. Pan fry on both sides in oil until crisp and brown. Prepare your burger with desired toppings. Makes 4 burgers.

Perfect Whole Foods: Use bread or buns that are unsweetened and 100% whole grain. Mayonnaise should have no sweetener added. Use a mustard with no sweetener or wine.
Percent Calories From Fat: 42 from tempeh and oil. Although this may sound high, it is much lower than even the leanest of ground beef.
Total Fat Grams In Recipe: 23

Turkey Treat Sandwich

This sandwich is even better if you make it ahead of time and refrigerate it for flavors to blend.

1 ounce roasted turkey, thinly sliced
1 ounce swiss cheese, thinly sliced
1 100% whole grain buns (unsweetened), sliced open or 2 slices bread
¼ tomato, thinly sliced
½ teaspoon olive oil
Seasoned Onions (p. 269)

Spread cut sides of bun with a thin layer of olive oil. Arrange turkey, cheese, tomato slices, and *Seasoned Onions* on bun, add bun top, and serve immediately or place in baggy and refrigerate to allow flavors to blend. Serves 1.

Perfect Whole Foods: Do not use turkey with sugar or starch added.
Percent Calories From Fat: 30
Total Fat Grams In Recipe: 13

Vegetarian Treat: Omit turkey.

Tuna Burgers

Make these burgers in a jiffy when you need a quick meal. Serve them on whole grain buns along with alfalfa sprouts or shredded lettuce.

6-ounce can water-packed tuna, not drained
1 egg, beaten slightly (or 2 whites)
¼ teaspoon granulated onion
1 tablespoon fresh lemon juice or 1 drop lemon oil, optional
¾ cup oat bran
⅛ teaspoon black pepper

Mix all ingredients together. Shape into 3 or 4 patties. Using a *SilverStone* griddle or one thinly coated with *Oil-Lecithin Combination* (p. 205), cook burgers on each side until browned.

Perfect Whole Foods: Select whole grain buns that are 100% whole grain and made without sweeteners. Also, omit lemon juice or use 1 drop lemon oil.
Percent Calories From Fat: 26
Total Fat Grams In Recipe: 16

WHOLE GRAINS AND CEREALS

In case you have little experience in cooking whole grains, I have included a variety of grain recipes including rice, oats, corn, barley, millet, and rye as well as lesser known ones like spelt, kamut, triticale, Job's tears, teff, quinoa, and amaranth. Try the unfamiliar! Don't limit yourself to rice, corn, and wheat when so many other grains are available. See the following list of grains that you can use like rice. You will quickly find that what was unfamiliar yesterday will be a regular in your diet tomorrow. Variety not only helps avert boredom but also helps prevent allergies to the frequently eaten grains like wheat and corn.

You Can Use Any One of These Cooked Grains in Place of Cooked Brown Rice

Millet	Spelt berries	Job's tears
Triticale berries	Kamut berries	

Various grains that are left in the whole state (not ground, flaked, or cut into pieces called grits) are called by different names. Whole wheat, rye, triticale, spelt, and kamut grains are called wheat, rye, triticale, spelt and kamut *berries*. Buckwheat and oat grains are called buckwheat and oat *groats*. Grains like brown rice, millet, quinoa, and amaranth are simply called by their names. Before cooking any whole grains, look them over for stones and dirt, just as you do dried beans. Rinse them in a strainer if they are dirty or dusty.

Methods of Preparing Whole Grains

Simmering in saucepan
Baking
Cooking in slow cooker
Sprouting
Soaking raw, whole grains or raw, flaked grains until they are soft
Pressure-cooking (follow manufacturer's directions)
Steaming
Toasting (previously cooked grains like rolled oats and wheat flakes or wheat germ)
Cutting into pieces or grinding before cooking
Uncooked (previously cooked grains like rolled oats or wheat flakes and wheat germ)

Adding salt while they are cooking toughens the grains and, therefore, lengthens the cooking time. Add salt after grains are cooked if salt is desired. Acid ingredients like tomato sauce and vinegar also should be added after cooking is almost completed since they, too, tend to toughen grains.

Whole Grain and Cereal Facts

Amaranth: (AM-a-ranth) A high-protein whole grain that can be cooked as a cereal or ground into flour for use in quick breads. Amaranth is not refined. Since amaranth is not a true cereal grain, it is particularly helpful to those allergic to grains.
Percent Calories From Fat: 14
Fat Grams In 1 Cup Cooked: 5

Barley: An easily-digested grain that grows with the inedible hull tightly attached to the bran. Barley is available in many forms; see the barley terms listed below. Use only hulled or whole barley or whole barley flour on the *Perfect Whole Foods* diet.
Percent Calories From Fat: 7
Fat Grams In 1 Cup Cooked: 2

Barley Flakes: If you find a brand of barley flakes made from hulled or whole barley, it can be used. *Arrowhead Mills* Barley Flakes are pearled or refined barley lightly cooked and rolled flat. Do not use these on *Perfect Whole Foods*.

Barley Grits: The hulled or pearled barley cut into small pieces. Barley grits cook much faster than barley that is not broken into pieces. Use only hulled barley grits on *Perfect Whole Foods*, not barley grits from pearled barley.

Barley, Hulled: Also called *whole barley*. Barley with only the hull mechanically removed. Hulled barley has more fiber, protein, and minerals than pearled barley. Hulled barley is delicious in soups. It takes longer to cook than the less nutritious pearled barley.

Barley, Pearled: Barley with various amounts of the bran chemically removed along with the hull. The whiter-looking the pearled barley, the more bran has been removed. (Lightly pearled barley has more fiber, protein, vitamins, and minerals than white pearled barley.) Don't use pearled barley on the perfect diet.

Barley, Pot: A lightly-refined barley that should not be used on the *Perfect Whole Foods* diet.

Barley, Quick: A lightly-refined barley that should not be used on the perfect diet.

Barley, Scotch: A lightly-refined barley that should not be used on the perfect diet.

Barley, Whole: See **Barley, Hulled**.

Berries: The whole grain (not ground, flaked, or cut) of wheat, rye, triticale, spelt, and kamut.

Bran: The outer part of a grain that is rich in fiber. The bran is part of the grain that's removed in refining. Bran may be used on the perfect diet since it contains many valuable nutrients.

Buckwheat: Buckwheat is a nutritious seed, not a true cereal grain, with a hard hull or shell that does not soften with cooking. When the hull is removed from the seed for cooking, it is called

whole, unroasted buckwheat or *buckwheat groats.* The groats are sometimes cut into small pieces or grits. Toasted groats are called *kasha,* a staple Russian food. Commercially ground buckwheat flour includes some of the hull or shell and is *dark* buckwheat flour. To make *white* buckwheat flour, grind unroasted buckwheat groats in a food processor into a flour. The *white* flour will be milder in flavor than the *dark.* Use any of these products on the perfect diet.
Percent Calories From Fat: 4
Fat Grams In 1 Cup Cooked: 1

Bulgur: A quick-cooking whole grain wheat product that has been parboiled, dried and then cracked. Bulgur is a staple food in the Middle East. It is usually interchangeable with *cracked wheat.*

Cereal, Toasted: Commercial cereals that have been cooked at high temperatures to produce a crunchy, toasted product should be avoided on the **Perfect Whole Foods** diet, even if they have no undesirable ingredients. The browning, called the *Maillard browning reaction*, denatures or changes the protein in the grain, especially the amino acid lysine, making it unavailable for use by the body. Minerals and vitamins in the grain are also changed to forms not useable by the body or destroyed by the high heat. (Puffed cereals, for instance, have been cooked at temperatures around 700° for two minutes.) Since cereals are so thin and crisply browned, the complete grain is affected nutritionally. Fortification does not correct this problem since only a few vitamins and minerals are added. In bread baking, the Maillard browning reaction occurs exclusively on the surface of the crust and, therefore, does not hurt the entire product. For optimal nutrition, use whole grains that you will cook or soak in water or rolled grains that were previously steamed.

Corn: A popular cereal grain that is often refined. Corn products may look like they are whole grains when they are not since even refined corn is coarse-looking, so don't be misled. The germ is often removed since it turns rancid quickly due to its high polyunsaturated fat content. Refined and whole corn are both ground into grits, meal, and flour from yellow, white, and blue corn. It's often difficult to determine if a specific corn product is unrefined by reading the package since the ingredient list doesn't usually state *whole* or *whole grain* as with whole wheat and whole rye. However, since many corn products are refined, assume that it is unless you find out otherwise from the manufacturer. Don't use products described on the package or ingredient list as *bolted, degerminated, enriched, fortified, hominy, hominy grits, corn flour,* or *masa* since these terms indicate refinement. Products made from corn kernels treated with lime (calcium hydroxide, not the fruit lime), lye, or wood ash to soften the grain may be whole grain, but check with the manufacturer to be certain. These products are richer in calcium and have more niacin available than corn not treated this way. Fresh whole grain corn meal and grits are likely to be available from small, local mills. Ask which corn products are 100% whole grain. Terms indicating that corn has not been refined include *whole grain* and *whole corn.* The terms *stone ground* and *water ground* do not specify whether or not corn has been refined. The term *unbolted* indicates that the bran has not been removed, but doesn't specify whether or not the germ is present. Also, sometimes a corn product will specify that the germ hasn't been removed, but doesn't mention the bran. Use only corn products that are *whole* on the **Perfect Whole Foods** diet.

Corn, Blue: A variety of corn that's blue in color. It is available in refined and whole forms. Use only the whole form on the perfect diet.

Corn Bran: The edible hull or bran layer of the corn kernel that's rich in soluble fiber.

Corn Flour: Corn that has been ground into a fine powder from bolted or refined cornmeal. *Masa corn flour* is popular in Mexican foods but is not a whole grain product and shouldn't be used on the perfect diet.

Corn Germ: The nutritious central core of the corn kernel that can be used like wheat germ—in baked goods, sprinkled on cereal or yogurt, and as a meat extender. Corn germ has a popcorn-like flavor. Since it's very perishable, store corn germ in the refrigerator and use quickly.

Corn Grits: Corn that is cut or ground into small particles. Most corn grits from the grocery store have been refined. Select only whole grain corn grits for the ***Perfect Whole Foods*** diet.

Cornmeal: Corn that is ground into a gritty, granular powder. Most cornmeal, both yellow and white, at the grocery store has been refined and will be labeled *bolted yellow cornmeal*, *bolted white cornmeal*, or *enriched cornmeal*. Make certain the cornmeal you use is *whole*. Read more details about corn in the previous listing on **Corn**.
Percent Calories From Fat: 10
Fat Grams In 1 Cup: 5

Couscous: A refined semolina wheat product that should not be used on the ***Perfect Whole Foods*** diet. Use whole wheat couscous on the perfect diet.

Dehulled: Dehulled is the same as hulled. In some grains like oats, barley, rice, and buckwheat, hard husks or hulls must be removed from grains before they can be cooked and eaten. The bran layer is under the hull. In other grains like corn, the edible hull *is* the bran layer. Removing the hull refines the grain. Therefore, the terms *dehulled* and *hulled* are used, in some instances, to denote whole grains and, in other instances, to denote refined grains.

Durum: A variety of wheat used in making pasta. Unless the ingredient list specifically states that it is *whole durum*, then the durum is refined. You may use whole durum on the perfect diet, but not durum.

Gluten: The protein protion of grains that allows bread dough to stretch and rise. For more information, see **Gluten** under **Yeast Bread Baking Terms** on page 195.

Grits: A grain cut into several small pieces. Grits are made from both refined and unrefined grains. Corn grits as well as soy and barley grits are available.

Groats: The term used for a grain with a tough hull that doesn't soften during cooking or soaking. The hulls are removed from these grains. Buckwheat and oat grains are called groats.

Hominy Grits: Corn grits made of highly refined corn.

Hull: The husk or outer covering of a grain. With some grains, the hull is inedible; with others the edible hull is actually the bran layer and must not be removed or the grain will be refined. Also see **Dehulled** on page 124.

Hulled: Hulls or hard husk removed from grain. Hulled is the same as dehulled. See Dehulled on page 124.

Job's Tears: An ancient, nutritious whole grain with a nut-like flavor. It has been grown in China for over 4,000 years. In Japan it is called hato mugi. Prepared alone or added to soups and stews, Job's tears should be cooked for at least an hour. It is never refined.
Percent Calories From Fat: 14
Fat Grams In ½ Cup Cooked: 2

Kamut: (Kah-MOOT) is a nutritious, ancient grain which, although it is closely related to wheat, can often be tolerated by those allergic to wheat. It can be used in baking yeast bread.
Percent Calories From Fat: 5
Fat Grams In 1 Cup Cooked: 1

Kasha: Toasted buckwheat groats which are stronger in flavor than the unroasted groats. See **Buckwheat** beginning on page 122.

Masa Harina: See **Corn Flour** in this list.

Milled: Ground into flour. This term is used with both refined and whole grains, so make certain you select only whole grains on the *Perfect Whole Foods* diet.

Millet: An easily-digested whole grain that's rich in iron. A tiny round seed, it is often found in bird feed. Millet can be cooked as a cereal or ground into flour for use in quick breads. Millet is never refined.
Percent Calories From Fat: 8
Fat Grams In 1 Cup Cooked: 1

Oat Bran: The outer coating of the oat groat that's rich in water-soluble fiber. Oat bran has been found to be helpful in lowering blood cholesterol. When baking with oat bran, you may need to adjust the amount of liquid ingredients or oat bran in the batter since various brands have different capacities to absorb liquid. 1 pound = approximately 4¼ cups.

Oat Flour: A flour made either from rolled oats or oat groats. To make oat flour from rolled oats, grind them in a blender or food processor. 1¼ cups rolled oats = approximately 1 cup oat flour.

Oat Groats: Whole oat grains with only the inedible hull removed.

Oats: A popular breakfast whole grain available at the grocery store as *oatmeal, rolled oats* and *quick oats*. Quick oats are cut into smaller pieces than rolled oats. Do not use instant oats on the perfect diet since they contain refined ingredients.
Percent Calories From Fat: 15
Fat Grams In 1 Cup Cooked: 4

Oats, Rolled: Oat groats are steamed before being rolled flat. Also called oatmeal. Available at grocery store as *Quaker* Oats. Don't use instant oats. 1 pound = approximately 4½ cups.

Oats, Scotch: Oat groats that have been cut into small pieces and are sometimes roasted to produce a nutty flavor. Similar to steel-cut oats.

Oats, Steel-cut: Oat groats cut into 2 or 3 small pieces.

Pasta, Corn: For those allergic to wheat products, corn pastas are available. They are not 100 percent whole grain, however, and should not be used on the **Perfect Whole Foods** diet.

Pasta, Soba: A pasta imported from Japan. Usually soba is made of a blend of white flour and buckwheat flour. However, a 100 percent buckwheat flour soba that can be used on the perfect diet is available. Check ingredient lists carefully.

Pasta, Whole Wheat: A variety of whole wheat pastas are available with or without vegetable powders added. Pasta is usually made of durum semolina flour, either whole grain or refined. If the durum flour is whole grain, the ingredient list will say *whole durum*. Do not use simply *durum* or *semolina* pasta on the perfect diet. Use only whole grains.

Phytic Acid: A naturally-occurring substance in the outer bran layer of grains and legumes that makes minerals unavailable for absorption. The phytic acid can be destroyed or decreased by sprouting, by fermenting the grain in the making of sourdough bread, by the action of yeast in yeast-risen bread, and by slow, moist cooking. These processes make the minerals more available for absorption. Quick breads should not be eaten regularly and in large quantities since the phytic acid is not destroyed or decreased.

Popcorn: A widely-available whole grain. Yellow kernels pop larger than white kernels; white kernels, however, are more tender. Don't use buttery-flavored powders and liquids that are available for seasoning since they usually contain unwanted ingredients. Most microwave popcorn and commercially-popped corn have large amounts of undesirable hydrogenated fats.

Quinoa: (KEEN-wa) A supergrain which was at one time a staple food of the ancient Incas. Quinoa is nutritious, quick-cooking, and has a light nut-like taste. Before cooking quinoa, make certain that you rinse it well. There are bitter-tasting substances called saponins that naturally occur on the quinoa seeds. By rinsing them away in a strainer, you will have a delicious dish. Quinoa is never refined.
Percent Calories From Fat: 17
Fat Grams in 1 Cup Cooked: 3

Rice, Aromatic: Rice that is very fragrant when cooked.

Rice, Basmati: A long-grain aromatic rice that is available as whole grain and refined. It originated in India. Use only brown basmati rice on the *Perfect Whole Foods* diet, not white basmati rice.

Rice, Brown: Whole grain rice that has only had the tough, inedible husk removed. Brown rice is available in short, medium, and long grain. Cooked short grain is somewhat sticky and chewy while long grain is drier and holds its shape. Medium grain is between the two. Experiment to determine which you like best. If a recipe does not specify the grain length, then use long grain. 1 pound = 2½ cups.
Percent Calories From Fat: 6
Fat Grams In 1 Cup Cooked: 2

Rice, Sweet Brown: A sticky, mildly-sweet rice that's short grain and used on the perfect diet.

Rice, Wehani: A long-grain, aromatic, whole grain rice that while cooking smells like nuts roasting or corn popping. The texture is similar to wild rice.

Rice, Wild: A gourmet treat that's not a true rice, but rather a seed. Wild rice can be mixed with other whole grain rices and cooked. Wild rice should be added to the water first and cooked a few minutes before adding other rices since it takes longer to cook. Do not use wild rice blends that are called *wild rice* if they include white rice. Read the ingredient list carefully.

Rye: A grain that can be cooked whole, steamed and rolled flat for cooking, or ground into flour for bread making. Make certain you use whole rye flour if you are on the perfect diet.
Percent Calories From Fat: 5
Fat Grams In ½ Cup Cooked Rye Berries: 1

Rye, Flaked: See **Rye, Rolled**.

Rye, Rolled: Whole rye that has either been cracked or left whole, briefly cooked, and then rolled flat. It is sometimes called flaked rye or rye flakes. The cooking time depends on the size of the flakes. See recipes for *Rye Flakes* on page 142.

Semolina: Refined durum wheat used to make pasta. Do not use on the perfect diet.

Sorghum: A cereal grain that can be eaten whole, cooked like rice, or ground into flour. The sweet syrup, made from the stalks of sorghum, should be eliminated on *Perfect Whole Foods*.

Spelt: An ancient, nutritious grain that has recently been revived and is available in several forms: whole grain, flaked, whole grain flour, and pasta. An important fact about spelt flour is that it can be used to make a delicious-tasting and good-textured yeast bread that, although it is closely related to wheat, most (but not all) people who are allergic to wheat can tolerate.
Percent Calories From Fat: 7
Fat Grams In 1 Cup Cooked: 2

Teff: A tiny whole grain that is very nutritious and versatile. It can be added, raw, to baked goods, used as a thickener in cooking, or cooked as a cereal. Teff was originally cultivated in Ethiopia thousands of years ago. Teff is never refined.
Percent Calories From Fat: 5
Fat Grams In 1 Cup Cooked: 1

Triticale: (trit-a-KA-lee) A nutritious hybrid grain that is a cross between wheat and rye. For those with allergies, it is neither wheat nor rye, but rather a different, although similar, grain. Triticale can be cooked whole or cracked, or flaked and cooked as a cereal, or ground into flour for breads. It is usually mixed with wheat flour for bread-making but can be made into flatter 100% triticale bread. Too much kneading is detrimental to its gluten. Triticale is never refined.
Percent Calories From Fat: 7
Fat Grams In 1 Cup Cooked: 2

Wheat: A popular grain that's used in many forms—flour, bulgur, flaked, cracked, whole berries, and sprouted. If an ingredient list reads *wheat, stone ground wheat*, or *organically-grown wheat* rather than *whole wheat, stone ground whole wheat*, or *organically-grown whole wheat*, the wheat ingredient is refined.

Wheat Berries, Hard: Whole wheat that is higher in gluten content than soft wheat berries. Hard wheat berries are ground into coarse or fine hard whole wheat flour for making yeast breads and sometimes muffins. 1 cup wheat berries = 1⅓ to 1½ cups flour.
Percent Calories From Fat: 7
Fat Grams In 1 Cup Cooked Wheat Berries: 2

Wheat Berries, Soft: Wheat that is lower in gluten content than hard wheat berries. Soft wheat berries are ground into a fine flour for use in quick breads such as biscuits, pancakes, cookies, and cakes. Flour ground from soft wheat berries is called soft or pastry whole wheat flour.

Wheat Bran: The coarse, edible, outer coating of the wheat berry that's rich in insoluble fiber and helpful in regulating the intestinal tract. When you eat whole wheat products, you are eating the bran as well as other parts of the wheat berry.

Wheat, Cracked: Whole wheat berries ground or cut into small pieces. Cracked wheat differs from *bulgur* in that cracked wheat is toasted rather than steamed. It is interchangeable with bulgur in most recipes.

Wheat Flakes: A commercial product made from whole wheat berries that are briefly cooked and then rolled flat.

Whole Barley: See **Barley, Whole**, in this list.

Whole Grain: A grain that has not had edible parts such as the bran and germ removed in its processing and is, therefore, a more nutritious food than refined grains. Only whole grains, not refined, are used on the ***Perfect Whole Foods*** diet. For information on why it's important to eat whole grains rather than refined, see the explanation beginning on page 23.

Whole Grain And Cereal Recipes

Basic Amaranth

Try amaranth if you have allergies to common grains like wheat and corn. Although it isn't a true grain, it cooks like one. Amaranth is also available ground into a flour.

6 tablespoons amaranth
1 cup cold water

Toast amaranth in a heavy dry saucepan for a couple of minutes or until many of the grains have popped. Do not burn. Remove from heat, add cold water, return to heat, bring to a boil, stir briefly, reduce heat, cover, and simmer for about 20 minutes or until water is absorbed. Makes almost 1 cup.

Percent Calories From Fat: 14
Total Fat Grams In Recipe: 5

Barley Stove-Top Casserole

1 onion, chopped
2 ribs celery, sliced plus chopped celery leaves
2 cups sliced mushrooms (about 6 large)
1 carrot, thinly sliced
1 or 2 cloves garlic, minced
2 teaspoons oil
½ cup hulled or whole barley, sorted, rinsed, and drained
1¾ cups fat-free chicken broth or water, boiling
1 teaspoon tamari or shoyu sauce (alcohol-free)
1 teaspoon dried dill weed

Sauté vegetables in oil for 3 to 5 minutes. Add barley and saute another minute or so. Add broth plus tamari and dill. Reduce heat when liquid returns to a boil, cover, and cook until liquid is absorbed and barley is tender or about 1 hour. Makes 3 cups.

Perfect Whole Foods: Do not use pearled barley since it is refined. If you use canned chicken broth, make certain no starches or sugars are included.
Percent Calories From Fat: 21
Total Fat Grams In Recipe: 13

Kasha

Kasha (toasted buckwheat groats) is a staple Russian food that's very nutritious. It is prepared here in one of the traditional Russian ways. Toasting makes the buckwheat have a flavor for which you may need to acquire a taste. If you prefer a milder flavor, use unroasted buckwheat.

2 teaspoons oil
1 small onion, chopped
2 mushrooms, chopped
1 carrot, thinly sliced
1 celery rib, thinly sliced
¼ green pepper, chopped
1 garlic clove, minced
1 cup kasha (toasted buckwheat groats) or unroasted buckwheat
1 egg, beaten
2 cups broth or water

Sauté vegetables in oil for a couple of minutes. Add buckwheat and sauté another minute. Add beaten egg, stirring to mix it with the other ingredients while it's cooking. Add broth or water to buckwheat mixture. Bring to a boil, reduce heat, cover, and simmer for about 8 to 10 minutes or until water is absorbed. Makes about 5 cups.

Percent Calories From Fat: 19
Total Fat Grams In Recipe: 18

Cream of Buckwheat

Pocono Cream of Buckwheat is a nutritious product available at many natural food stores. Because it is not toasted like kasha, Cream of Buckwheat has a rather mild flavor.

¼ cup *Pocono* Cream of Buckwheat
1 cup water

Bring water to a boil, sprinkle cereal over water, stir briefly, reduce heat, and cook for about 10 minutes, stirring occasionally. Remove from heat, cover, and let sit for a few minutes. Makes 1 cup.

Percent Calories From Fat: 4
Total Fat Grams In Recipe: 1

Whole Grain Corn Grits

Most grocery store corn grits are refined. Terms that indicate refinement include bolted, degerminated, *and* partially degerminated. *(The term* stone ground *doesn't indicate whether a product is whole or refined.) Even if these terms are not used on the label, the grits are likely to be refined unless the ingredient list or a statement on the package states that they are truly* whole grain. *Do not settle for refined corn grits on the perfect diet.*

1 cup whole grain yellow or white corn grits
3 cups water
Salt, optional

On separate burners, heat 3 cups of water in the upper pan of a double boiler and bring water to a boil in the lower pan. The water in the lower pan should not hit the upper pan when the two are put together. Stir the grits into the hot water in the upper pan. Cover and cook over the boiling water for about 30 minutes, until grits are thickened, stirring occasionally. Grits can also be cooked without a double boiler if you have a heavy pan. Salt if desired. Makes 3½ cups.

Perfect Whole Foods: Use whole grain grits.
Percent Calories From Fat: 10
Total Fat Grams In Recipe: 4

Cheesy-Garlic Grits: Before serving, stir in ½ cup shredded low-fat cheese, ½ teaspoon garlic powder, plus salt and pepper to taste.

Popcorn

The most nutritious way to prepare popcorn is to pop it in an air popper and serve it plain. However, many people prefer it buttered and salted. Here's a method of getting a little salt to stick to the corn without adding butter.

Locate a glass jar (preferably dark in color) with a pump spray, wash and dry the bottle, and partially fill it with fresh flax oil, unrefined corn oil, or unrefined safflower or sunflower (not high-oleic) oil. Store it in the refrigerator, as you do other oils, and spray your popped corn with a little oil just before salting. Another good seasoning for popcorn, instead of salt, is good-tasting nutritional yeast. Just sprinkle it on the popped corn that has been sprayed lightly with one of the oils already mentioned. 1 cup corn makes 8 cups popped corn.

Percent Calories From Fat: 12 (for air-popped, no oil added)
Total Fat Grams In Recipe: 1 in 3 cups air-popped, no oil added. One teaspoon oil adds 5 grams of fat.

Basic Job's Tears

Job's tears is an ancient, nutritious whole grain with a nut-like flavor. Prepare it alone, as in this basic recipe, or substitute it for other grains in recipes such as Country Garden Rice *(p. 139), using 2½ cups water per cup of grain and cooking it 1 hour.*

½ cup Job's tears, sorted, rinsed, and drained
1¼ cups boiling water

Add Job's tears to boiling water, reduce heat, cover, and simmer for 1 hour. Remove from heat and let sit for about 10 minutes. Makes about 1¾ cups.

Percent Calories From Fat: 14
Total Fat Grams In Recipe: 7

Basic Kamut Berries

Kamut as well as spelt are excellent alternatives to wheat if you have allergies or are trying to eat a wider variety of foods. Use the cooked berries as a breakfast cereal or as a whole grain in place of brown rice.

1 cup kamut berries, sorted, rinsed, and drained
3 cups boiling water

Add kamut berries to boiling water, reduce heat, cover, and simmer for 1½ to 2 hours or until water is absorbed. Makes 2½ cups.

Variation: To shorten cooking time, soak berries overnight or all day in cold water, then cook for about 30 to 40 minutes, or until water is absorbed and kamut berries are tender.

Percent Calories From Fat: 5
Total Fat Grams In Recipe: 2

Basic Kamut Flakes

½ cup kamut flakes
1 cup boiling water

Stir kamut flakes into boiling water, reduce heat, cover, and simmer for 15 to 18 minutes. Remove from heat and let sit for a few minutes. Add your favorite toppings. Makes 1 cup cereal.

Percent Calories From Fat: 5
Total Fat Grams In Recipe: 1

Basic Millet

Serve this for dinner in place of brown rice or at breakfast topped with a sprinkle of nuts, cinnamon, and skim milk. Always prepare millet just before serving as it tends to solidify upon standing.

1 cup millet, sorted, rinsed, and drained
3 cups boiling water

Sprinkle millet into boiling water slowly while water continues to boil, reduce heat, cover, and simmer for 40 to 45 minutes, until water is absorbed. Do not stir while cooking. Makes 3½ cups.

Percent Calories From Fat: 8
Total Fat Grams In Recipe: 3

Broccoli-Millet Casserole

½ cup millet, sorted and rinsed
1 teaspoon olive oil
1 cup mushrooms, coarsely chopped
1 large onion, chopped
1½ cups broccoli cut into tiny pieces
1 cup frozen whole kernel corn
¼ cup English walnut pieces
¼ cup shredded cheese
Salt, to taste

Slowly add millet to 1½ cups of boiling water. Reduce heat, cover, and simmer until water is absorbed, about 40 to 45 minutes. While millet is cooking, sauté onion, and mushrooms in oil for a few minutes. Oil an 8 x 12-inch flat casserole dish with *Oil-Lecithin Combination* (p. 205). Preheat oven to 350°. Layer ingredients in casserole by beginning with half of the cooked millet, half of the cooked onions and mushrooms, half of the broccoli and corn. Sprinkle salt on first layer. Repeat layers with remaining half of ingredients. Salt again. Top with nuts and cheese. Bake for 20 to 30 minutes without a lid. Makes about 6 cups.

Percent Calories From Fat: 48
Total Fat Grams In Recipe: 33

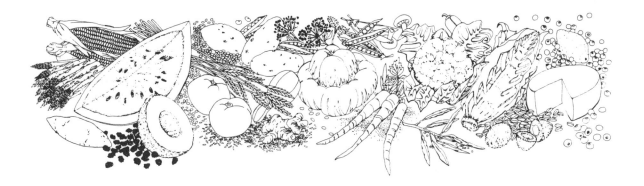

Oatmeal

Oatmeal is one of the few unsweetened whole grain cereals that is available at all grocery stores. Buy the regular or quick-cooking rolled oats, not instant varieties which have sweeteners or refined starches added.

½ cup rolled oats or ⅓ cup quick oats
1 cup boiling water

Sprinkle oats into boiling water, reduce heat, and simmer 5 to 10 minutes (3 or 4 minutes for the quick oats). Remove from heat, cover, and let sit for a few minutes for the oatmeal to thicken. For a creamier cereal, combine oats and cold water, bring to a boil, and cook as instructed above. Makes 1 cup.

Percent Calories From Fat: 15
Total Fat Grams In Recipe: 4

Breakfast Chow

½ cup raw rolled oats
Fruit, such as sliced banana, chopped apple or raisins
½ teaspoon fresh lemon juice
1 tablespoon raw seeds or nuts such as sunflower, pumpkin, or almonds (if you use tiny seeds like flax seeds, then grind them in a nut or seed grinder)

Mix all ingredients in cereal bowl and serve. Serves 1, the quantity depending on the amount of fruit added.

Perfect Whole Foods: Omit lemon juice and use fresh fruit rather than raisins.
Percent Calories From Fat: 21
Total Fat Grams In Recipe: 8

Oat Bran Cereal

Oat bran is one of the high-fiber foods used by Dr. James Anderson in research at the University of Kentucky in Lexington. His studies show that the soluble fiber found in oat bran, oatmeal, dried beans, and apples is helpful in lowering blood cholesterol as well as reducing insulin need in diabetics.

⅓ cup oat bran
1 cup cold water

Combine cold water and oat bran in saucepan. Heat until cereal starts to boil and thicken, stirring constantly. Remove from heat, add lid, and let sit for few minutes. Makes 1 cup.

Percent Calories From Fat: 16
Total Fat Grams In Recipe: 2

Basic Steel-Cut Oats

Cooked steel-cut oats are much creamier than rolled oats. They also have more texture and lots of taste.

½ cup steel-cut oats

Add oats to 2½ cups of boiling water, reduce heat when cereal comes to a boil, cover, and cook until water is absorbed and oats are tender, or about 30 minutes. Remove from heat and let sit, covered, for a few minutes. Makes 2 cups.

Percent Calories From Fat: 15
Total Fat Grams In Recipe: 7

Basic Oat Groats

If you're looking for a nutritious, cooked breakfast cereal with some texture, then try oat groats.

1 cup oat groats

Sprinkle the oat groats into 2½ cups of boiling water. Reduce heat, cover, and simmer for 30 minutes, stirring occasionally. Pour into serving bowls and add your favorite breakfast toppings. Makes 2 cups.

Percent Calories From Fat: 15
Total Fat Grams In Recipe: 14

Overnight Oats: Add 1¼ cups oat groats and 5 cups of water to a slow cooker and cook on low for approximately 8 hours. Makes 5 cups.

Company Oats

Prepare this in the slow cooker and let it cook overnight. Next morning, breakfast will be a breeze.

2 cups oat groats, steel-cut oats, or rolled oats
2 cups unsweetened applesauce
¼ cup raisins or currants
1 tablespoon sesame seeds
1 tablespoon raw sunflower seeds
¼ cup chopped nuts (such as walnuts, almonds, or pecans)

Place all ingredients in slow cooker with 5½ cups of water and stir. Turn on low and cook for approximately 8 hours. Stir well and serve with skim milk. Makes 9 cups.

Perfect Whole Foods: Omit raisins and currants or substitute fresh chopped fruit. Use Homemade Applesauce *(p. 275).*
Percent Calories From Fat: 25
Fat Grams In 1 Cup: 5

Basic Quinoa

If you are allergic to common grains such as wheat and corn, try quinoa (pronounced KEEN-wa). Quinoa is a grain-like food that doesn't actually belong to the grain family. It's quick-cooking, is not heavy as are some grains, has a mild flavor, and is easy to digest. Try it!

½ cup quinoa, rinsed in strainer and drained
1 cup boiling water

Add rinsed quinoa to boiling water, reduce heat when water has returned to a boil, cover, and simmer for 10 to 15 minutes or until water is absorbed. Makes 1¼ cups.

Percent Calories From Fat: 17
Total Fat Grams In Recipe: 4

Herbed Quinoa: Add the following ingredients to the quinoa and water, cooking as directed above: 2 minced garlic cloves, 1 small chopped onion, 1 chopped carrot, and ¼ teaspoon dried dill weed.

California Quinoa

Here's a light and tasty side dish. It's an excellent way to try quinoa.

¾ cup quinoa, rinsed in a strainer, drained, and then toasted in dry skillet for several minutes
1½ cups boiling water
1 teaspoon olive oil
¼ cup sun-dried tomato flakes
½ teaspoon dried basil
1 clove garlic, minced
2 tablespoons pinenuts or sunflower seeds

Add quinoa and vegetables to boiling water, reduce heat when water returns to a boil, cook for a minute without lid, then cover, and simmer for 10 to 15 minutes or until water is absorbed. Stir in oil, tomato flakes, basil, garlic, and nuts. Makes about 3 cups.

Percent Calories From Fat: 35
Total Fat Grams In Recipe: 19

Perfect Brown Rice

Use this recipe for long, medium, or short grain brown rice, basmati brown rice, or sweet brown rice. Basmati is my favorite since it has a wonderful fragrance while cooking and a nutty flavor.

1 cup brown rice, sorted, rinsed, and drained
2 cups boiling water

In a dry pan, heat drained brown rice over medium-high heat until grains are dry and only slightly browned. Add boiling water and reduce heat to medium-low so that rice will continue to boil faster than a simmer. Do not stir. Cover and cook for 35 minutes. Check for unabsorbed water by removing the lid and tilting the pan slightly. Cover and continue cooking until all water is absorbed. Makes 3 cups. Reheat leftovers in a stainless steel steaming basket over hot water.

Quick-Cooked Brown Rice: Prepare as above, cooking only 5 minutes. Remove from heat. Let stand overnight or all day. Just before serving, cook over moderate heat 10 minutes or until water is absorbed and rice is tender.

Percent Calories From Fat: 6
Total Fat Grams In Recipe: 6

Baked Brown Rice

Use this recipe if you are going to be gone all day and will arrive back home at dinner time. By taking just a few minutes in the morning, your rice will be cooked and ready to eat. Have dried beans cooking in the slow cooker too, and your last minute preparation will be a vegetable, salad, and perhaps some kind of bread. Use any of the brown rices: long, medium, or short, basmati, or sweet brown.

1 cup brown rice, sorted and rinsed
2½ cups water

Combine rice and water in a 1½-quart casserole and cover. Place in cold oven and set timer so that oven comes on to 350° one hour before dinner time. Set timer to go off after cooking 45 minutes so rice can sit in oven for about 15 minutes. The water will be absorbed if you have soaked the rice all day. Makes 3 cups.

Variation: If you want to bake brown rice without soaking it, add 2 cups boiling water to rice in casserole, cover, place in oven, and bake for about 40 minutes or until water is absorbed.

Percent Calories From Fat: 6
Total Fat Grams In Recipe: 6

Seasoned Baked Brown Rice: Chop 1 onion and 1 clove garlic, place in casserole along with rice and water, and cook as above.

Mixed Rice

Here's a simple, yet delicious, combination of whole grain rices. The wild rice takes a little longer to cook than the others.

¼ cup wild rice, sorted, rinsed, and drained (keep separate from the other rices)
½ cup long grain brown rice, sorted, rinsed, and drained
¼ cup sweet brown rice, sorted, rinsed, and drained (or ¼ cup additional long grain brown rice)
2 cups + 2 tablespoons boiling water

Slowly sprinkle the wild rice into the boiling water so that the water continues to boil. Reduce heat, cover, and cook (faster than a simmer) about 10 minutes. Remove lid, sprinkle other rices in slowly, add lid again, and cook for about 35 minutes more or until water is absorbed. Makes 3 cups.

Percent Calories From Fat: 5
Total Fat Grams In Recipe: 4

Gooey Brown Rice

This makes a tasty, quick breakfast and is a good way to use left-over rice.

¾ cup cooked brown rice
¼ cup shredded low-fat cheese
A few sesame or sunflower seeds, optional
Tamari or shoyu (alcohol-free), optional

Oil pan with *Oil-Lecithin Combination* (p. 205). Add cooked rice and cheese to pan, stirring gently while heating the two. Sprinkle with sesame or sunflower seeds, and a little alcohol-free tamari or shoyu, if desired. Makes almost 1 cup.

Percent Calories From Fat: 22 (without seeds)
Total Fat Grams In Recipe: 6 (without seeds)

Country Garden Rice

Adding vegetables to brown rice while it is cooking is an easy and delicious way to increase the vegetables in your diet.

1 cup brown basmati or long grain brown rice, sorted, rinsed, and drained
2 cups boiling water
1 to 2 cups assorted chopped vegetables such as onion, carrots, mushrooms, summer squash, green pepper, celery, broccoli flowers or stalks

In a dry pan, heat drained brown rice over medium-high heat until grains are dry and only slightly browned. Add boiling water and reduce heat to medium-low so that rice will continue boil faster than a simmer. While rice is cooking, prepare vegetables and then add to rice, increasing heat briefly to keep mixture boiling. Do not stir. Cover rice for a total of about 35 minutes or until water is absorbed. Check for unabsorbed water by removing the lid and tilting the pan slightly. Cover and continue cooking until all water is absorbed. Do not stir until rice is cooked. Makes about 4 cups.

Percent Calories From Fat: 6
Total Fat Grams In Recipe: 5

Broccoli-Brown Rice Deluxe

Easy to prepare and delicious, too! Stir in a can of tuna packed in water or leftover turkey pieces just before serving for a simple main dish casserole.

1 cup long grain brown rice, sorted, rinsed, and drained
2 cups boiling water
¼ teaspoon granulated onion
⅛ teaspoon granulated garlic
10-ounce package frozen cut broccoli
¼ cup shredded low-fat cheddar cheese
1 tablespoon sliced almonds

In a dry pan, heat drained brown rice over medium-high heat until grains are dry and only slightly browned. Add granulated onion and garlic to boiling water and then add boiling water to the rice, reduce heat, cover, and cook (faster than a simmer) for 15 minutes. Add remaining ingredients, increasing heat until rice comes back to a full boil. Do not stir. Reduce heat and cook about 20 minutes longer or until most of liquid is absorbed. Stir and serve. Makes about 4 cups.

Percent Calories From Fat: 15
Total Fat Grams In Recipe: 15

Brown Rice Stuffing

Here's the taste of old-fashioned stuffing without the turkey.

1 teaspoon oil
1 onion, chopped
1 rib celery, thinly sliced
½ cup chopped mushrooms
2 cloves garlic, minced
½ teaspoon dried sage
½ teaspoon dried thyme
1 cup short grain brown rice, sorted, rinsed, and drained
2 cups boiling water or broth

Sauté vegetables in oil for a couple of minutes. Add seasonings and rice, cooking for another minute while stirring. Add water, return to a full boil, reduce heat, cover, and cook (faster than a simmer) until water is absorbed or about 35 minutes. Do not stir while cooking. Makes 3½ to 4 cups.

Percent Calories From Fat: 9
Total Fat Grams In Recipe: 8

French-Style Brown Rice

This is a favorite of Dr. Robert Barnes, a chiropractor practicing in Winchester, Kentucky. After you try it, you'll know why he likes it so much. Delicious!

1 cup long grain brown rice, sorted, rinsed, and cooked in 2 cups water
10-ounce package frozen French-style green beans, steamed about 10 minutes
1 recipe *Cheesy Tamari Sauce* (p. 267)
Black pepper, optional

Oil a 8 x 12-inch flat casserole with *Oil-Lecithin Combination* (p. 205), spread cooked rice on bottom and then the green beans. Top with the sauce, sprinkle with pepper if desired, and serve. Makes about 5½ cups.

Percent Calories From Fat: 16
Total Fat Grams In Recipe: 21

Spanish Brown Rice

My friend Margie Duncan doubles this recipe, takes it to pot luck suppers, and says that she usually brings her casserole dish back home empty!

2 teaspoons oil
1 onion, chopped
1 or 2 clove garlic, minced
1 cup short grain brown rice, sorted, rinsed, and drained
1¾ cups boiling water
¼ green pepper, diced
1 cup tomato purée
¾ teaspoon chili powder
¼ teaspoon oregano
¼ teaspoon basil

Heat oil in pan and sauté onion and garlic for a couple of minutes. Add rice and cook for a minute or two longer. Add boiling water, reduce heat when water has returned to a boil, cover, and cook (faster than a simmer) until most of water is absorbed or about 30 minutes. Add remaining ingredients, stir gently, and simmer until most of liquid is absorbed. Makes about 3½ cups.

Percent Calories From Fat: 13
Total Fat Grams In Recipe: 11

Basic Rye Berries

1 cup rye berries, sorted and rinsed
3 cups boiling water

Sprinkle rye berries into boiling water, reduce heat when water has returned to a boil, cover, and simmer until water is absorbed, about 1½ hours. Makes 3 cups.

Percent Calories From Fat: 5
Total Fat Grams In Recipe: 4

Rye Flakes

For a hearty breakfast that will stick with you until lunchtime, try rye flakes, rolled rye, or ConAgra's Cream of Rye. The flakes vary in size according to the brand; the cooking time is determined by the size of the flakes. When the rye berries have been cracked into small pieces before being rolled, they take only about 8 minutes to cook. Rolled whole rye berries take up to 20 minutes to become tender and creamy.

⅓ cups rye flakes
1 cup boiling water

Add rye flakes to boiling water, reduce heat when water has returned to a boil, and cook for 8 to 20 minutes, until tender and creamy. Remove from heat, cover, and let sit for a few minutes. Good with a sprinkle of pecan meal and skim milk. Makes 1 cup.

Percent Calories From Fat: 5
Total Fat Grams In Recipe: 1

Basic Spelt Berries

Use spelt occasionally in place of brown rice or potatoes. Or serve it for a satisfying breakfast cereal.

1 cup spelt berries, sorted and rinsed
2 cups boiling water

Add spelt berries to boiling water. Reduce heat when water has returned to a boil, cover, and simmer for 50 to 60 minutes or until liquid is absorbed. Makes 3 cups.

Percent Calories From Fat: 7
Total Fat Grams In Recipe: 6

Spelt Flakes

⅓ cup spelt flakes
1 cup boiling water

Add spelt flakes to boiling water, reduce heat when water has returned to a boil, and simmer for 10 minutes. Add lid and let sit for a few minutes to thicken. For a creamier cereal, combine spelt flakes and cold water, bring to a boil, and cook as instructed above. Makes 1 cup.

Percent Calories From Fat: 7
Total Fat Grams In Recipe: 2

Basic Teff

Teff is a tiny whole grain that's packed with nutrients. It has been cultivated for several thousands of years but is unknown to most Americans. Teff is especially useful for those allergic to common grains like wheat and corn.

¼ cup teff
1 cup water

Toast teff in a heavy, dry pan over medium heat for a few minutes, being careful not to burn it. There should be a fragrant aroma. Add water, bring to a boil, reduce heat, cover, and simmer for 20 to 25 minutes or until water is absorbed. Stir occasionally to keep teff from sticking. Serve as a breakfast cereal. Makes ⅞ cup.

Percent Calories From Fat: 5
Total Fat Grams In Recipe: 1

Cream of Teff Cereal

⅜ cup teff flour (¼ cup + 2 tablespoons)
1 cup water

Toast the teff flour in a heavy pan for 2 to 3 minutes, being careful not to burn it. There should be a fragrant aroma. Cool the teff and pan. Add water, stirring constantly. Continue to stir, bring the water to a boil, reduce heat, cover, and simmer for 5 minutes. Stir occasionally to prevent sticking. Makes 1 cup.

Percent Calories From Fat: 5
Total Fat Grams In Recipe: 1

Overnight Wheat Berries

1 cup wheat berries
3½ cups water

Combine ingredients in slow cooker and cook on low for 8 to 10 hours. Makes 2⅔ cups.

Percent Calories From Fat: 5
Total Fat Grams In Recipe: 4

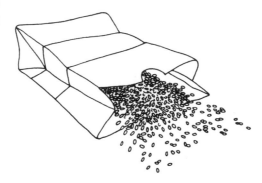

Calico Wheat Crunch

½ cup hard whole wheat berries
1½ cups boiling water
½ teaspoon oil
1 onion, chopped
1 carrot, coarsely chopped
¼ green pepper, diced
1 clove garlic, minced
⅛ teaspoon salt

Add wheat berries to boiling water, reduce heat when water returns to a boil, cover, and simmer for one hour or until berries are tender but still crunchy. Drain, if necessary. Sauté vegetables in oil for 3 or 4 minutes and stir into berries along with salt.   Makes about 3 cups.

Wheat-Free Calico Grain Crunch: Substitute any whole grain berries like spelt, rye, kamut, or triticale for the wheat berries.

Percent Calories From Fat: 9
Total Fat Grams In Recipe: 5

Creamy Breakfast Wheat

½ cup wheat flakes
1 cup boiling water

Stir wheat flakes into boiling water, reduce heat, cover, and cook for about 15 minutes. Remove from heat and let sit, covered, for a few minutes before serving. Good with a dash of cinnamon and a some dairy, soy, or nut milk. Makes 1 cup.

Percent Calories From Fat: 4
Total Fat Grams In Recipe: 1

Toasted Wheat Flakes

3 cups wheat flakes (or other flaked grain)

Preheat oven to 325°. Look over flakes carefully, removing any whole wheat berries that did not get rolled. Place flakes in a colander. Pour water over them, getting all of the flakes wet. Drain and, using an 11 x 15-inch baking sheet with sides, toast the wheat flakes in oven for 20 to 30 minutes, stirring every 10 minutes. If you have a smaller pan, use fewer flakes, so that there will be a thin layer in the pan. After cooking, cool and serve with milk or yogurt. Store in airtight container. Makes 3 cups.

Percent Calories From Fat: 5
Total Fat Grams In Recipe: 7

Wheatena

*Wheatena is a whole grain cereal available at many grocery stores and co-ops. Since once a grain is ground or cracked, the fats in it quickly begin to deteriorate, check the date on the box for freshness. Because the expiration date is given approximately two years after the cereal is processed, don't buy Wheatena if the date is almost current. Also, don't confuse Cream of Wheat with Wheatena. Cream of Wheat is highly refined and should be not be used on the **Perfect Whole Foods** diet.*

¼ cup *Wheatena* cereal
1 cup boiling water

Stir *Wheatena* into boiling water, reduce heat when water returns to a boil, and cook for 4 to 5 minutes. Remove from heat, cover, and let sit for a few minutes. Makes 1 cup.

Percent Calories From Fat: 7
Total Fat Grams In Recipe: 1

Cooked Bulgur Cereal

⅓ cup bulgur or cracked wheat
1 cup boiling water
Pinch of cinnamon

Sprinkle bulgur into boiling water. Add cinnamon. Reduce heat when water returns to a boil, stir, cover and cook over low heat until all water is absorbed or about 10 minutes. To serve, sprinkle with a few nuts on top and add milk if desired. Makes 1 cup.

Percent Calories From Fat: 3
Total Fat Grams In Recipe: 1

Easy Bulgur Breakfast

This is a good hot-weather breakfast. But don't forget to prepare it the night before you want to serve it. Easy Bulgur Breakfast is good topped with a sliced banana at breakfast time.

⅓ cup bulgur
⅔ cup skim milk, soy milk, or nut milk

In a covered bowl or jar, soak bulgur in milk overnight in the refrigerator. It can be soaked for as little as 1½ to 2 hours for a crunchy cereal. Makes 1 cup.

Perfect Whole Foods: Make sure soy or nut milk is unsweetened.
Percent Calories From Fat: 4, using skim milk
Total Fat Grams In Recipe: 2, using skim milk

Tabouli

Tabouli is a traditional Middle Eastern salad. Serve it one night for dinner and take the leftovers, if you have any, to work the next day in a wide-mouth thermos.

1 cup bulgur or cracked wheat
¾ cup chopped fresh parsley
1 green pepper, diced
1 cucumber, diced
2 tomatoes, diced
3 green onions, sliced in thin diagonals
¼ cup lemon juice
¼ cup olive oil
1 teaspoon tamari or shoyu soy sauce (alcohol-free)
Black or green olives, optional

Soak bulgur or wheat in 2 cups hot water 15 minutes to soften. Drain using cheese cloth to squeeze out moisture. Toss vegetables and soaked wheat together. Combine lemon juice, olive oil, and tamari. Add to wheat and vegetable mixture, mixing well. Chill. Serve on a lettuce leaf. Garnish with olives, if desired. Makes 8 cups.

Perfect Whole Foods: Include pulp with the lemon juice. Or substitute cider vinegar for the lemon juice.
Percent Calories From Fat: 33
Total Fat Grams In Recipe: 59

Quinoa Tabouli: To make a wheat-free tabouli, thoroughly rinse 1 cup quinoa in a strainer, drain, and add it to 2 cups boiling water, reduce heat, cover, and cook for 15 minutes. Cool quinoa and substitute it for the soaked and drained bulgur.

Spanish Bulgur Salad

Here's another delicious salad using bulgur wheat.

¾ cup bulgur
2 cups canned tomato purée
2 cups water
⅛ to ¼ teaspoon cayenne or red pepper
1 large fresh tomato, chopped
2 green peppers, chopped
2¼-ounce can sliced black olives (about ½ cup)

Toast bulgur in a dry skillet over low heat for a few minutes. Add tomato purée and water and bring to a boil while stirring frequently. Stir in cayenne pepper and cool slightly. Put bulgur/tomato mixture in a bowl along with remaining ingredients. Mix well and chill for several hours so that mixture will thicken and flavors will blend. Makes about 8 cups.

Percent Calories From Fat: 16
Total Fat Grams In Recipe: 15

Whole Wheat Couscous

If you are new to whole foods and find most whole grains a bit too heavy, try whole grain couscous. It's made from whole durum wheat which is lighter than most other whole wheat products. Here are the basic directions for cooking whole wheat couscous. Try topping it with a variety of sautéed vegetables.

1 cup whole wheat couscous
1¾ cups boiling water

Add couscous to boiling water, reduce heat, cover, and cook for 4 minutes or until water is absorbed. Makes 3 cups.

Percent Calories From Fat: 4
Total Fat Grams In Recipe: 4

Whole Wheat Breakfast Couscous: Top cooked couscous with cinnamon or *Cinnamon Spice Blend* (p. 256), a few chopped nuts, and skim milk or soy milk (unsweetened if on the perfect diet).

Whole Grain Pasta

Most pastas (not flat noodles) double in volume when cooked. Use this rule of thumb when deciding how much spaghetti or macaroni to cook. To reheat leftover pasta (without the sauce), place it in a steamer basket over boiling water until hot. When buying whole grain pasta, don't go by the name on the package. Read the ingredient list carefully since sometimes a whole grain will be combined with a refined grain or starch.

4 quarts water per pound of pasta
Whole grain pasta (whole wheat, spelt, kamut, brown rice, or buckwheat)
½ teaspoon oil, optional
¼ teaspoon salt, optional

Bring water to a boil. Add oil and salt, if desired. Oil helps keep pasta from becoming sticky. It's important to add the pasta slowly to the water, making certain the water continues to boil. If you don't, the pasta will become sticky and gummy. Cook at gentle boil, with lid on, until pasta is tender, but still firm. It takes a little longer to cook whole grain pasta than the refined ones. The exact time depends on the thickness of the pasta. Noodles take about 7 minutes; lasagna cooks in about 18 minutes. (Overcooking will also produce a gummy pasta.) Drain in colander immediately. If you don't have a colander and want to drain it while holding the lid loosely over the pan, blow into the steaming water while draining to keep the steam from burning your hand. 1 pound whole wheat spaghetti makes about 7 cups cooked spaghetti.

Perfect Whole Foods: Don't use corn pasta or pastas with corn flour as an ingredient since corn flour is refined. Also, don's use semolina pastas since the term semolina refers to a refined wheat product.
Percent Calories From Fat: 4 (pasta made without eggs)
Total Fat Grams In Recipe: 7 in one pound (pasta made without eggs)

California Pasta

½ pound whole grain pasta, cooked, drained and left in pan
2 teaspoons olive oil
¼ cup sun dried tomato flakes
¼ cup fresh basil, chopped
2 tablespoons pinenuts or sunflower seeds
2 garlic cloves, minced

Add olive oil to pan with cooked pasta. Toss to coat the pasta. Add other ingredients, gently mix, and serve immediately.   Makes about 4 cups.

Percent Calories From Fat: 18
Total Fat Grams In Recipe: 23

Breakfast Quick

Prepare this granola-type recipe (that's lower in fat than commercial granolas) and store it in the refrigerator for a quick hot or cold breakfast. If you have food allergy tendencies, especially allergies to grains, avoid this and other recipes that include several grains. It's best to eat just one grain at a time to help prevent additional allergies.

5 cups rolled oats
1 cup wheat flakes
½ cup raw sunflower seeds
2 teaspoons cinnamon
1½ cups fresh, raw wheat germ
¼ cup almonds, chopped
¼ cup cashew pieces
¼ cup date pieces
½ cup raisins

Heat oven to 300°. Combine oats, wheat flakes, sunflower seeds, and cinnamon in an 8½ x 11-inch baking dish or pan. Using the center shelf of the oven, toast for 30 minutes, stirring every 10 minutes. In 2 smaller pans, toast the wheat germ and the nuts for about 10 or 15 minutes. To keep the wheat germ from burning, stir it often and away from the sides of the pan. While still hot, combine toasted ingredients with dried fruit. Cool cereal before transferring it to an airtight container. Store in the refrigerator. To serve, top with one of the following: hot or cold skim milk or nut milk; plain, nonfat yogurt;, or boiling water. Each results in a completely different yet tasty cereal. Makes 9 cups.

Perfect Whole Foods: Omit the dates and raisins.
Percent Calories From Fat: 26
Fat Grams In 1 Cup: 13

Carob Breakfast Quick: Substitute ¼ cup carob powder for the cinnamon. Also, vary the nuts and fruits as desired.

Instant Breakfast Mix

This is an unusual recipe. If you're looking for something other than cooked cereal for breakfast, why not try this mix? It makes a quick breakfast since it's prepared ahead of time and stored in the refrigerator. One recipe makes enough for several days. You can make half a recipe the first time to see how well you like it. If you don't have all of the ingredients, you can easily improvise and make your own combination.

½ cup rolled oats, raw
4 tablespoons wheat, spelt, or kamut berries, raw
4 tablespoons hulled barley, raw
4 tablespoons millet, raw
4 tablespoons buckwheat, raw
4 tablespoons rye berries, raw
2 tablespoons sesame seeds
2 tablespoons pumpkin seeds
2 tablespoons raw sunflower seeds
2 tablespoons fine, unsweetened coconut, optional

Look over the whole grains for rocks and debris and then wash and drain if they appear dirty. Place all ingredients in a quart jar and mix. Add 1½ cups water, stirring to mix ingredients with the water. Soak at room temperature for 15 to 18 hours (less in a warm kitchen). Store, covered, in the refrigerator. To serve, place ¼ to ½ cup in cereal bowl and top with sliced fresh fruit or plain, nonfat yogurt. Makes 3 cups.

Perfect Whole Foods: Do not use coconut.
Percent Calories From Fat: 24, without coconut
Fat Grams In ¼ Cup: 3, without coconut

Margie's Breakfast Special

1 cup oat bran
1 cup thick rolled oats
1 cup steel cut oats
1 cup rye flakes

Mix together and store in airtight container. For each serving, add ¼ cup mixture to ¾ cup boiling water. Reduce heat and simmer for 5 to 7 minutes. Remove from heat, cover, and let sit for a few minutes. Top each serving with:
1 teaspoon blackstrap molasses
2 tablespoons plain, nonfat yogurt
1 or 2 teaspoons raisins

Perfect Whole Foods: Omit molasses and raisins, adding your favorite nuts or seeds instead.
Percent Calories From Fat: 14, cereal only; 12, with topping
Fat Grams In 1 Serving: 2, with or without topping

Mixed Berry Cereal

⅓ cup wheat berries
⅓ cup spelt berries
⅓ cup rye berries

The evening before you plan this for breakfast, sort and rinse the berries. Bring 3 cups water to a boil. Add the berries, reduce heat when water has returned to a boil, cover, and cook for 15 minutes. Turn heat off and let it sit overnight. Next morning, bring to boil, reduce heat, and cook until tender and most of water is absorbed or about 20 to 30 minutes. Makes 3 cups.

Variation: Use 1 cup of a single grain rather than the mixture.

Percent Calories From Fat: 5
Total Fat Grams In Recipe: 4

Mixed Berry Cereal—Slow Cooker Style

⅔ cup wheat or triticale berries
⅔ cup spelt berries
⅔ cup rye berries

The evening before you plan this for breakfast, sort and rinse the berries. Combine them in your slow cooker, add 6 cups of hot water, and cook on low for 8 to 10 hours. Makes 6 cups.

Variation: Use 2 cups of a single grain rather than the mixture.

Percent Calories From Fat: 5
Total Fat Grams In Recipe: 8

Berry Breakfast Delight

Start with any kind of cooked whole grains you like - from wheat, rye, or triticale berries to spelt or kamut berries. Next, use whatever fresh fruit that's in season and you'll have a delightful cereal that will keep you energized until lunchtime!

¾ cup cooked wheat, rye, triticale, spelt, or kamut berries
1 piece or ¾ cup of fresh fruit (like a banana, a peach, strawberries, or blueberries), sliced
½ cup plain, nonfat yogurt

Top cooked cereal berries with fresh fruit and yogurt. Makes 1 hardy serving.

Percent Calories From Fat: 6, using wheat berries and strawberries
Total Fat Grams In Recipe: 1, using wheat berries and strawberries

VEGETABLES

If you're like most people, you should be eating more vegetables. Include at least three servings, preferably more, in your diet each day. If you are eliminating fruits temporarily due to *Candida* treatment, then make certain you eat even more vegetables. Include fresh and frozen vegetables in your diet—both raw and cooked.

Loss of nutrients before vegetables ever reach the dinner table can be a problem. Handle vegetables carefully and cook them properly to preserve their nutrients. Purchase fresh vegetables that are fresh-looking. Bruised, limp vegetables that are starting to decay and are reduced for clearance are no bargain. Many of their nutrients have been destroyed before you buy them. Select crisp vegetables that are free from bruises and skin punctures. Growing many of your vegetables or going to farms where you can pick them will assure you of really fresh vegetables. Organically grown vegetables are preferable to those grown with chemical fertilizers, pesticides, and fungicides.

Store most vegetables in a cool place, usually in the refrigerator. Fresh vegetables displayed in grocery stores should also be stored this way. If you cannot buy all of your vegetables fresh, then frozen and dried are good choices as long as you read the ingredient lists carefully. Don't use frozen vegetables with sauces, breading, and preservatives, and always cook frozen vegetables from the frozen state. Thawing before cooking causes a greater loss of nutrients and makes vegetables watery.

Do not use canned vegetables on the **Perfect Whole Foods** diet. The canning process destroys more of the food's nutrients than does freezing or drying. There is one exception concerning canned vegetables on the perfect diet. You may use canned tomato products in cooked foods like soups, stews, and pasta sauces. Read ingredient lists carefully so you won't buy canned tomato products with added sugar or starch. Also, don't crowd other fresh or frozen vegetables from your diet by filling up on a bowl of canned tomatoes or a glass of tomato juice. Use canned tomato products for flavoring, not as your vegetable source.

Peeling vegetables removes valuable nutrients, especially fiber and minerals. Just under the skin, especially in root vegetables like potatoes and carrots, lies a mineral ring that's partially removed when the vegetable is peeled. By scrubbing these vegetables with a stiff non-metal brush or plastic scouring pad rather than peeling them, you'll benefit from the nutrients in the whole vegetable. Peel wax-coated vegetables to avoid eating the wax as well as insecticides and fungicides under the coating. Cucumbers are often waxed to make them stay fresh-looking longer.

Avoid the practice of soaking cut-up vegetables in ice water to freshen them and make them crunchier. Water-soluble vitamins dissolve in the water and will be thrown away when the vegetables are drained. Also, don't soak most vegetables in water while cleaning them. (Sometimes green leafy vegetables must be soaked briefly to get the sand and dirt off.)

Methods of Cooking Vegetables

Steaming	Braising	Pressure cooking
Stir-frying	Baking	Boiling*
Sautéing		

*Boil vegetables only if you're going to eat the liquid in which they're cooked as in soups and stews. You'll waste valuable water-soluble vitamins and minerals that dissolve in the liquid if you pour it down the drain.
I have not listed microwaving above since microwave ovens are not used on the Perfect Whole Foods diet.*

Use stainless steel baskets for steaming vegetables. Put the adjustable basket into a pan with an inch or so of water. Add a lid to the pan and let the steam cook the vegetables in the basket. Since the vegetables don't actually touch the water, you won't throw valuable water-soluble vitamins and minerals down the drain.

To Retain a Green Vegetable's Natural Color

Cook vegetables for a minute or two without a lid at the beginning. Then add a lid and continue cooking. This simple step allows the volatile acids that dull the green color to escape.

Stir-frying is a frying of cut-up ingredients in a very small amount of oil with medium heat and constant stirring. Don't use high heat as recommended in most cook books since it causes all oils to form toxic trans-fatty acids. Monounsaturated, unrefined sesame oil and expeller-pressed high-oleic safflower oil (the safflower oil label must say high-oleic in order for it to be monounsaturated rather than polyunsaturated) are good to use for stir-frying at medium temperatures since they don't smoke or break down as easily under heat as polyunsaturated oils do. (See more information about selecting and handling oils on page 44.) Cut vegetables for stir-frying so they cook quickly. You can dice them or slice them wafer thin. Shred leafy vegetables or tear them into bite-size pieces. Use a wok or skillet to stir-fry. (See recipe for *Stir-Fried Vegetables* on page 177.)

Sautéing is similar to stir-frying except that the ingredients are not stirred continuously while cooking. If you need to eliminate added fat in your diet, you can sauté vegetables in a nonstick *SilverStone* skillet with either nothing or a sprinkle of water or broth added to the skillet. Mushrooms and onions are easily cooked this way.

Braise vegetables by cooking them, covered, in a small amount of flavorful liquid like broth or tomato juice. When the vegetables are almost tender, remove the lid and continue cooking to boil the liquid down without burning the vegetables or letting them stick. The pan should be large enough so that the vegetables are arranged in one layer. Root vegetables are especially good braised.

Baking a vegetable in its skin will retain much of its food value. Root vegetables and winter squash are especially good when baked. For optimum nutrition, always preheat the oven and don't overcook the vegetable. If you are on the perfect diet, be certain to eat the skin of both potatoes and sweet potatoes since the peeling provides fiber. Other valuable nutrients are also located just under the skin and they are discarded if the potatoes are peeled. (While on the perfect diet, select small to medium-size potatoes rather than large ones.)

Pressure cooking is another good method of cooking vegetables. Follow directions that come with your pressure cooker.

Whatever method of cooking you use, don't overcook vegetables since more nutrients will be destroyed than necessary. Most vegetables should be cooked until tender-crisp or tender yet crunchy, not soggy. Some people have a difficult time digesting overcooked vegetables of the cabbage family (like cabbage, cauliflower, and broccoli). If you have trouble digesting them, then try reducing their cooking time and steaming or stir-frying them at a lower than usual temperature. High cooking temperatures break down sulfur compounds in these vegetables, causing gasses to form in the intestinal tract during digestion.

Cook vegetables just before serving them. Don't cook them too soon and then keep them hot until mealtime. Don't let them sit for a long time at room temperature and then reheat them when it's time to eat. Each time you reheat vegetables, more nutrients are lost. It's best to cook only enough vegetables for one meal. However, you may find that it's not always practical to cook vegetables this way. If you like fixing a big pot of vegetable soup or beans with vegetables that can be served for several meals, be certain to refrigerate the leftovers immediately after the meal. Also serve a fresh vegetable or salad with each meal.

As you eliminate refined foods from your diet, your taste will change and you should be able to enjoy the flavor of plain vegetables rather than vegetables highly seasoned with fats and salt. The flavors of steamed broccoli, baked acorn squash, and stir-fried green beans are all unique and, when cooked correctly, should be mild and pleasant. Should you want to add more flavor to your vegetables, try sprinkling them with a little granulated garlic or granulated onion (not garlic or onion salt) or a dash of salt. You may also want to try placing a clove of garlic or a sliced onion in the water before steaming vegetables. This will add flavor to the vegetables. Save the water and use as stock in soups. Sprinkling cooked vegetables with dill weed or nutritional yeast also makes a tasty addition.

Because vegetables are so important in the diet, I have included a variety of basic recipes. Some readers may not need instructions for steaming broccoli or carrots, yet others do. I have included a number of soup recipes. For those who have not yet learned to eat vegetables, soups are an easy way to include them in the diet.

Sea Vegetables

Sea vegetables are like gold from the sea. Often called seaweeds, they deserve a much better sounding name than weed. These nutritious vegetables have been used for centuries by the peoples of Japan, Ireland, Scotland, Russia, and the South Pacific.

Sea vegetables are excellent sources of many nutrients, especially minerals including calcium, phosphorus, magnesium, iron, sodium, iodine and others. (Including sea vegetables in your diet will assure you adequate iodine since the *Perfect Whole Foods* diet don't use iodized salt.) All minerals in sea vegetables are in forms that the body can easily use.

As more Americans become interested in good nutrition, they are turning to sea vegetables for part of their nourishment. These foods definitely belong in the whole foods diet. If you are not accustomed to using sea vegetables, then do make an effort to use them. Experiment and decide how you best like to use these vegetables. Food co-ops usually have a variety of sea vegetables available.

The milder tasting sea vegetables include dulse, kombu, nori, Irish Moss, agar, and arame. Kelp, wakame, and hijiki have more flavor. Learn to use these milder tasting vegetables before going on to the stronger ones.

In general, sea vegetables have a salty taste so you should add less salt to food you season with sea vegetables. Sprinkle powdered sea vegetables like dulse or kelp on foods as you would salt and pepper. You might want to include a special shaker at your table filled with ground sea vegetables. That way, you'll remember to use it along with or in place of salt and pepper. Or, you can add some to the salt shaker.

Add flaked sea vegetables to soups and stews. An excellent soup recipe that includes dulse flakes (a reddish sea vegetable) is *Mushroom-Miso Soup* (p. 183). You can also sprinkle dulse on vegetable salads.

You can add another sea vegetable, kombu, to dried legumes while they are cooking to enhance their flavor, shorten their cooking time, improve their nutrition, and, also importantly, improve their digestibility. Try adding a 3 or 4-inch strip of kombu per cup of beans next time you cook them.

Nori is a nutty-flavored sea vegetable that is cultivated in Japan. Nori, dried into sheets and toasted, is one of the ingredients in sushi. Toasted nori, also available shredded, is delicious sprinkled over cooked brown rice and other cooked grains.

Both Irish moss (sometimes called carragheen) and agar have gelling properties. Irish moss produces a softer gel than agar and is used for puddings and jellies. Agar is used to make a traditional Japanese gelatin dessert called kanten which is made with apple juice and fruit. If you like, you can substitute agar for gelatin in aspic and fruit gelatin recipes. Agar is available as a powder, flaked, or in bar form (also called kanten.)

To Gel 2 Cups of Liquid with Agar

Use one of these in place of 4 teaspoons gelatin
2 teaspoons powder
2 tablespoons flakes
1 bar kanten

The liquid will set either at room temperature or in the refrigerator. For a fruit dessert recipe using agar flakes, see page 282.

Arame, a slightly sweet-tasting sea vegetable, is good in soups or cooked and served as a vegetable with grains. Soak it briefly before using it as a vegetable. The recipe *Arame with Brown Rice and Vegetables* (p. 164) is an excellent way to try arame. Once you try it this way, you may want to create your own recipes using it. You can substitute wakame, a large dark brown sea vegetable, in soups, as a vegetable, or in place of arame in *Arame with Brown Rice and Vegetables*.

Soups

I've always found that serving soups often (as well as salads) is an easy way to get my family to eat more vegetables. I've included my family's favorites, *Vegetable-Barley Soup* (p. 186) and *Broccoli-Potato Soup* (p. 178). You may never be tempted to buy another can of soup when you discover the goodness of homemade ones. See recipes for heavier soups in the **Main Dish** section of this book.

Several recipes for soups (as well as some other recipes) call for flavorful chicken broth or vegetable broth as a base rather than water. If you don't have these broths available, refer to the chart that follows for other substitutions.

When A Recipe Calls for Broth

Consider These Options
• Homemade chicken or turkey broth (chill before using to remove hardened fat)
• *Pritikin* Canned Chicken Broth
• *Homemade Vegetable Broth* (p. 179)
• One teaspoon *Gaylord Hauser's* Vegetable Broth powder per cup of water
• Pinch of granulated onion, granulated garlic, and cayenne pepper in water
• One teaspoon miso per cup of water
• Few drops of tamari or shoyu soy sauce (alcohol-free) per cup of water
• Water left from steaming vegetables (don't use potato water)

*Pay close attention to the ingredient lists of all products if you are on **Perfect Whole Foods**.*

Raw Vegetables

Include raw vegetables in your daily diet. Most are naturally low in fat as well as calories; they also provide nutrients that are destroyed in cooking. If you notice the *Percent Calories From Fat* in many of the following salad recipes, you'll see that salads are *not always* so low in fat. In fact, some are quite high. Dressings made of oil, mayonnaise, or avocados are very high in fats and calories. When you add even a little high-fat and high-calorie dressing to a low-fat and low-calorie raw vegetable, you automatically get a high percentage of calories from fat. By using fats and oils that provide essential fatty acids rather than saturated fats, the fat in salad dressings will be beneficial and not just a source of unnecessary calories and fat. Oils with the most beneficial Omega-3 essential fatty acid (the one hardest to get in the diet) include fresh flax oil, unrefined safflower oil (not high-oleic), and unrefined sunflower oil (not high-oleic). Always store oils in the refrigerator. Oils freshly pressed by methods that exclude light, oxygen and excessive heat are preferable since these factors are destructive to the oil. For more information on oils, see page 44.

If you are on an extremely low-fat diet, there are several good low-fat dressings as well as dips that can be used as dressings (see *Creamy Spinach Dip*, *Claire's Famous Yogurt Dip*, *Herbed Buttermilk Dressing*, and *Zero Dressing* recipes on pages 260 through 263). Consider, also, adding a sprinkle of lemon or lime juice (not on the perfect diet), raw cider vinegar, or Balsamic vinegar plus a pinch of herbs. Or try using low fat cottage cheese, plain nonfat yogurt, or water-packed tuna to top your salads in place of a dressing. Don't forget about serving such vegetables as carrot sticks, celery sticks, and cucumber slices with or without a low fat dip. You have many low-fat options!

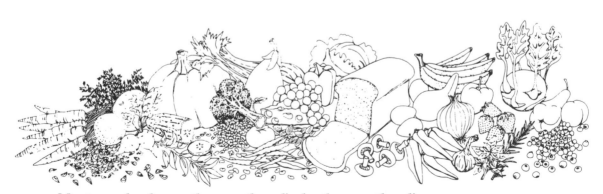

Most people choose the way they die by the way they live.

Vegetable Salad Ingredients

Use your imagination and creativity to come up with different salads every day. Don't settle for salads of only iceberg lettuce, carrots, and tomatoes day after day. Vary not only the salad ingredients, but also the way you cut the vegetables. Carrots, for example, can be cut into coins, match sticks, sticks for dipping, or shredded for an entirely different appearance and texture.

If you have a difficult time getting your family to eat raw vegetables, you might want to experiment with how you serve them. I found that my children, when younger, ate more salad if I served it in individual bowls or on plates rather than in a large bowl where they helped themselves. They would eat all that I served them, whereas they would take only a small helping from the large bowl. Don't overwhelm them the first time you do this with a large serving. Gradually increase the salad size. I still often serve vegetables or some other food this same way. If it's on their plate when they come to the table, they are more likely to eat it. Often, after children have eaten something several times, they develop a taste for the particular food.

Consider Some of These Ingredients for Salads

Greens: Choose those with deep colors more often than iceberg lettuce. Other salad greens such as spinach, leaf lettuce, romaine, endive, and watercress generally have more nutrients than iceberg.

Cabbage: Use, in addition to green cabbage, some of the more unusual cabbages. Savoy, bok choy, and nappa are usually available at large grocery stores. Red cabbage makes a pretty addition to salads.

Raw Vegetables: Select from green peas, snow peas, tender green beans, mushrooms, zucchini and yellow squash, avocados, beets, scallions, green onions, broccoli, cauliflower, tender asparagus, garlic, red peppers, alfalfa sprouts, parsley, chives, and cherry tomatoes, in addition to the traditional celery, onions, green peppers, carrots, radishes, cucumbers, and tomatoes.

Grains: Cooked whole grains, like brown rice, wheat berries, and whole barley make good additions to salads. Use leftovers as a garnish, or with larger amounts, add several chopped raw vegetables and a dressing.

Protein Foods: Make your salad into a main dish by including some cheese (preferably low fat), hard cooked egg, cooked beans (kidney, pinto, garbanzo), sliced lean meat, sunflower seeds, fresh wheat germ, almond slices, plain nonfat yogurt, or tuna canned in water.

Other Foods: Try dried sea vegetables (dulse flakes and kelp flakes, for example) and fruit (orange sections, grapes, apple chunks, and other fresh fruits).

Sprouts

Almost any grain, bean, or seed can be sprouted. It's an easy way to have really fresh vegetables available all year around. Sprouts are economical, nutritious, and a crunchy, refreshing treat. Sprout only seeds that were meant for human consumption since seeds for planting are often treated with toxic chemicals. Also, be aware that sprouts from certain seeds are themselves toxic. For instance, don't eat tomato or potato sprouts. Soybean sprouts should always be cooked for at least five minutes to destroy their protein-inhibiting enzymes.

Alfalfa sprouts are the most popular of all the sprouts. Use them on sandwiches and in salads. Alfalfa sprouts are usually available in the produce department of food co-ops and grocery stores. Before buying them, check to make certain their condition is good. Wilted and soggy sprouts will quickly turn you against them.

There are many ways to sprout seeds. Some people use ziplock bags, fine baskets, or special equipment for sprouting. Most use a Mason jar with a canning ring or rubber band and a fine net or cheese cloth. I used this method for years yet sometimes my alfalfa sprouts were not as crisp, green, and fresh-tasting as I like them. Several years ago, I started using a 1-quart clear food storage container with a plastic lid. My husband drilled holes in the lid for draining. Having two of these containers, with holes in only one lid, allows me to seal and refrigerate my finished sprouts using the lid without holes. I can then start sprouts in the other container again using the lid with holes. This way, sprouts seem to be fresher tasting, as they should be.

Alfalfa Sprouts Grown in a Plastic Container

2 tablespoons alfalfa seeds
1-quart clear food storage rectangular container with ⅛" holes drilled 1 inch apart in lid
A fine meshed strainer

- Place seeds in the container, adding 1 cup lukewarm spring water. Soak overnight or 8 hours.
- Drain water from the container using the strainer. Rinse the seeds with more lukewarm water and let them drain again, this time for at least 10 minutes to eliminate excess water.
- Place well-drained seeds back into the container and attach the lid with holes. Place the container in a dark, warm place, such as inside a kitchen cabinet.
- Rinse seeds 2 times a day for about 5 days. Use the strainer until sprouts are large enough to keep them from falling through the holes in the lid. After that, drain through the lid.
- Sprouts are ready for sunlight when leaves are well-formed. Place the container upside down (over a plate) near a window where the light can shine through the bottom of the plastic container. Continue to rinse and drain twice a day. The leaves will become very green.
- When sprouts are intertwined and will hold together, turn over entire mass of sprouts so that the sprouts on the other side can become green.
- Before serving, float out the hulls and non-sprouted seeds by filling the container with cool water and draining hulls and seeds out with the water. Repeat until most hulls are removed.
- Drain well, place airtight lid on container, and refrigerate. Use within 4 days.

Alfalfa Sprouts Grown in a Mason Jar

- Place 2 tablespoons alfalfa sprouts in a quart jar. Secure netting on the jar with a rubber band or canning ring. Add 1 cup lukewarm spring water to the jar. Soak overnight or about 8 hours.
- Drain water from the jar through the net. Add more lukewarm water, rotate the jar so all seeds are rinsed. Drain for at least 10 minutes to eliminate excess water.
- Place the jar in a dark, warm place, such as inside a kitchen cabinet. Rinse the seeds 2 times a day for about 5 days until leaves are well-formed.
- Sprouts are now ready for sunlight. Place the jar near a window, turning the jar occasionally so that all the leaves that receive the light become very green. Continue to rinse and drain twice a day.
- When sprouts are the desired length and the leaves are green, pour the entire jar of sprouts into a large bowl and add cool water. Hulls and unsprouted seeds will float and can be discarded while water is drained. Repeat until most of hulls and seeds are removed. Drain well.
- Fill quart jar with sprouts and use an airtight lid. Refrigerate, and use within 4 days.

Mung beans can be sprouted by either of the above methods. They are good in stir-fried vegetables. Add them to cooked foods just before serving to preserve their crispness and nutritive value.

When Sprouting Mung Beans

- Rinse and sort ½ cup beans for a 1-quart container.
- Soak in 2 cups of lukewarm spring water for 18 to 24 hours, changing the water during soaking at least once to prevent fermentation.
- Rinse twice a day and sprout for 3 to 4 days or until sprouts are at least ½-inch long.

Vegetable Facts

Agar: A substance extracted from sea vegetables that is used to produce a gel. Agar can be used in place of gelatin in recipes for aspic and fruit gelatin recipes. (See page 155 for substitution amounts.)

Alfalfa Seeds: The seeds usually used in the kitchen for sprouting. (See pages 158 through 159 for seed sprouting sechniques.)

Arame: A fibrous sea vegetable that needs to be soaked before using.

Avocado: Very high in fat, mostly monounsaturates. Ripen a hard avocado at room temperature in a loosely-closed paper bag and check it daily. It is ripe when you can press it gently with your thumb. Use a stainless steel knife to cut avocados. Carbon steel knives will cause them to discolor. If you cut the avocado in half, remove its seed, then cut it into strips, you will be able to peel the skin easily. If you use only part of an avocado, storing the remainder along with the seed will help keep it from browning so fast. California avocados have a rougher and darker green skin than Florida avocados which are usually large, smooth, and bright green.
Percent Calories From Fat: 88 in California variety; 72 in Florida variety
Total Fat Grams: 30 in California variety; 27 in Florida variety

Cabbage: 1 pound = 4 to 5 cups (shredded).

Canned Food: Canning, whether commercially processed in a metal can, glass jar, or home canned, destroys more nutrients than do other methods of food preservation. Canned foods, therefore, should not be eaten when on the **Perfect Whole Foods** diet. Exceptions include canned tomato products used in cooking and canned tuna and salmon. Occasionally, small amounts of canned condiments like black and green olives can also be used. Other foods should be either fresh, dried, or frozen.

Carrots: 1 pound = 6 medium-sized carrots.
4 medium-sized carrots = 1 cup fresh carrot juice.

Cruciferous Vegetables: Vegetables in the cabbage family, including broccoli, cabbage, cauliflower, Brussel sprouts, kale, rutabaga, and turnips. These vegetables are thought to protect against some kinds of cancer.

Cucumbers: Peel cucumbers before eating only if they have been waxed since the peeling provides beneficial fiber. By peeling wax-coated cucumbers, you'll avoid eating the wax as well as insecticides and fungicides under the coating.

Dulse: A reddish-colored sea vegetable that is a good source of trace minerals. Use flakes to season and to add nutrition to soups and salads.

Garlic, Dried: Although fresh is best, when using dehydrated garlic, use the following information for substituting:
1 garlic clove = ⅛ teaspoon granulated garlic or garlic powder (*not* garlic salt).
1 garlic clove = ⅛ teaspoon dehydrated minced garlic.

Garlic, Fresh: A clove of garlic is one section of the entire bulb or head. Garlic varies greatly in size of cloves and strength. The method of cutting garlic also determines its strength. For cooked garlic, whole cloves are mildest, minced next, and then pressed are strongest. Also, raw garlic is stronger than cooked garlic. Considering these facts as well as your personal taste, you might want to adjust the amount of garlic in a recipe. A hint for removing the peel of fresh garlic cloves is to press the clove gently between your fingertips to loosen the peel. Then, remove the peel and mince or chop as desired. I find it easier to mince garlic using a small paring knife rather than a long knife.

Garlic, Granulated: Dried garlic powder.
⅛ teaspoon granulated garlic or garlic powder = 1 clove fresh.

Greens, Fresh: In general, greens are a good source of calcium as well as beta carotene and C and should be eaten often and regularly. Yet many people never give them a try. Some greens are stronger than others, but, as with other foods, you can learn to like them if you cook them properly. Mild-flavored ones to try first include kale, collards, beet greens, chicory, escarole, and spinach. Others are dandelion, mustard, swiss chard, and turnip greens. If you've tried canned or frozen greens and didn't like them, try them fresh. There's no comparison! Some green leafy vegetables should not be eaten often because of their oxalic acid which combines with the calcium and keeps it from being utilized. Greens containing oxalic acid include spinach, beet leaves, and swiss chard.

Herbs: 1 teaspoon fresh herbs = ⅓ to ½ teaspoon dried leaf herbs.
1 teaspoon dried leaf herbs = ½ teaspoon powdered herbs.

Hijiki: A very flavorful sea vegetable.

Kelp: A sea vegetable that contains many trace minerals. Use the powdered form as a seasoning.

Kombu: A sea vegetable that is cooked with legumes to tenderize them, to improve their digestibility, and to provide trace minerals, especially iodine.

Leek: A member of the onion family, leeks are milder than onions. To prepare, remove roots, the outer layer, and the tops of tough leaves, keeping 2 to 3 inches of the green leaves. Wash thoroughly to remove sand and dirt.

Mung Beans: Small, green dried beans which sprout easily and are good when sprouted in stir-fried dishes and salads.

Mushrooms: 6-ounce jar, drained = ½ pound fresh mushrooms, sliced and cooked. Use fresh mushrooms on the perfect diet.

Nori: A mild-flavored sea vegetable. It is available dried in thin sheets and shredded.

Onions, Dried: Although fresh is best, when using dehydrated onions or powder, use the following information for substituting:
1 medium onion = ½ to ¾ cup chopped fresh onion.
1 medium onion = 2 tablespoons dehydrated onion flakes.
1 medium onion = 1½ teaspoons granulated onion (*not* onion salt).

Onion, Fresh: Chopping onions can be a messy, slow chore if you don't know the simple way to do it. First, cut the ends off and peel the onion. Then, cut it in half lengthwise. One at a time, place each half with cut-side down on the cutting board and slice in strips lengthwise, keeping pieces together. Finally, turn the onion 90 degrees and slice crosswise in a similar manner. Onion will be chopped in uniform pieces.

Onion, Granulated: Dried onion powder.
1½ teaspoons = 1 medium onion.

Oxalic Acid: A naturally occurring substance in certain foods (rhubarb, cocoa, sesame seed hulls, Swiss chard, spinach, beets, and beet greens) that combines with calcium from the food and makes the calcium unable to be used by the body. Don't count on these foods as a main source of calcium.

Potatoes: Avoid eating green potatoes. Potatoes grown above the ground or stored in light develop a green color on the skin due to the toxic alkaloid solanine.

Sea Vegetables: Usually available in dried form only (unless you're lucky enough to live close to the sea). Sea vegetables have an abundance of minerals as well as some vitamins. (See also pages 154 and 155.)

Sprout: A germinated seed or grain which is an easily-grown, nutrient-rich, fresh vegetable.

Squash: Squashes are usually classified according to whether they are *summer* or *winter*. This does not refer to the season in which they are grown, but rather their stage of maturity when harvested. See below.

Squash, Summer: Immature, soft-shelled, and small when picked. The shell or skin as well as the seeds are eaten unless they are allowed to develop into mature, hard-shelled vegetables. In this case, they may need to be peeled and seeds removed. Summer squashes includes yellow (straightneck and crookneck), zucchini, pattypan, and cocozelle.

Squash, Winter: Mature when picked. The shells are hard, the seeds are tough, and the size may vary from small to large. Usually winter squashes are cut open, seeds removed, and then baked until tender. Examples are acorn, butternut, buttercup, hubbard, pumpkin, marblehead, turban, banana and, spaghetti squashes. Winter squashes are plentiful in late summer and fall and are often inexpensive then. Stock up and store them in a cool, dark, dry place. They will keep for 4 to 6 months.

Tomato: Tomatoes are best stored at room temperature, away from sunlight. However, they will keep that way only a day or so once they have ripened. If you need to refrigerate ripe tomatoes, then store them in the warmest part of the refrigerator and, for a better flavor, let them sit at room temperature before serving. To speed the ripening process of tomatoes, place them in a paper bag with an apple or banana and check them daily. The gas given off by the fruit encourages ripening of the tomato.
1 pound fresh tomatoes = 1½ cups cooked.

Tomato Paste: A salt-free concentrated product. Use in place of salted tomato juice, *V-8 Juice*, or tomato sauce if you need to restrict your sodium intake.
6-ounce can tomato paste + 3 cans water = 24-ounce can tomato juice.
6-ounce can tomato paste + 1 can water = 12-ounce can tomato sauce.

Tomato Purée: Since tomato purée is usually a salt-free product, use it (read label carefully) in place of tomato sauce if you need to restrict your sodium intake.

Tomato Sauce: For *Perfect Whole Foods*, read labels carefully so you won't buy those with sweeteners added. (See page 22 for words denoting refined sugars.)

Vegetable Juice from the *Vita Mix*: Although it would seem likely that fresh vegetable juice made from the *Vita Mix* appliance would be preferable on the *Perfect Whole Foods* diet to juice in which the fiber is eliminated, this is not so when you consider several facts. Most recipes for juices made in a *Vita Mix* require either fruit juice or a food with high water content like tomatoes as a base. Firm vegetables like carrots and celery cannot be juiced alone but are rather puréed in other liquids. Recipes using fresh tomatoes plus other ingredients that are allowed on the perfect may be used. However, since good quality, fresh tomatoes are available only in the summer months, since large quantities of canned tomatoes are not recommended, and since fruit juice is eliminated on the perfect diet, the *Vita Mix* is not practical as a juicer. If you already have one, use it to make unsweetened whole grain bread dough while you're on the perfect diet.

Vegetable Juice, Raw, Freshly Squeezed: These juices, like carrot and celery, are concentrated in nutrients and, compared to fruit juice, contain relatively little carbohydrates. Limit your intake of carrot juice to 1 cup serving per day while on the perfect diet since carrot juice has a greater concentration of carbohydrates than other vegetable juices.

Wakame: A large, dark brown sea vegetable. (See page 154.)

Vegetable Recipes

Arame with Grains and Vegetables

1 ounce arame (about 0.06 pound)
1 teaspoon oil
1 onion, chopped
1 garlic clove, minced
1 carrot, thinly sliced
1 celery rib, sliced
2 to 3 teaspoons tamari or shoyu soy sauce (alcohol-free)
1 cup raw whole grain such as brown rice or millet, cooked

Rinse and then soak arame for 3 to 5 minutes in cold water. It will expand to about 2 cups. Drain, reserving soaking liquid for later use. Heat oil in skillet, add fresh vegetables, and stir until vegetables are evenly combined. Top with arame and ½ cup of the reserved liquid. Do not stir. Bring to a boil, reduce heat, cover, and simmer for about 1 hour. Add tamari and cook 15 minutes longer. Serve over cooked grains such as brown rice or millet. Use the remaining soaking liquid for watering house plants. Makes about 4 cups.

Percent Calories From Fat: 10
Total Fat Grams In Recipe: 10

Wakame with Grains and Vegetables: Substitute wakame for the arame, cooking only 30 minutes

Fresh Steamed Asparagus

Wash fresh asparagus quickly under running water. Break the woody portion from the more tender part. Split the very thick part of the stem lengthwise with a sharp knife, stopping before you get to the tender part. Steam the asparagus in a covered steaming basket over boiling water until just tender, 6 to 14 minutes. Serve immediately. Good seasoned with fresh lemon juice or minced dill weed. One pound makes about 2 cups cooked.

Perfect Whole Foods: Do not use lemon juice.
Percent Calories From Fat: 9
Fat Grams In 12 spears: 1

Green Beans Gourmet

1 pound fresh, tender green beans, cleaned and broken
½ teaspoon oil
1 small onion, chopped
1 cup sliced fresh mushrooms
1 tablespoon sliced almonds
Salt, optional

Steam fresh green beans in a covered steaming basket over boiling water until tender-crisp, about 20 minutes. While beans are cooking, sauté mushrooms, onions, and almonds for about 5 minutes. Top beans with sautéed mixture, salt, and serve. Makes about 3 cups.

Percent Calories From Fat: 31
Total Fat Grams In Recipe: 7

Mixed Bean Salad

This dish is a hit at pot luck suppers. It's not only nutritious, but also colorful and flavorful!

1 cup each fresh or frozen green beans, yellow wax beans, limas, and peas
2 cups cooked dried beans such as kidney, pinto, or black beans
1 small or ½ large red onion, chopped
3 ribs celery, sliced
½ red pepper, diced
2 tablespoons olive oil
¼ teaspoon granulated onion
⅛ teaspoon granulated garlic
⅛ teaspoon black pepper
¼ teaspoon salt
2 tablespoons Balsamic vinegar

If using fresh vegetables, prepare and steam until tender-crisp. Steam frozen vegetables to defrost. Add seasonings to olive oil and drizzle over cooked vegetables, beans, and raw vegetables, stirring gently. Drizzle vinegar and stir again. Serve either hot or at room temperature. Makes about 6 cups.

Percent Calories From Fat: 20
Total Fat Grams In Recipe: 28

Fresh Steamed Beets

Scrub fresh beets. Cut off tops, leaving about 1 inch of the stem. Save tops if they are crisp and green; cook separately. (See directions for *Fresh Steamed Greens* on page 169.) Steam whole beets in covered steaming basket over boiling water until beets are tender. The time depends on size and age of beets. Cool slightly and remove stem with knife and skin with fingers. Dice, slice, shred, or leave whole if small and uniform in size. Season, if desired, with grated lemon or orange peel, minced parsley, or vinegar. One pound makes about 2 cups diced beets.

Percent Calories From Fat: 2
Fat Grams In 20 Medium Beets: 1

Fresh Steamed Broccoli

Wash fresh broccoli. Cut off the end of stalks and peel away any tough part of stalk. You may also want to split the stalk lengthwise part of the way up so it will cook faster and be tender when the broccoli flowers are cooked. Arrange broccoli in a stainless steel steaming basket over boiling water and, to retain bright green color, cook without lid for a minute. Cover and cook until broccoli is tender-crisp, about 8 to 15 minutes. Do not overcook. Top with a pinch of crushed red pepper, minced garlic, or grated lemon peel for variety. One large bunch serves 4 to 6.

Percent Calories From Fat: 10
Fat Grams In 3 Stalks: 1

Fresh Steamed Brussels Sprouts

Wash fresh brussels sprouts in cold water and cut off stem. Remove wilted and discolored leaves. Cut an *X* into the stem ends to make the sprouts cook faster. Place in stainless steel steaming basket over water. Bring water to a boil, and, to retain bright green color, leave lid off pan for a minute or so. Cover and steam until just tender, about 8 to 10 minutes. Overcooking makes the sprouts harder to digest. Season, if desired, with a dash of onion powder or some fresh chives. One pound makes about 2½ to 3 cups.

Percent Calories From Fat: 10
Fat Grams In 15 Brussels Sprouts: 1

Steamed Fresh Cabbage

Wash and cut fresh cabbage either into wedges or shreds. Place in stainless steel steaming basket over boiling water. Cook for a minute without lid to retain the green color. Cover and steam until tender-crisp for about 10 to 15 minutes. Season with a sprinkle of caraway seeds or grated lemon peel and minced parsley, if desired. One pound (½ small head) makes about 3½ cups of cooked cabbage.

Percent Calories From Fat: 8
Fat Grams In 5 Cups Shredded Cabbage: 1

Braised Cabbage

1 green pepper, coarsely chopped
1 onion, chopped
1 teaspoon oil
1 small head cabbage, sliced into ½-inch strips
Fresh lemon juice or grated lemon peel

Sauté peppers and onions in oil in a large skillet for a couple of minutes. Add cabbage, cover, and cook until cabbage is lightly wilted, removing lid and stirring occasionally. Do not burn. Drizzle with lemon juice or grated lemon peel. Makes 4 to 5 cups.

Perfect Whole Foods: Omit lemon juice.
Percent Calories From Fat: 25
Total Fat Grams In Recipe: 6

Fresh Steamed Carrot Coins

Scrub fresh, young carrots with a vegetable brush or a plastic scrubber. Cut into thin slices and cook in stainless steel steaming basket over boiling water, using lid, until carrots are tender or about 20 minutes. If desired, season carrots with toasted sesame seeds, lemon juice, parsley, cumin, or dill, chives, mint, tarragon, coriander. One pound package makes about 2½ cups cooked carrots.

Perfect Whole Foods: Do not use lemon juice to season carrots.
Percent Calories From Fat: 5
Fat Grams In 8 Medium Carrots: 1

Fresh Steamed Cauliflower

Cut fresh cauliflower into uniform pieces, about 2 inches in size, and wash. Cook in stainless steel steaming basket over boiling water, using a lid, until tender-crisp or about 10 to 15 minutes. Do not overcook or cauliflower will be hard to digest. A dash of paprika or minced parsley makes a colorful garnish. One pound makes about 1½ cups cooked cauliflower.

Percent Calories From Fat: 7
Fat Grams In 5 cups: 1

Corn on the Cob

There are several good ways to prepare corn on the cob.

• Steam husked corn (fresh or frozen) until tender, using a covered stainless steel steaming basket over boiling water. Young, fresh corn takes only 15 or 20 minutes of cooking.

• Place fresh husked corn on ends in a slow cooker (cut to fit if necessary). Add ½ cup water, cover, and cook on low for about 4 hours.

Percent Calories From Fat: 5
Fat Grams In A 6-Inch Piece Of Corn: 1

Ratatouille

The fresh cilantro in this vegetable stew gives it a unique flavor.

1 teaspoon olive oil
3 to 4 garlic cloves, chopped
1 small onion, chopped
1 large eggplant, cut into 1-inch cubes (peeling is not necessary)
1 medium zucchini, cut into ½-inch slices
6 to 8 mushrooms, sliced
16-ounce can whole tomatoes with juice (coarsely chop the tomatoes)
1 tablespoon dried basil
½ cup fresh cilantro, snipped with scissors
½ cup shredded low-fat cheese

In a large, heavy skillet, sauté the garlic, onion, and eggplant for a minute or two. Add other vegetables and juice from tomatoes, cook for a couple of minutes, then cover, and cook for about 30 minutes longer or until vegetables are tender. Add the basil and cilantro, stirring to mix. Top with optional cheese, cover, and simmer for 5 minutes longer. Makes about 5 to 6 cups.

Percent Calories From Fat: 29, with cheese; 13, without
Total Fat Grams In Recipe: 16, with cheese; 5, without

Fresh Steamed Greens

Some greens like spinach wilt down to almost nothing when cooked. Buy and prepare plenty of these in order to have a sufficient amount of cooked greens.

Fresh greens such as kale, collards, spinach, beet greens, or mustard greens
Lemon juice or raw apple cider vinegar, optional

Wash greens carefully to remove any sand or dirt. If stems are thick, remove them by folding the leaf together in one hand and pulling stem off with the other hand. If you like, cut or tear into bite-size pieces. Either cook in a covered steaming basket over boiling water or cook in pan using the water that clings to the greens, watching carefully to make certain that all the moisture doesn't evaporate. To retain the bright color of the fresh greens, cook for 1 minute without the lid, then cover and cook for 5 to 20 minutes depending upon the maturity of the greens. Many people like to season greens at the table with lemon juice or cider vinegar. One pound makes approximately 2 cups. (This varies greatly according to the variety and cooking time.)

Perfect Whole Foods: Do not use lemon juice.
Percent Calories From Fat: 10-23, depending on type
Fat Grams In 1 Cup Cooked: 1

Stir-Fried Spinach

1 pound fresh spinach
½ teaspoon oil

Wash leaves carefully to remove dirt or sand. Dry with a clean cloth or paper towel. Remove thick stems by folding a leaf together in one hand and pulling stem off with other hand. Heat oil in a wok or skillet. Add spinach and stir-fry only until leaves are coated with oil. Serve immediately. Makes about 2 cups.

Percent Calories From Fat: 24
Total Fat Grams In Recipe: 4

Garden Fresh Okra Creole

Fresh, young okra, washed, ends removed, and cut into ½-inch pieces
Fresh tomatoes, cored and cut into chunks
Green pepper, cored and coarsely chopped (seeds and white pith are edible, too, and are rich
  in vitamin C)
Onion, chopped

Place all ingredients in a heavy pan. The amounts will depend upon your supply and preference.
Bring to a boil, reduce heat, add some water if tomatoes are not juicy, and cover. Cook until
vegetables are tender, about 15 minutes.

Percent Calories From Fat: Approximately 6
Total Fat Grams In Recipe: Approximately 2 grams in 4 cups of creole

Parsnip Pureé

Fresh parsnips
Salt, pepper, and ground nutmeg

Remove ends and scrub parsnips. Cut into chunks, steam, reserve steaming water, and mash
parsnips with an electric mixer until smooth. Add some of reserved water to make the
consistency of mashed potatoes. Season to taste with salt, pepper, and nutmeg.

Percent Calories From Fat: 3
Fat Grams in 5 Cups: 1

Herbed Peas

2½ cups fresh or frozen peas
1 tablespoon chopped fresh herbs or 1 teaspoon dried herb flakes (see below for suggestions)

Steam peas until they are slightly tender. Fresh, tender peas cook in about 8 minutes. Just
before serving, sprinkle with herbs such as tarragon, dill, chives, mint, basil, or parsley. Or add
a little grated lemon peel. Makes about 2 cups.

Percent Calories From Fat: 6
Total Fat Grams In Recipe: 2

Whole Mashed Potatoes

Make certain you mash potatoes with the skins while you are on the perfect diet. You'll probably get used to potatoes this way and want to continue even after you liberalize the perfect diet.

White potatoes, well-scrubbed, sliced, and steamed until tender (do not peel)
Skim milk or water reserved from steaming potatoes
Salt, pepper, and butter to taste

Using an electric mixer, whip potatoes. Add warmed skim milk or water used in steaming the potatoes and continue whipping until the potatoes are smooth and skins are in small pieces. Season with salt, pepper, and a little butter, if desired.

Percent Calories From Fat: 1 (mashed with skim milk, no butter)
Fat Grams in 6 To 7 Cups: 1 (mashed with skim milk, no butter)

Baked Potatoes

Preheat oven to 350-375°. The temperature may vary depending upon what else you want to bake in the oven at the same time. Scrub and make a slash into the potatoes with a knife or fork. (This will prevent steam build-up inside the potato which can cause it to explode in oven.) Bake for approximately 1 hour or more, the time depending upon size of potato and oven temperature. Test potatoes for doneness by squeezing gently while holding a potholder to protect your fingers. If potatoes are still hard, bake longer. If they give slightly, they are done. Sweet potatoes are baked according to the above directions, but because they often ooze out of their skin as they bake, place them on a cookie sheet to keep the oven clean.

Perfect Whole Foods: Select a small to medium-size potato rather than a large one. Eat the skin of sweet potatoes as well as white potatoes.
Percent Calories From Fat: 1
Fat Grams In 10 Medium Potatoes: 1

Slow-Cooked Baked Potatoes

Scrub potatoes and place them in a slow cooker. Do not add water. You may cook as many as 10 or 12 medium-size potatoes at once. Cook on low for 8 to 10 hours.

Perfect Whole Foods: Select a small to medium-size potato rather than a large one and eat the skin along with the starchy portion.
Percent Calories From Fat: 1
Fat Grams In 10 Medium Potatoes: 1

Basil Potato Salad

I like to use yellow finn potatoes when they're available. Otherwise, I like to use either red potatoes or new potatoes for this delicious potato salad.

4 medium-size potatoes (about 1½ pounds), scrubbed, cut into ½ to ¾-inch chunks, steamed until barely tender, and cooled
1 shallot, finely chopped (or use a green onion if shallots are not available)
¼ cup finely chopped green pepper
¼ cup fresh parsley, snipped with scissors
½ teaspoon dried basil
2 tablespoons mayonnaise
3 tablespoons plain, nonfat yogurt
Salt to taste

Gently combine all ingredients except mayonnaise and yogurt. Mix mayonnaise and yogurt together and stir into potato mixture. Add salt to taste. Cover and refrigerate until ready to serve. Makes 4 cups.

Perfect Whole Foods: Do not peel the potatoes. Make certain mayonnaise is not sweetened and contains no starches.
Percent Calories From Fat: 21
Total Fat Grams In Recipe: 21

Dairy-Free Potato Salad: Omit yogurt and use more mayonnaise.

Oven Fries

If you like French fries but avoid them because of the fat they contain, try these baked fries. They are great! If you double or triple the recipe, make certain you leave space on the cookie sheet between the potato sticks so they can become crisp and brown. If you don't leave space, they will be soggy.

1 very large baking potato, scrubbed and cut into ½-inch sticks
1 teaspoon oil
Salt, to taste

Preheat oven to 450°. Oil pan (preferably one without sides) with *Oil-Lecithin Combination* (p. 205). Place potato pieces in a plastic bag and add oil. Toss potatoes in the bag to coat them with the oil. Arrange them in a single layer on cookie sheet. Do not let potatoes touch. Bake for 15 minutes. Turn them over using tongs or a pancake turner and bake about 15 minutes longer. Sprinkle with salt. Serves 2, about 10 to 12 pieces each serving.

Perfect Whole Foods: Do not peel potato.
Percent Calories From Fat: 11 (compared to 48 percent in fast food fries)
Total Fat Grams In Recipe: 4 (compared to 24 grams in 2 small orders of fast food fries)

Golden Potatoes

My mother-in-law, Dorothy Loiselle, prepared this dish years ago while we were visiting her in Canada.

2 parts potatoes, scrubbed and sliced
1 part carrots, scrubbed and thinly sliced
Salt, if desired

Steam carrots for about 10 minutes, add potatoes, and steam until both carrots and potatoes are very tender. Pour into mixing bowl, reserving liquid in the bottom of steamer. Mash with mixer, adding some of the reserved liquid if necessary to make potatoes fluffy. Season with salt, if desired.

Perfect Whole Foods: Do not peel potatoes.
Percent Calories From Fat: 2
Total Fat Grams In Recipe: 1 in about 5 cups of Golden Potatoes

Betty's Greek Potatoes

Here's a recipe that is best if put together in the morning, refrigerated during the day so the flavors blend, and baked just before serving. It's a great company dish!

4 cups potatoes, scrubbed, thinly sliced, and steamed until tender
3 garlic cloves, minced
1 large onion, chopped
2 teaspoons olive oil
1 cup low-fat cottage cheese
2 fresh tomatoes, sliced
1 teaspoon dried sage
½ cup shredded low-fat cheese

Oil a 1¾-quart casserole with *Oil-Lecithin Combination* (p. 205). Sauté the onion and garlic in oil for about 5 minutes. Stir in sage. Arrange in layers in the casserole: ⅓ potatoes, ½ onions, ½ cottage cheese, and ½ tomatoes. Repeat layers and top with remaining third of potatoes and all of shredded cheese. Cover and refrigerate until almost ready to bake. If casserole dish is still cold, don't preheat oven. Remove lid, place in cold oven, set to 350 °, and bake about 1 hour. Makes about 6 cups.

Perfect Whole Foods: Do not peel potatoes. Select a cottage cheese with no starches or sugars added.
Percent Calories From Fat: 24
Total Fat Grams In Recipe: 22

Hash Brown Potatoes

These potatoes are good served for Sunday brunch along with fresh fruit, scrambled eggs or Scrambled Tofu *(p. 89), and* Whole Wheat Yeast Biscuits *(p. 212).*

3 or 4 medium-size potatoes, scrubbed and cut into 1½-inch chunks
1 or 2 onions, quartered
Oil-Lecithin Combination (p. 205), about 1 teaspoon
Salt and black pepper, to taste

Steam potatoes in a covered stainless steel basket over boiling water for 5 to 8 minutes. Cool slightly and then shred in food processor along with onions. Oil heavy griddle or skillet with *Oil-Lecithin Combination*, using a little more oil than when oiling pans for baking. Heat griddle; cook potatoes and onions until tender and browned, turning with a pancake turner occasionally to make certain they all are cooked. Add salt and pepper, to taste. Makes 4 servings.

Perfect Whole Foods: *Do not peel potatoes.*
Percent Calories From Fat: 15
Total Fat Grams In Recipe: 5

Baked Acorn Squash

Keep in mind that adding butter significantly increases the fat content.

1 acorn squash, scrubbed, cut in half lengthwise, and seeds removed
Cinnamon Spice Blend (p. 256) or ground cinnamon
Salt, to taste
1 teaspoon butter

Preheat oven to 350°. Oil baking dish with *Oil-Lecithin Combination* (p. 205). Place squash cut sides down in dish and bake for 30 to 45 minutes or until pulp is tender. Turn cut side up and rub butter over the hot surface. Sprinkle with *Cinnamon Spice Blend* and a little salt. Makes 2 servings.

Percent Calories From Fat: 12 with butter, 2 without butter
Fat Grams In Recipe: 5 with butter, 1 without butter

Hubbard Squash

Since this is higher in fat than most vegetable recipes in this book, serve it with a very low fat main dish such as dried beans.

1 hubbard squash, peeled and cut into 1-inch cubes
2 teaspoons butter
½ teaspoon ground nutmeg or cinnamon
1 tablespoon pecan meal

Sauté squash in butter for a few minutes in a large skillet. Cover and steam until squash is tender, about 20 to 30 minutes, removing lid and stirring occasionally to make certain squash does not stick or burn. Add a little water if necessary while cooking. Pour into serving bowl and sprinkle with nutmeg or cinnamon and pecan meal. Makes 2½ to 3 cups.

Percent Calories From Fat: 29
Total Fat Grams In Recipe: 14

Pumpkin Purée

When our children were young, my husband Jim and the children, Heather and Keith, made a jack-o-lantern each fall. Since we didn't want to waste the pumpkin inside, Jim scraped out much of the flesh. I steamed it, puréed it in the food processor, and then either used it immediately or froze it for a Thanksgiving pie. Here's a simple way to prepare pumpkin purée for freezing when you don't need a jack-o-lantern. Use it in Pumpkin Soup, Pumpkin Muffins, *or* Pumpkin Pie *or substitute pumpkin for the squash in* Squash Rolls.

If the pumpkin is small or medium in size: Cut off top including stem as in making a jack-o-lantern. Scoop seeds and stringy material out and replace top. Place the pumpkin on cookie sheet.

If the pumpkin is large: Cut it in half crosswise and scoop seeds and stringy material out of each half. Place the 2 pumpkin halves cut side down on cookie sheets with sides to collect the juice that will form while baking.

Preheat oven to 350°. Bake until pumpkin is tender. Medium-sized pumpkins will take about 1½ hours. Large pumpkins will probably need to be baked one half at a time. Check while baking to see if you need to remove liquid as it collects in the cookie sheet. Cool, spoon liquid out of the whole pumpkin, and purée flesh in food processor or blender. Package in 1 or 2 cup portions and freeze. Each pound of pumpkin will yield ¾ to 1 cup of pulp.

Percent Calories From Fat: 4
Fat Grams In 5 Cups: 1

Spaghetti Squash

1 spaghetti squash
Commercial spaghetti sauce or *Quick Pasta Sauce* (p. 268)
Steamed or stir-fried vegetables (onions, garlic, mushrooms, broccoli, green peppers, celery, and carrots are good)
Shredded low-fat cheese or grated parmesan cheese, optional

Preheat oven to 350°. Cut squash lengthwise and remove seeds and stringy material. Bake with cut sides down on a cookie sheet for about 45 minutes to 1 hour or until skin is tender. To serve, cut into individual portions, release spaghetti-like strands with a fork, and top with hot spaghetti sauce, vegetables, and optional cheese. Serves 2 to 4.

Perfect Whole Foods: If you use commercial spaghetti sauce, make certain it is unsweetened.

Zucchini Casserole

Here's a casserole using fresh vegetables from the garden. It's very juicy and good served over cooked brown rice. The amounts are approximate. Try adding other vegetables like fresh mushrooms, yellow summer squash, celery, broccoli, cauliflower, and garlic for variety. If you like, substitute low fat cottage cheese or ricotta cheese for the shredded cheese.

3 cups sliced zucchini
2 fresh tomatoes, sliced
1 green pepper, coarsely chopped
1 onion, sliced and separated into rings
6 tablespoons shredded low-fat cheese
Dash of dried oregano
Salt and pepper

Preheat oven to 350°. Oil 1¾-quart baking dish with *Oil-Lecithin Combination* (p. 205). In casserole, layer the ingredients until bowl is almost full. Cover and bake for about 1 hour. Makes about 5 or 6 cups.

Percent Calories From Fat: 25
Total Fat Grams In Recipe: 11

Skillet Squash

¼ to ½ teaspoon oil
Zucchini squash and yellow squash
Granulated onion and granulated garlic in shaker
Parmesan cheese

Sauté vegetables in a very small amount of oil for about 5 minutes, sprinkling liberally with granulated onion and garlic while cooking. Just before serving, top with a little Parmesan cheese. For a lower fat dish, use a *SilverStone* skillet and omit the oil.

Stir-Fried Vegetables

The possibilities for stir-frying are endless. By including a source of protein like tofu cubes or chicken, you will have an easy-to-prepare, nutritious main dish.

1 to 2 teaspoons oil
2 to 4 cups fresh vegetables, cleaned and thinly sliced, diced, shredded, or julienned (such as celery, carrots, mushrooms, broccoli, cauliflower, onions, garlic, green beans, green peppers, zucchini, cabbage, summer squash, whole peas, and spinach pieces)
Cooked brown rice or other cooked whole grain

Optional Ingredients:
Fresh mung bean sprouts
Snow peas
Nuts (sliced almonds, walnut halves, pine nuts)
Seeds (sunflower seeds, toasted sesame seeds)
Tofu cut in cubes (I usually use *Mori-Nu* tofu)
Small pieces of meat or poultry–already cooked or cooked thoroughly before adding vegetables and then removed from skillet or wok

Sauce: (Combine ingredients in small bowl. Use the small amounts if you are preparing 2 cups of vegetables and the larger amounts if you are preparing 4 cups.)
1 to 2 tablespoons tamari or shoyu soy sauce (alcohol-free)
2 to 4 teaspoons arrowroot, cornstarch, or kuzu or 1 to 2 tablespoons whole grain flour
½ to 1 cup water

Heat oil using medium heat in skillet or wok. Do not let oil smoke or become very hot. Add vegetables (don't add sprouts or snow peas yet) in order of cooking time, longest cooking vegetables first (such as carrots and celery). Stir while cooking until vegetables are tender-crisp. Reduce heat and stir in optional ingredients. Add sauce ingredients, gently stirring until it thickens and ingredients are glazed. If using arrowroot or kuzu, remove vegetables from heat before adding sauce ingredients. If vegetables are too hot, arrowroot or kuzu sauce will thicken before you stir it into vegetables. Do not bring to a complete boil if using arrowroot. Serve immediately over cooked brown rice.

Perfect Whole Foods: Use whole grain flour rather than other thickeners.
Percent Calories From Fat: about 30 (using 1 teaspoon oil)
Total Fat Grams In Recipe: 5 (using 1 teaspoon oil)

Variation: Use unsweetened soy milk in place of water.

Broccoli-Potato Soup

Children who resist eating green vegetables often find this soup appealing. Once they develop a taste for broccoli in the soup, they might be more willing to give steamed broccoli a try. The recipe can easily be cut in half if you want to make less. Or, freeze leftovers in individual serving-size containers.

1 bunch fresh broccoli, including stalk, cut into chunks
4 medium-sized potatoes, scrubbed and sliced
3 or 4 garlic cloves, halved
2 large onions, sliced
½ to 1 teaspoon salt, optional

In a large pot, bring vegetables and 8 cups of water to a boil, remove lid for a minute or so to retain the bright green color of the broccoli. Reduce heat, cover, and simmer until vegetables are tender. Cool slightly and then purée with food processor, hand blender, or blender. Season with salt, if desired. Makes about 1 gallon.

Perfect Whole Foods: Do not peel potatoes.
Percent Calories From Fat: 11
Total Fat Grams In Recipe:

Borscht

Borscht or beet soup is a traditional Russian soup. Full of vegetables, it makes a healthy and colorful addition to a meal.

4 large beets, scrubbed, steamed for 20 to 25 minutes, cooled slightly, peeled, and cubed
1 onion, chopped
2 garlic cloves, minced
2 ribs celery, thinly sliced
3 or 4 carrots, sliced
1 teaspoon oil
2 or 3 potatoes, scrubbed and diced
2 cups shredded cabbage
2 tablespoons apple cider vinegar or lemon juice
¼ teaspoon salt, optional

While beets are steaming, sauté onion, garlic, celery, and carrots in oil for 2 to 3 minutes. Add potatoes and 4 cups of water. Bring to a boil, reduce heat, cover, and simmer for about 15 minutes. Add cubed beets, cabbage, and vinegar or lemon juice. Simmer about 15 minutes longer. Season with salt, if desired. Makes about 8 cups.

Perfect Whole Foods: Do not peel potatoes. Use vinegar or 1 or 2 drops lemon oil in place of lemon juice.
Percent Calories From Fat: 11
Total Fat Grams In Recipe: 6

Homemade Vegetable Broth

This broth can be used in recipes calling for chicken broth. You can vary the vegetables by using whatever you have on hand.

1 onion, chopped
3 or 4 garlic cloves, each cut in half
2 or 3 mushrooms, sliced
2 tablespoons chopped fresh parsley
2 carrots
4 ribs celery with leaves
1 small parsnip or turnip, optional
½ teaspoon peppercorns
1 bay leaf
¼ teaspoon dried basil
¼ teaspoon dried thyme
1½ teaspoon salt

Coarsely chop the carrots, celery, and optional parsnip or turnip in food processor. Add all vegetables and seasonings to soup pot along with 8 cups of water. Bring to a boil, reduce heat, cover, and cook for about 45 minutes or until vegetables are very tender. Strain. Makes about 8 cups.

Perfect Whole Foods: If you vary the vegetables, do not use potatoes since straining would exclude the skin.
Percent Calories From Fat: 0
Total Fat Grams In Recipe: 0

Rich Vegetable Broth: Sauté vegetables in 2 teaspoons olive oil before adding water.

Nature is the living, visible garment of God.   *Goethe*

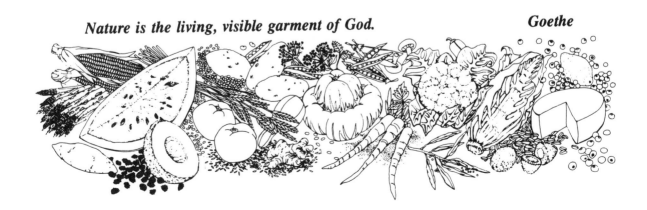

Cabbage Soup Olé

1 teaspoon oil
4 cups shredded cabbage
1 onion, chopped
3 garlic cloves, minced
3 large ripe tomatoes
2 teaspoons tamari or shoyu soy sauce (alcohol-free)
1 to 2 teaspoons chili powder, or more to taste
¼ to ½ teaspoon ground cumin
Salt, optional
Chopped jalapeno peppers, optional

Sauté cabbage, onions, and garlic in oil, using medium heat, until vegetables are limp. Blend 2 tomatoes with tamari until smooth. Add to cabbage mixture, along with chili powder, cumin, third tomato that has been chopped, and 4 cups of water. Cook until cabbage is tender, 5 to 10 minutes. Add salt and peppers, if desired. Makes 9 cups.

Variation: If ripe tomatoes are not available, substitute a 14-ounce can of tomatoes canned in juice, blending half of the tomatoes with the juice and chopping the remaining.

Percent Calories From Fat: 19
Total Fat Grams In Recipe: 7

Chicken-Noodle Soup

Children like this recipe, so make plenty! Select a commercially-canned chicken broth, bouillon cubes, or broth powder without sugar, starch, or fruit juice in the ingredient lists, or use homemade chicken broth. Adding left-over chicken pieces will make this soup into a simple main dish.

1 teaspoon olive oil
1 small onion, chopped
1 carrot, coarsely chopped
1 rib celery, sliced
2 or 3 mushrooms, chopped
1 garlic clove, minced
½ teaspoon dried basil
4 cups liquid, preferably part fat-free chicken broth or vegetable broth and water or 4 cups water
1¼ cups whole wheat noodles, uncooked
Salt and pepper to taste
Small pieces of cooked chicken, optional

Sauté vegetables in oil for a minute or two. Add basil and broth and bring to a boil. Add noodles, cooking until vegetables and noodles are tender, about 10 minutes. Add salt, pepper, and cooked chicken pieces, if used. Makes 5 cups.

Perfect Whole Foods: Make certain broth does not have sugar or starch added if you use a commercially canned one.
Percent Calories From Fat: 22
Total Fat Grams In Recipe: 7

Chicken-Rice Soup: Substitute 1½ cup cooked brown rice for noodles, adding it when the vegetables are almost tender.

Please Read These Important Notes:
If you have strictly followed the **Perfect Whole Foods** diet for at least two weeks, but you are not feeling dramatically better, see page 35 for additional steps that may be necessary.

If you are allergic to wheat, do not substitute spelt or kamut without first determining that you can tolerate them.

If you are being treated for *Candida*, please see specific guidelines on page 315, Appendix A: If You Have Candidiasis.

Eggdrop Soup

1 teaspoon oil
3 or 4 green onions, thinly sliced
2 ribs celery, thinly sliced
4 or 5 mushrooms, thinly sliced
3 to 6 plump garlic cloves, minced (more if they are small)
½ teaspoon minced fresh ginger
4 cups chicken broth or *Homemade Vegetable Broth* (p. 179)
1½ teaspoon tamari or shoyu soy sauce (alcohol-free)
1 egg, beaten with 1 tablespoon water

Sauté vegetables in oil for about 2 minutes. Add broth and tamari and bring it to a boil. Cook with a lid until vegetables are tender-crisp. Turn off heat and add egg-water mixture, 1 teaspoon at a time, while constantly stirring. Makes about 5 cups.

Percent Calories From Fat: 30
Total Fat Grams In Recipe: 13

Gazpacho

Fresh tomatoes blended to equal 2 cups
1 small onion
Pinch of cayenne pepper
2 tablespoons raw apple cider vinegar or lemon juice
1 garlic clove
1 small green pepper, chopped
1 rib celery, chopped
1 cup chopped mushrooms
½ small cucumber, chopped

Place onion, cayenne pepper, vinegar or lemon juice, and garlic in blender with tomato purée. Process on medium speed until smooth, scraping down the sides of the container when necessary. Pour into 3 or 4 serving bowls. Divide the green pepper, celery, mushrooms, and cucumbers and stir into the bowls of soup. Chill until serving time. Makes about 4½ cups of soup with the vegetables.

Perfect Whole Foods: Do not use lemon juice. If you can't use vinegar, then substitute 1 or 2 drops of lemon oil.
Percent Calories From Fat: 6
Total Fat Grams In Recipe: 1

Mushroom-Barley Soup

2 or 3 garlic cloves, minced
1 onion, chopped
2 ribs celery, chopped
1 teaspoon oil
½ cup hulled barley
1 large carrot, sliced
8 cups water or part fat-free chicken broth or *Homemade Vegetable Broth* (p. 179)
¾ pound fresh mushrooms, coarsely chopped (about 4 cups)
Salt and pepper, to taste

In a soup pot, sauté garlic, onion, and celery in oil for a minute. Add barley and sauté 1 or 2 minutes longer. Add carrot slices, mushrooms, and liquid. Bring to a boil, reduce heat, add lid, and simmer until barley is tender, about 1 hour. Season with salt and pepper if desired. Makes about 10 cups.

Perfect Whole Foods: If you use broth, use homemade chicken broth or Pritikin *brand canned broth plus water. Do not use most other commercially canned chicken broths, bouillon cubes, and broth powders since they contain sugar and starch. Use hulled or whole barley rather than pearled.*
Percent Calories From Fat: 19
Total Fat Grams In Recipe: 15

Mushroom-Miso Soup

If you've been wanting to try miso and sea vegetables, here's a recipe using both. It is simple to prepare and tastes delicious.

½ teaspoon oil
½ cup sliced mushrooms
1 small onion, thinly sliced
¼ green pepper, cut into strips
1 tablespoon miso
1 tablespoon or more dulse, torn into bite-size pieces
Parmesan cheese, optional

Sauté mushrooms, onions, and green pepper in oil for 3 or 4 minutes. Add 2 cups of water and bring to a boil. Reduce heat. Add miso stirred into a little of the hot vegetable broth. Add dulse. Heat briefly but do not allow to boil after miso is added. If desired, sprinkle with Parmesan cheese. Makes about 3 cups.

Perfect Whole Foods: Read ingredient list of miso carefully to make certain only whole grains are used, not refined ones. Don't use white miso since it is always made with refined grains.
Percent Calories From Fat: 23 (without cheese)
Total Fat Grams In Recipe: 3 (without cheese)

Celery-Carrot Miso Soup: Use thinly sliced carrots and celery in place of mushrooms and peppers.

Potato-Leek Soup

3 large potatoes, scrubbed and diced
2 large leeks
1 garlic clove, minced
2 ribs celery, sliced
2 carrots, thinly sliced
1 teaspoon dried dill weed
½ teaspoon salt, optional

To prepare leeks, remove outer layer of bulb, wash thoroughly, and slice thinly, including 2 to 3 inches of the green leaves. In large saucepan, cook potatoes, leeks, and garlic in 2½ cup of water about 20 minutes or until potatoes are tender. In a smaller pan, cook celery, carrots, dill weed, and salt in 1 additional cup of water until vegetables are barely tender. With a fork or potato masher, mash potatoes slightly and add celery-carrot mixture. Heat slightly and serve. Makes about 6 cups.

Perfect Whole Foods: Do not peel potatoes.
Percent Calories From Fat: 2
Total Fat Grams In Recipe: 1

Potato-Onion Soup: Substitute 2 medium-sized onions for leeks.

Pumpkin Soup

2 cups cooked, puréed pumpkin
2 teaspoons oil
1 small onion, finely chopped
1 garlic clove, minced
1 tablespoon whole grain flour
2 cups water or broth
¼ teaspoon ground cinnamon
½ teaspoon fresh grated ginger
¼ teaspoon salt, optional
1 apple, coarsely chopped
Ground nutmeg

Sauté onion and garlic in oil for 2 to 3 minutes. Stir flour into onions and garlic. Add all remaining ingredients (except apple and nutmeg) and stir while bringing soup to a boil to thicken slightly. Garnish each bowl of soup with a sprinkle of nutmeg and chopped fresh apples. Makes about 4½ cups.

Percent Calories From Fat: 29
Total Fat Grams In Recipe: 10

Sunshine Soup

2 teaspoons olive oil
1 onion, chopped
1 rib celery, sliced
1 medium-large sweet potato (about ½ pound), scrubbed and diced into ½-inch pieces
2 teaspoons paprika
½ teaspoon turmeric
1 teaspoon dried basil
⅛ teaspoon ground cinnamon
Pinch of cayenne pepper
1 tomato, diced
1 large green pepper, coarsely chopped
¼ to ½ teaspoon salt

In a medium to large soup pot, sauté the onion, celery, and sweet potato in the oil for 5 minutes. Add 3 cups of water and seasonings. Bring to a boil, reduce heat, cover, and simmer the soup until potatoes are tender or about 15 minutes. Add tomatoes and green peppers and simmer for 5 or 10 minutes longer. Makes about 6 cups.

Perfect Whole Foods: *Do not peel the sweet potato.*
Percent Calories From Fat: 21
Total Fat Grams In Recipe: 10

Oriental Vegetable-Miso Soup

1 teaspoon oil
1 carrot, thinly sliced
1 small onion, sliced
1 or 2 garlic cloves, minced
3 or 4 mushrooms, sliced
4 cups water or broth
2 tablespoons sliced water chestnuts, optional
10 to 20 snow peas, ends and strings removed and halved
4 leaves nappa (Chinese cabbage), coarsely chopped
2 tablespoons miso
Nori, toasted and shredded

Sauté carrot, onion, garlic, and mushrooms in oil for a minute or two. Add water and optional water chestnuts. Simmer until vegetables are tender-crisp, about 5 minutes. A few minutes before serving, add snow peas and nappa. Remove a little of the cooking water, cream miso into the small amount of water and stir back into the soup. Heat briefly, but do not boil. Pour into soup bowls and sprinkle with nori. Makes 6 to 7 cups.

Perfect Whole Foods: Read label of miso carefully to make certain only whole grains are used, not refined ones. Do not use white miso since it is made with refined grains.
Percent Calories From Fat: 26
Total Fat Grams In Recipe: 6

Vegetable-Barley Soup

Here's a family favorite. If you don't want so much soup, then use a 24-ounce can of V-8 Juice and half the amount of remaining ingredients. My mother makes a concentrated soup by using less than 5 cups of water and then diluting just the amount she's ready to use—that way the soup takes less storage space in the refrigerator or freezer.

2 cups thinly sliced celery
2 cups frozen mixed vegetables
46-ounce can *V-8 Juice*
1 large onion, chopped
½ cup hulled barley (or other whole grain)
2 cups sliced cabbage

In a large pot, combine 5 cups of water plus all ingredients except cabbage and simmer for 45 minutes. Add cabbage and simmer 15 minutes longer or until barley is tender. Stir occasionally. Makes 1 gallon.

Perfect Whole Foods: Use a brand of frozen mixed vegetables that does not contain potatoes since they would be peeled. Use hulled or whole barley rather than pearled.
Percent Calories From Fat: 5
Total Fat Grams In Recipe: 5

15-Minute Soup

1 small carrot, cut into matchsticks
1 small celery rib, sliced into thin diagonals
2 fresh mushrooms, thinly sliced
1½ teaspoons dried onion flakes
2 tablespoons whole wheat couscous
Pinch of dulse flakes
Pinch of dried basil
Salt, to taste

Cook carrot, celery, mushrooms, and onion flakes in 1¾ cups water for 10 minutes. Add couscous, dulse, and basil, then cook five minutes longer. Add salt to taste. Makes 2 cups.

Percent Calories From Fat: 4
Total Fat Grams In Recipe: 1

Dressing a Salad

You don't have to buy expensive bottled salad dressings or go to the trouble of preparing and storing dressings in the refrigerator. A good way to have a fresh salad dressing each time you fix a tossed salad is to dress it with oil and vinegar just before you serve it. Here's how to do it. Make certain you use an oil that contains the essential fatty acids. Fresh flax oil is an excellent choice.

Wash and thoroughly dry vegetables for your salad. Your oil won't cling to them if the vegetables are wet. In a large bowl, put your cleaned, cut-up vegetables. Tear the lettuce rather than cut it. Vary the combination of vegetables each time to give variety to your salads. Save juicy vegetables such as tomatoes and add to the completed salad.

Pour 1 teaspoon to 1 tablespoon unrefined oil on salad. The amount depends on the size of the salad. Toss about 20 times or until all surfaces shine with oil.

If you are not ready to serve the salad, stop here and refrigerate it. A few minutes before serving, add 1 teaspoon to 1 tablespoon raw cider vinegar or lemon juice. Add seasonings such as granulated garlic, granulated onion, kelp, celery seeds, dill seeds, herbs, salt, and pepper. For variety, change the seasonings each time you dress a salad. Toss 10 to 12 times and add any garnishes such as cheese, tomato wedges, and fragile sprouts. Serve immediately.

Perfect Whole Foods: Do not use lemon juice.
Percent Calories From Fat: Varies. Remember that 100% calories come from fat in oil. The vegetables are very low in fat as well as calories.
Total Fat Grams In Recipe: Varies. Remember that 1 teaspoon oil contains 5 grams of fat.

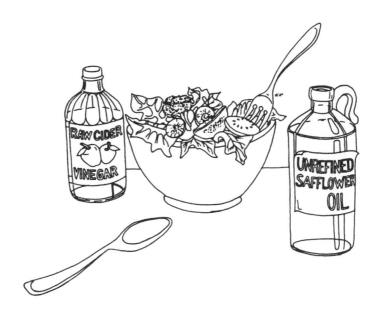

Shredded Beet Salad

This is simply delicious!

Fresh beets, peeled and shredded in a food processor
Fresh lemon juice or your favorite dressing
Leaf lettuce

Arrange lettuce leaves on salad plates. Top with a mound of shredded beets. Drizzle lemon juice or your favorite dressing over the beets and serve.

Perfect Whole Foods: Don't use lemon juice.
Percent Calories From Fat: 3 (using lemon juice)
Fat Grams In 5 Cups: 1 (using lemon juice)

Chinese Slaw

Gently combine the following ingredients in desired proportions and sprinkle with your favorite homemade oil and vinegar dressing:

Thinly sliced cabbage   Thinly sliced onion
Thinly sliced celery   Shredded carrots
Minced green pepper   Mung bean sprouts

Percent Calories From Fat: Varies. Remember that almost 100% calories come from fat in oil and vinegar dressings. The vegetables are very low in fat as well as calories.
Total Fat Grams In Recipe: Varies. Remember that 1 teaspoon oil contains 5 grams of fat.

Imperial Slaw

½ small head cabbage
1 green pepper
2 or 3 carrots
3 or 4 radishes
2 or 3 ribs celery
1 cup *Creamy Coleslaw Dressing* (p. 264)
Salt, to taste

Using metal blade, finely chop vegetables separately in food processor. Combine vegetables with *Creamy Coleslaw Dressing*. Season with salt if desired. Makes 5 to 6 cups.

Percent Calories From Fat: 65
Total Fat Grams In Recipe: 45

Broccoli-Cauliflower Salad

Drizzle cauliflower and broccoli flowers with a small amount of *Herb Dressing* (p. 265). Refrigerate for several hours, stirring occasionally.

Percent Calories From Fat: Varies. Nearly 100% calories come from fat in the dressing.
Total Fat Grams In Recipe: Varies. Remember that 1 teaspoon oil contains 5 grams fat.

Carrot Salad

2 medium-size carrots, scrubbed and shredded in food processor
1½ teaspoon oil
1½ teaspoon lemon or lime juice
Salt to taste

Toss carrots with oil. Add juice and salt, mixing well. Serves 2 to 3.

Perfect Whole Foods: Use raw cider vinegar in place of lemon or lime juice.
Percent Calories From Fat: 46
Total Fat Grams In Recipe: 7

Jiffy Corn Salad

2 cups fresh corn cut from cob or frozen whole kernel corn, thawed
⅔ cup coarsely chopped peppers, assorted colors (green, red, and yellow)
¼ cup fresh parsley, chopped
½ purple onion, coarsely chopped
1½ teaspoons olive oil
Juice from 1 lime

Toss vegetables together. (Do not cook the fresh corn.) Drizzle the olive oil over the vegetables, toss, drizzle the lime juice, and toss again. Makes about 3½ cups.

Perfect Whole Foods: Substitute 1 tablespoon raw apple cider vinegar for the lime juice.
Percent Calories From Fats: 15
Total Fat Grams In Recipe: 7

Green Pea Salad

10-ounce package frozen peas, thawed and drained
¼ cup nuts (sliced almonds or whole pine nuts are good)
½ cup chopped celery
1 small onion, chopped
¼ cup chopped green pepper
Plain, nonfat yogurt or a little mayonnaise mixed with yogurt, as a dressing

Mix all ingredients together gently and stir in dressing. Refrigerate for a couple of hours before serving. Makes about 2½ cups.

Percent Calories From Fat: 41 (using plain, nonfat yogurt for dressing)
Total Fat Grams In Recipe: 17 (using plain, nonfat yogurt for dressing)

Spinach Salad

4 cups fresh spinach, cleaned, dried, rib removed, and broken into bite-size pieces
1 cup thinly sliced mushrooms
1-inch cube (1 ounce) blue cheese, crumbled
1 teaspoon oil
1 teaspoon raw apple cider vinegar

In large salad bowl, combine spinach, mushrooms, and cheese. Pour oil over salad and toss gently. Now sprinkle vinegar on the salad and toss again.   Makes 5 cups.

Percent Calories From Fat: 52
Total Fat Grams In Recipe: 13

Alfalfa's Monkey Salad

Here's a delicious recipe from Alfalfa Restaurant, a natural foods restaurant near the campus of the University of Kentucky in Lexington.

Green or purple cabbage, chopped
Raw sunflower seeds
Shredded carrots
Chopped celery
Romaine or endive lettuce, finely shredded
Alfalfa sprouts
Herb Dressing (p. 265)

Toss vegetables and sunflower seeds together and add desired amount of *Herb Dressing*.

Percent Calories From Fat: Varies. Keep in mind that Herb Dressing *has 98 percent calories from fat.*
Total Fat Grams In Recipe: Varies. Herb Dressing has 7 grams of fat per tablespoon.

Summer Salad

1 home grown tomato, diced
⅛ to ¼ avocado, cut into small pieces
Pinch dried basil
Pinch celery seeds
1 or 2 lettuce leaves

Mix together all ingredients except lettuce. Serve on lettuce leaf. Serves 1 or 2, depending on the size of the tomato.

Percent Calories From Fats: 44 (using ⅛ avocado)
Total Fat Grams In Recipe: 19 (using ⅛ avocado)

Tomato Relish Salad

2 home grown tomatoes, cut in chunks
½ green pepper, cut in chunks
1 small onion, sliced and separated into rings
2 celery ribs, sliced
¼ cucumber, thinly sliced
1 clove garlic, minced
1 carrot, sliced
2 or 3 radishes, sliced
1 tablespoon chopped fresh parsley
Approximately 2 tablespoons *Herb Dressing* (p. 265)

Combine all ingredients, mixing gently. Refrigerate for several hours before serving. Makes 4 to 5 cups.

Percent Calories From Fat: 54
Total Fat Grams In Recipes: 19

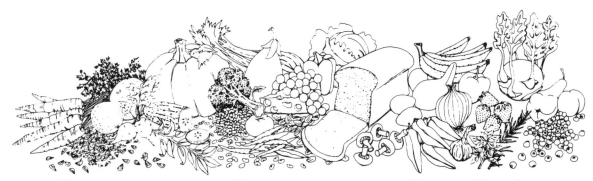

The doctor of the future will give no medicine, but will interest his patients in the care of the human frame, in diet, and in the cause and prevention of disease.
Thomas Edison

Pasta Salad

This salad can be varied each time you prepare it. Use whole grain elbow macaroni or spiral pasta with or without dried vegetables added. Vary the vegetables according to what's in season and what you have on hand. Make a main dish salad by adding protein-rich ingredients. You'll enjoy each variation. I have found that by stirring just a little mayonnaise into the salad first, the pasta doesn't absorb the dressing and, therefore, less dressing is needed.

Whole grain pasta: cooked until tender and drained
Raw vegetables, chopped, shredded, or sliced (select several with a variety of colors): onions, carrots, green peppers, zucchini, cucumber, peas, snow peas, celery, cabbage, mung bean sprouts, broccoli, whole or halved cherry tomatoes
Protein-rich ingredients (for main dish salad, select one or two): cooked legumes such as garbanzo beans or kidney beans; chopped hard cook eggs; water-packed tuna, drained; cooked turkey pieces; nuts or seeds; cubed or shredded cheese
Dressing: Mayonnaise, *Herb Dressing* (p. 265) or *Newman's* Own Olive Oil and Vinegar Dressing
Seasonings: dried herbs, salt, and black pepper to taste

Gently mix pasta with selected vegetables and protein ingredients, if used.   Mix a very small amount of sugar-free mayonnaise into salad. Next, drizzle dressing onto salad, add salt and pepper, and toss. Taste and add more seasonings if necessary. Refrigerate several hours before serving.

Perfect Whole Foods*: Use whole grain pasta and a dressing with no sugar or lemon juice. Do not use* Newman's *Own Olive Oil and Vinegar Dressing.*

Nancy's Potato Salad: Substitute steamed potato cubes (scrubbed, then diced with skin left on) for the pasta.

Spaghetti Salad

This tasty pasta salad recipe was originally high in fat, high in sodium and contained refined pasta. One of my weight-control clients and I converted it to this more nutritious version.

½ pound whole grain spaghetti, cooked and drained
4 or 5 cups vegetables steamed until tender-crisp (I like chopped onion, sliced mushrooms, zucchini and yellow squash slices, and green pepper chunks.)
⅓ to ½ bottle *Pritikin* Herb Vinaigrette Fat Free, Sodium Free Dressing
2 ounces feta cheese, crumbled
1 fresh tomato, cut into chunks

Combine all ingredients and refrigerate several hours before serving. Makes 7 or 8 cups.

Perfect Whole Foods*: Select a dressing with no sugar, starch, or juice. Don't use* Pritikin *dressings since they contain fruit juices.*
Percent Calories From Fat: 13
Total Fat Grams In Recipe: 15

WHOLE GRAIN BREADS

There are many types of whole grain breads. In general, breads are either leavened or risen with yeast (using baking yeast or a sourdough starter), chemicals (using baking soda or baking powder), eggs, or unleavened. I have included recipes for all of these basic types, including yeast breads, sourdough bread, pizza crusts, bagels, muffins, cornbread, crackers, flat breads, crepes, pancakes, and waffles.

When buying commercially prepared breads, pay careful attention to ingredient lists to eliminate undesirable ingredients from your diet.

For the Perfect Whole Foods Diet, Select Only Breads That Are

- 100% whole grain (no refined flour or starch added)
- Unsweetened (diastatic malt is allowed)

Other usual ingredients are yeast, oil, baking soda, dairy products, eggs, and salt. Whole grain flours are designated by such terms as 100% whole wheat, whole wheat, unbleached whole wheat, whole rye, and brown rice flour. Spelt, kamut, millet, triticale, amaranth, and quinoa flours are almost always whole grain. Don't buy any product that includes part whole grain and part refined grain, as a bread with whole rye flour *and* rye flour *in it.*

Typical Terms That Indicate a Flour Is Refined

Barley flour	Patent flour
Corn flour	Potato flour or starch
Durum	Rice flour
Enriched flour	Rye flour
Flour	Semolina flour
Gluten flour	Sifted rye flour
High gluten flour	Sifted whole wheat flour
Light rye flour	Unbleached flour
Medium rye flour	Wheat flour
Organically grown wheat flour	White rye flour
Partially-refined flour	Whole wheat with 80% (or any) extraction

Read ingredient lists carefully and check the **Quick Reference for Foods** *(p. 349) if you find an ingredient about which you are not sure.*

Always examine the ingredient list, not the name of the product. *Whole wheat* in a title does not necessarily denote *100% whole wheat.* In fact, it doesn't indicate that any of the grain is *whole.* One brand of crackers on the market has a title of Whole Rye Crackers. The single flour in the crackers, according to the ingredient list, is *organically grown rye flour* which is not *whole* at all. It's refined. The ingredient list would read *whole rye flour* to indicate that the rye flour is *whole.* The same company that makes those crackers has a variety that's called Wheat and Rye

Crackers. This product is 100% whole grain, according to the ingredient list, and can be used on the **Perfect Whole Foods** diet. The ingredients include *whole wheat flour, whole rye flour,* yeast, and salt.

If you live in the Central Kentucky area, you'll appreciate *Great Harvest Bread Company* which bakes whole grain breads daily from freshly ground wheat berries. Several years ago, they began making, at Dr. Stoll's request, a delicious unsweetened 100% whole wheat bread using diastatic malt. As it turned out, they have a great demand for the bread in addition to Dr. Stoll's patients on the **Perfect Whole Foods** diet. Since several other *Great Harvest* bakeries are now making the unsweetened version, check with your nearest *Great Harvest* to see if they too make the unsweetened bread or could begin making it. Make certain the bakery uses diastatic malt (grain that is sprouted, dried, and ground), not other types of malt.

Nokomis Farms Bakery in East Troy, Wisconsin (1-800-367-0358) makes several unsweetened sour dough breads using whole grains (wheat, rye, spelt, and kamut as well as combinations). Call to order their products. Always ask about ingredients so you won't buy bread made with unbleached wheat flour and refined rye flour if you are on the perfect diet.

Yeast Breads

Yeast breads are leavened or risen by baking yeast or by naturally fermented dough as in sourdough. If you have never baked yeast breads or whole grain yeast breads before, don't be frightened at the length of the recipes, especially the *Whole Wheat Bread (Unsweetened, 100% Whole Grain)* recipe on page 208. I have given detailed instructions so you will succeed each time you bake. Terms and ingredients that might be unfamiliar to you appear in bold letters in the recipe. I've explained these words in **Yeast Bread Baking Terms** beginning on the next page. Other bread terms not used in the recipe are explained in **Whole Grain Bread Facts** (p. 202 to 207). Even bread that is not perfect is usually edible and good-tasting. To help you improve your bread-baking skills, I have included a chart on **How to Improve Your Whole Grain Yeast Breads** (p. 197). Nothing is better-tasting than a loaf of freshly-baked, whole grain bread. So go on and give it a try!

Authentic sourdough bread is made from a starter that's composed of flour, water, and wild yeast from the air. Sourdough bread has a slightly acid, rich flavor and can be made of 100% whole grain flour without sweeteners, making it great for the perfect diet. An advantage of sourdough over yeast-risen bread and quick breads is that it's easier to digest since the process of fermentation partially digests the grain. Also, much of the naturally-occurring phytic acid of whole grains is destroyed during the fermentation process, making more minerals available to the body than with most other kinds of breads and cooked grains. Some people who cannot tolerate yeast risen bread due to allergies or sensitivities can eat sourdough bread. The recipes for making sourdough starters from several kinds of flour and bread from the starters begin on page 213.

Yeast Bread Baking Terms

Ascorbic Acid Powder: An optional ingredient in yeast bread-baking. It helps develop and strengthen the gluten as kneading also does. Those with little experience in baking with whole grains have a tendency to under-knead the dough; the ascorbic acid powder compensates for the under-kneading. It prevents dry, crumbly bread. Make certain you use ascorbic acid powder or crystals, not buffered, ester C, or sodium ascorbate which are not acidic.

Diastatic Malt Powder: Is an unrefined malt product that is used in making unsweetened breads. Active enzymes in diastatic malt convert some of the starch from the flour into sugar—as a food source for the yeast. Yeast must have sugar rather than starch to make it grow, which in turn makes the bread rise. Many bread bakers in Europe use diastatic malt routinely. Diastatic malt is made by sprouting a grain, drying the sprouts, and grinding them into a powder. Diastatic malt has many advantages over sugar. Since it is a whole food, it is not rapidly absorbed by the body and does not cause blood sugar fluctuations. Using too much will result in a gummy dough because of the enzyme activity. Begin with ¼ teaspoon per loaf and experiment each time you bake. If the dough is gummy, use a little less next time. Diastatic malt's enzyme activity varies according to the specific grain used, the length of time the grain was sprouted, and the exact temperature at which it was dried. It is easily made from wheat berries. See recipe for *Diastatic Malt* on page 209. Beware of commercial diastatic malt powders which, more than likely, also contain refined ingredients like sugar and wheat flour.

Done: Bread is fully baked when it has pulled away slightly from the sides of the pan, is somewhat brown and, when tapped on the top, has a hollow sound. Another test for doneness is to remove the bread from its pan and insert a small knife into the bottom. If the knife comes out sticky, the bread needs to be baked longer. Unsweetened baked bread will not become as golden brown as will bread made with sugar or honey since the caramelizing of sugar in bread helps give more color than the browning of the flour. If you bake unsweetened bread until it's golden brown, it will probably be too dry inside.

Gluten: Is the protein substance of grains that allows the dough to stretch and rise. Beating and kneading strengthens the gluten, thus allowing the dough to stretch and produce a high-rising bread. Hard whole wheat flour contains much more gluten than soft whole wheat (whole wheat pastry flour). Hard wheat flour should be used for yeast breads; soft or pastry flour for most quick breads, cakes, and cookies. Other grains containing appreciable gluten include rye, spelt, kamut, and triticale. Oats and barley also contain gluten, enough that gluten-sensitive people need to eliminate them, but not enough to make a yeast-risen bread. If you are allergic to wheat and are looking for an alternative to whole wheat yeast bread, spelt and kamut flours just might be your answer. Some, but not all, people with wheat allergies can tolerate spelt and kamut. (If you are gluten-sensitive, see page 330 for information about spelt and gluten sensitivity.) Yeast bread made with all whole rye or triticale flour, although possible, is more difficult to make.

Knead Dough: Fold the farthest edge of the dough to the center, press or knead it with the palm of your hands. Repeat this motion, turning the dough 90 degrees each time you knead. Add flour as necessary to prevent sticking, but don't add more than is specified or the bread will be too heavy and dry.

Lecithin Granules: An optional ingredient in yeast bread that helps keep the bread fresh for several days. Since lecithin is a soy product, omit it if you are allergic to soy.

Oil-Lecithin Combination: See **Whole Grain Bread Facts** on page 205.

Punch the dough down: Moisten your hand with water and, using your fist, carefully press the center and the edges of the risen bread dough to release the tiny gas bubbles. Gently remove the dough from the bowl, shape it into a ball again, and return the dough to the bowl. The term *punch* is actually a misnomer since you should be very gentle and avoid breaking the dough's gluten strands during this step. Keeping the gluten strands intact will help produce a higher loaf of bread.

Rise: Bread dough should rise in a warm place free from drafts. The temperature should be somewhere between 70 and 80 degrees. Good places to put the dough to rise: on top of the refrigerator, on top of the stove while something else is baking (make certain it isn't too hot), on the kitchen counter on a hot day, and inside a styrofoam cooler next to a jug of hot water.

Shape a loaf of bread: Press it into a small rectangle. Roll or fold it into a loaf shape, pinching the seams together. Place in pan with smooth side up.

Soft Dough: Term used for yeast-water-flour mixture in which just enough flour is added so that it holds together and becomes a solid yet moist dough.

Test 1: To see if you have *kneaded the dough enough*, form dough into a ball and press your finger into it. If the hole fills up almost immediately, you have kneaded sufficiently.

Test 2: To see if the dough has *risen enough*, gently insert a finger into the dough, near the side of the bowl, about ½-inch deep. If the hole remains more or less intact, the dough has risen adequately. Be gentle or air may be released from the dough and the test will not work.

Warm Water: 85 to 100°—use a thermometer if possible. Or test with finger. Water should feel only slightly warm, about the temperature of a baby's bath water. If it is too warm, it will kill the yeast; if it is too cold, the yeast will take a long time to begin to grow.

How to Improve Your Whole Grain Yeast Breads

If you have a **dense, heavy loaf**, you may have:
• let it rise too long before baking
• not let it rise long enough before baking
• not kneaded enough
• killed the yeast by using too hot a liquid
• used too cold a liquid so the yeast wasn't activated
• used old yeast
• kneaded in too much flour
• used the wrong kind of flour (flour with insufficient gluten)
• not pre-heated the oven
• baked the bread in too hot an oven—400° is usually maximum
• let the dough rise in a cool place

If your bread is **hard and dry**, you may have:
• baked it in too hot an oven
• baked it too long
• used too much yeast
• used the wrong kind of flour (flour with insufficient gluten)

If you have a **moist, gummy loaf**, you may have:
• undercooked it
• not baked it in hot enough oven—325° is usually minimum
• not used enough flour
• used too much diastatic malt

If your bread has a **sour, yeasty smell**, you may have:
• allowed it to rise too long without punching the dough down
• let it rise in too warm or too cool a place (70 to 100° is okay, around 85° is best)
• used too much yeast

If your bread **does not brown**, you may have:
• baked it in too large a pan
• not baked it in a hot enough oven—325° is usually minimum
• not baked it long enough (unsweetened bread will not brown as well as sweetened bread)

If your bread is **mushroom-shaped**, you probably:
• baked it in too small a pan

If your bread **crumbles**, you may have:
• not kneaded it enough
• let the dough rise too long
• used the wrong kind of flour (flour with insufficient gluten)

If your bread is **flat instead of rounded on top**, you may have
• placed pans too close together in the oven
• cooled the bread in a draft
• added too much flour during kneading
• let the bread dough rise too much in the pan before baking

If your bread has a **large hole** under the crust, you may have:
• let the shaped bread dough rise too long in the pan before baking
• let the shaped bread dough rise in too hot a place

Walt Stoll, M.D.
Aerobic exercise, skilled relaxation, and nutrition are the three primary
stress reducers that pay dramatic dividends to everyone in our society.

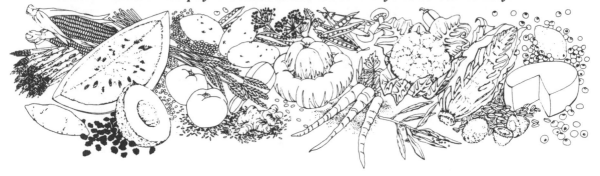

Quick Breads

Breads using baking powder or baking soda for leavening are called quick breads and are made more quickly than yeast-risen breads. Quick breads include muffins, pancakes, waffles, and cornbread. Baking powder should not be used on the **Perfect Whole Foods** diet since it contains cornstarch or potato starch, both refined carbohydrates. When baking powder is used on the liberal whole foods diet, *Rumford* Baking Powder should be used since it contains no aluminum as most other brands do.

Baking soda is used to make quick breads rise on the perfect diet. However, baking soda (for the perfect or liberal diet) and baking powder (for the liberal diet) should be used infrequently for several reasons. First, both products are very high in sodium. One teaspoon soda contains more than 1000 milligrams of sodium; one teaspoon of baking powder contains approximately 400 milligrams. (It takes more baking powder to replace baking soda in a recipe.) Another reason to limit these chemical leavening agents is that the phosphates in baking powders upset the calcium-magnesium-phosphorus balance of the body. Regular use could contribute to osteoporosis. Also, foods leavened with these chemicals are poorer sources of minerals than those leavened with yeast because of the phytic acid naturally occurring in flour. The action of yeast partially destroys the phytic acid, making the minerals in the flour more available.

When you use baking soda as a leavening agent, you must also use an acid ingredient to react with the sodium bicarbonate (the chemical term for baking soda) to produce the carbon dioxide gas which makes the bread rise. You can use any of these acid ingredients: buttermilk, yogurt, apple cider vinegar, lemon juice, cream of tartar, ascorbic acid powder, molasses, and honey. Buttermilk or apple cider vinegar is used in most recipes in this book since these are common ingredients that may be used on the perfect diet. The chart below will help you develop your own whole grain recipes by using baking soda and an acid ingredient in place of baking powder. Or use the chart if you must avoid vinegar or buttermilk and want to alter recipes in this book.

One Teaspoon Baking Powder Is Equivalent to Any of These

- ¼ teaspoon baking soda + ½ cup buttermilk (use to replace other liquid)
- ¼ teaspoon baking soda + 1½ teaspoon cider vinegar (mix vinegar with other liquids)
- ¼ teaspoon baking soda + 1½ teaspoon lemon juice (mix lemon juice with other liquids) (Do not use lemon juice on the perfect diet.)
- ¼ teaspoon baking soda + ½ teaspoon cream of tartar (mix powder into other dry ingredients)
- ¼ teaspoon baking soda + ⅛ teaspoon Vitamin C or ascorbic acid powder or crystals* (mix powder into other dry ingredients)

When mixing flour and baking soda, make certain you thoroughly combine the soda or you will get a bitter taste when eating the finished bread.

*Do not use buffered or ester C since these would not provide the acidity to react with the baking soda.

If you need to limit the sodium in your diet, potassium bicarbonate can be used in place of baking soda (sodium bicarbonate). Before doing so, check with your doctor to make certain that potassium-containing chemicals are okay for you to use. Potassium bicarbonate is available at some pharmacies. And don't forget to eliminate the salt in bread recipes as well as the baking soda if you need to restrict your sodium intake.

Be aware that hard whole wheat and pastry (or soft) whole wheat flours are usually not interchangeable. (See **Whole Wheat Bread Facts** on page 207 for an explanation.) Use the type each recipe calls for to assure success. Pastry or soft whole wheat flour is usually used in quick breads. I've adapted the muffin recipes for using hard whole wheat flour. Because wheat is such an over-used grain, it's a good idea to use other flours when possible, especially if you have allergy tendencies. Most recipes in this book provide variations using other flours.

For any product using flour, small amounts of additional flour or liquid may sometimes be needed because of variations in the flour's absorbency due to coarseness of grind and moisture content of the flour. You may also need to vary the exact amount of flour or liquid depending on the type of liquid you use. Since buttermilk thickens with age and since sour milk (p. 244) is rather thin, a batter will vary in consistency according to which liquid is used. As you cook and gain experience, you will realize when a pancake batter is slightly too thick or a biscuit is too sticky.

Approximate Substitutions for Whole Wheat Flour in Making Quick Breads

- Equal amount of whole barley flour as whole wheat pastry flour
- ¾ as much spelt flour as whole wheat pastry flour
- ¾ as much triticale flour as whole wheat pastry flour
- ⅝ as much kamut flour as whole wheat pastry flour

When calculating the amounts for substitutions, remember that 1 cup = 16 tablespoons.
Batters made from some of these flours thicken upon standing and will need to be thinned down with liquid if they are not cooked immediately after being mixed. Other flours such as oat, buckwheat, corn, brown rice, millet, soy, and chickpea flours can change the texture and the flavor of the product considerably and are not as successfully interchanged with whole wheat pastry flour. Recipes should be formulated especially for these flours.

Muffins

Muffins are popular quick breads. Besides being quickly made, they can be varied from time to time by adding such ingredients as cinnamon, chopped nuts, fruit, or shredded cheese.

Whereas most quick breads are best made with whole wheat pastry flour, you may use either hard whole wheat flour or whole wheat pastry flour when making muffins. I prefer the hard and have formulated the recipes using it.

Don't over-mix muffins when you combine the wet and dry ingredients. Stir them only until the dry ingredients are moistened. If you over-mix, you'll have tough, heavy muffins that are not rounded or symmetrical on top. Fill the muffin cups (greased with *Oil-Lecithin Combination,* page 205) almost full of batter unless a recipe says otherwise. When you're making oat or wheat bran muffins, if your recipe makes more muffins than you can bake at one time, you'll probably need to add a little more liquid before baking the second batch. The bran, upon sitting, will absorb liquid in the batter and become dry. Just gently stir in water or more of the liquid you originally used until the consistency seems right.

Also remember to half fill any unused muffin cups with water before baking. This will prevent the dry metal of the muffin tins from scorching. If you need to reheat leftover muffins, a good way to do it is to place them in a paper bag and warm them in a preheated 200° oven for 10 to 12 minutes. The bag keeps the muffins from drying out.

If you find recipes in other books for muffins with more fat than you want to use, you can decrease the fat by substituting unsweetened applesauce for some or all of the oil (use *Homemade Applesauce*, page 275, if you are on the perfect diet). I have found that since applesauce is less liquid than oil, it takes about 1½ times as much applesauce as oil. Another way to reduce the fat (and cholesterol) in muffin recipes calling for whole eggs is to substitute 2 egg whites for each whole egg. If you use *Now* Eggwhite Powder, you won't have to discard leftover yolks.

An Important Reminder

You May Need to Alter the Amount of Liquid or Flour in Quick Bread Recipes
• If you use an very thick liquid like buttermilk that has been in the refrigerator for a week or so.
• If you use a liquid that's very thin like sour milk (milk plus vinegar).
• If you let the batter sit while baking as you do in making pancakes and waffles.
• If you use flour that was packed down while being measured.

Whole Grain Bread Facts

Baking Powder: A mixture usually of baking soda, an acid ingredient, and a starch. In the presence of a liquid and heat, the soda reacts with the acid producing carbon dioxide gas which leavens or raises quick breads or baked desserts. Many baking powders have an aluminum salt as one of the ingredients. Since aluminum is a toxic metal that should be avoided, *Rumford* Baking Powder is a better choice than one of those with aluminum. All commercial baking powders should be eliminated on the **Perfect Whole Foods** diet because of the starch they contain. Even aluminum-free baking powders should be limited on a liberal whole foods diet because of the phosphates they contain. Phosphates upset the calcium-phosphorus-magnesium balance in the body and contribute to osteoporosis. See also **Baking Soda**, below.

Baking Soda: Use baking soda in place of baking powder with just a few changes. When you use soda, also use an acid ingredient like buttermilk, yogurt, vinegar, lemon juice, or cream of tartar. The acid will react with the soda to produce carbon dioxide. It's the carbon dioxide that leavens or raises the quick bread or dessert. For information on substituting one acid ingredient for another, see page 199.

Barley Flour: You may use whole barley flour in place of whole wheat pastry flour in many recipes. Since most commercial barley flour is made from pearled or refined barley (*Walnut Acres* barley flour is whole grain), you may want to grind hulled barley into whole barley flour with a grain grinder. (Do not attempt to use your blender or food processor; the barley grain is too hard.) Barley flour packs down easily so handle it carefully before measuring or you will use too much in your product.

Bran: The outer part of a grain kernel that is rich in fiber plus other nutrients. The bran is part of the grain that is removed in the refining process.

Bread: When you buy commercial yeast or sourdough bread, pay special attention to the ingredient list on the label. Buy 100% whole grain breads rather than the ones with part whole grain and part refined. Breads that are called *wheat bread* include refined flour since *wheat flour* does not indicate that it is *whole* wheat flour. Also, rye flour is not *whole* unless the label says *whole* rye flour or *whole* grain rye. Don't use products whose ingredient lists name *wheat flour* or *rye flour* as an ingredient if you are on the perfect diet. Also don't buy breads that have hydrogenated fat as an ingredient. These are sometimes called *vegetable shortening* or *pure vegetable shortening*. If you are on the **Perfect Whole Foods** diet, don't select breads with sweeteners added. Diastatic malt may be used since it is whole and not refined. (See pages 195 and 209.)

Buckwheat Flour: Commercially ground buckwheat flour has dark specks in it since the buckwheat groats have some of the dark hull included. *Dark* buckwheat flour is stronger in flavor than *light* buckwheat flour. Prepare *light* buckwheat flour at home by grinding unroasted buckwheat groats into a flour using a food processor. The word *whole* doesn't have to appear next to the word *buckwheat* in commercial flour since buckwheat is not refined.

Chapatis: (pronounced cha-PAT-ees) Unleavened flat bread. You can buy chapatis made with whole wheat flour in some stores. Read the ingredient list carefully and don't buy flat breads leavened with baking powder if you are on the perfect diet.

Chickpea Flour: A flour made from the legume chickpeas (also called garbanzo beans). It is often toasted. Chickpea flour is sometimes used in baked goods to add protein but cannot generally be substituted for other flours in recipes. Toasted chickpea flour is good used as a thickener for sauces and gravies.

Corn Tortillas: Soft corn tortillas are made with either refined or whole grain corn. However, the word *whole* or *whole grain* will probably not be on the ingredient list if it is whole grain. Check with the manufacturer. If you cannot find whole grain corn tortillas, you can substitute whole wheat flour tortillas in some recipes.

Cornmeal: Corn that is ground into a gritty, granular powder. Most commercial cornmeals, both yellow and white, have been refined. Read more about corn on page 123. Select whole grain corn meal. 1 pound = 3 to 4 cups, depending upon fineness.

Cornmeal, Bolted: Cornmeal in which some or all of the bran has been removed by sifting. The term doesn't describe whether or not the germ is present. Always buy whole grain cornmeal rather than bolted if you're on the perfect diet.

Cornmeal, Degerminated: Cornmeal in which both the germ and bran have been removed. Always buy whole grain cornmeal rather than refined.

Cornmeal, Unbolted: Cornmeal in which the bran has not been removed. The term doesn't describe whether or not the germ is still present. If you're on the perfect diet, always make certain you buy whole grain cornmeal with neither bran nor germ removed.

Crackers: There are many brands of commercial whole grain crackers. However, when you read their ingredient lists, you'll often discover such ingredients as white flour; sugar, honey, or malt syrups; hydrogenated oils; or preservatives added to the whole grain flour. For the *Perfect Whole Foods* diet, look for whole wheat flour (or whole rye flour) and salt, with or without baking yeast. Commercial crackers are easier to find for the perfect diet than yeast bread. You can make *Basic Crackers* (p. 236) using almost any whole grain flour or develop your own cracker recipes, as my friend Sheri Focke did, using small amounts of leftover cooked cereals and mixing in enough whole grain flour to make a dough that can be rolled, cut, and baked.

Cream of Tartar: An acid ingredient, potassium hydrogen tartrate, that can be used along with baking soda to leaven quick breads and baked desserts.

Dark Buckwheat Flour: See **Buckwheat Flour** on page 202.

Gluten: A protein part of grains, especially wheat, that gives bread doughs cohesiveness. When bread dough rises, it's the gluten that allows the bread to stretch without breaking. Grains containing gluten include wheat, rye, and triticale. Oats, millet, barley, amaranth, and quinoa also have gluten—enough gluten that gluten-sensitive people may need to avoid them, but not enough gluten to make a yeast-risen bread.

Gluten Flour: A grayish-white, high protein flour made from the gluten portion of wheat. It is sometimes added to whole grain yeast breads to make them less heavy and dense than 100% whole grain breads. Gluten flour is not used on the *Perfect Whole Foods* diet since it includes some refined starch.

Graham Flour: A flour named after Sylvester Graham, a clergyman who in the early nineteenth century recognized the fact that refined flour is not as nutritious as unrefined. Graham crackers are named after him. Most graham crackers today, however, would not be approved of by Sylvester Graham since they are almost entirely made of white flour along with sugar and hydrogenated fat. Some graham crackers from food co-ops and health food stores are appropriate for a liberal whole foods diet. Read the ingredient list carefully. Also, some graham flour has part of the bran removed, so pay special attention to the label information before using graham flour on the perfect diet to make certain it is 100% whole grain.

Kamut Flour: (Kah-MOOT) Flour made from the grain kamut. Although it is a form of wheat, kamut can sometimes (but not always) be tolerated by those sensitive or allergic to wheat. If you must avoid wheat, you should not substitute kamut (or spelt) unless you know or determine that you can tolerate it. An important fact about kamut flour is that it can be used to make a delicious-tasting and good-textured yeast bread. See recipe for *Kamut Bread (Unsweetened, 100% Whole Grain)* on page 209. Since kamut, at this point in time, is not refined, the word *whole* doesn't have to appear with the word *kamut* to denote a whole grain.

Lecithin, Liquid: (LESS-a-thin) A fatty, liquid substance produced from soybeans and sometimes used as a food supplement. Lecithin is used in combination with oil to grease pans so they won't stick. (See **Oil-Lecithin Combination** on page 205.)

Light Buckwheat Flour: See **Buckwheat Flour**.

Masa: A refined corn flour sometimes used in making tortillas. It should not be used on the *Perfect Whole Foods* diet.

Miller's Bran: Another name for pure wheat bran.

Millet Flour: A whole grain flour. It does not substitute well for whole wheat pastry in quick breads. Since millet flour is never refined, the word *whole* doesn't have to appear with the word *millet*.

Oat Flour: A whole grain flour made from either rolled oats or oat groats. To make approximately 1 cup oat flour, grind 1¼ cups rolled oats in the blender or food processor to make a fine powder.

Oil-Lecithin Combination: A mixture of oil and *liquid* lecithin—used to grease baking pans and skillets. To prepare *Oil-Lecithin Combination*, combine ¼ cup oil with 2 tablespoons liquid lecithin, mixing well. Refrigerate in a jar with an air-tight lid. Baked goods will not stick to pans greased with this liquid. If you use only oil to grease the pans, the baked products will absorb the oil, causing them to stick. Liquid lecithin is available in a 16-ounce bottle which will last for months if you store it in the refrigerator. Avoid the mint-flavored variety to prevent all your baked goods from tasting like mint! Don't use non-stick cooking sprays on the perfect diet since they contain alcohol. (Many people on a liberal whole foods diet like the convenience of using non-stick cooking sprays.) Avoid shortening since it contains undesirable hydrogenated fat.

Pancakes: Light, flat hot cakes usually associated with lots of butter, maple syrup, and honey. Pancakes are also delicious topped with fresh whole or sliced fruit, plain nonfat yogurt, Homemade Applesauce, and even a fruit syrup made by blending ripe bananas, fresh strawberries, or blueberries and a little orange juice if you are on the liberal diet. For a syrup recipe that's made with diastatic malt and may be used on with the **Perfect Whole Foods** diet, see page 258.

Patent Flour: Refined wheat flour. Do not use on the perfect diet.

Pita Bread: (pronounced PEE-ta) A round, flat bread (4 to 8 inches in diameter) that forms a pocket when baked. Cut pita bread in half to form 2 pockets and stuff the halves with sandwich fillings. Unsweetened 100% whole wheat pita bread is sometimes available at grocery stores and natural foods stores. Read the ingredient list with care if you're on the perfect diet.

Rice Cakes: Crunchy round cakes made of puffed rice. They are available at most grocery stores. Nut butters such as almond butter, cashew butter, peanut butter, tahini, and sunflower butter are delicious spread on rice cakes. Because of their high degree of processing, even though they are whole grain, don't use rice cakes often in your diet. Read the ingredient list carefully, eliminating those with degerminated corn, malt syrups, or any other refined products if you are on **Perfect Whole Foods**.

Rice Flour, Brown: A flour made from brown rice. Although it is permitted on the perfect diet, it tends to produce crumbly products and does not substitute well for whole wheat pastry flour.

Rumford Baking Powder: A baking powder that is free of aluminum. Baking powder is not used on the perfect diet due to its corn starch content. Because it contains phosphates, Rumford Baking Powder (as well as other baking powders) should not be used often on a liberal whole foods diet. Phosphates upset the mineral balance in the body and contribute to osteoporosis.

Rye Breads: Because rye has less gluten than wheat, 100 percent whole rye bread is difficult to make. Most commercial rye breads are made with refined ingredients, usually refined rye flour and refined wheat flour. On **Perfect Whole Foods**, eliminate products containing refined forms of rye such as *white rye, rye flour, organically grown rye flour, stone ground rye, light rye,* or *sifted rye*. The word *whole* should be included with the word rye on the ingredient list.

Rye Flour, Whole: Make certain the rye flour you buy is whole grain. If the label says simply *rye flour*, *white rye*, *light rye*, *sifted rye*, or *organically grown rye flour*, then it is not whole grain. It must say whole rye, whole rye flour, or whole grain rye for the perfect diet.
1 pound whole rye flour = approximately 6 cups.

Soy Flour: A flour made from soybeans. It is used to add moisture and extend shelf life to baked goods as well as add protein. Using too much results in a bitter taste. Use soy flour in products that are cooked well to make the soy protein more digestible. Three types of soy flours are available: full-fat, low-fat, and defatted. Low-fat and defatted soy flours are both by-products of soybean oil production. Full-fat soy flour, the best choice since it is less processed, must always be stored in the refrigerator to maintain freshness.

Soy or Soya Milk Powder: A heat-treated soy powder that can be used to make an instant soy milk. It can also be used in other recipes that don't require cooking. (Raw soy bean products should not be eaten since they are poorly digested.) *Soya* is the commonly used British term for soy. To reconstitute soy or soya powder into soy milk, combine ½ to 1 cup (or to taste) of soy milk powder with 2 cups of water and stir or blend for about 10 seconds. Pour into a jar, add lid, and refrigerate. Use in cooking.

Spelt Flour, Whole: Whole grain flour from an ancient, nutritious wheat-related grain which has recently been revived in use. An important fact about spelt flour is that it can be used to make a delicious-tasting and good-textured yeast bread that is tolerated by some people who are allergic to wheat. (See recipe for *Spelt Bread (Unsweetened, 100% Whole Grain)* on page 209.) If you are allergic to wheat, use spelt (as well as kamut) only after you have determined that you can tolerate it. If you are following the *Perfect Whole Foods* diet, the word *whole* must appear with the word *spelt flour* to denote a whole grain flour since refined spelt flour is also available.

Sprout Bread: An unleavened bread made from sprouted, ground, and baked grains. It is available commercially or can be homemade. Commercial brands include *Essene* Bread and *Manna* Bread. *Ezekiel* Bread is another excellent sprouted grain bread, but it must be avoided while on the perfect diet because one ingredient, *malted barley*, is not a whole food. Since it is readily available at health food stores and natural food groceries, you might want to make it your daily bread after you can liberalize your diet.

Stone Ground: This term describes a desirable method of grinding grain into flour, not whether or not the flour is refined. Although the method is often used for grinding whole grain flours, sometimes the grains are refined. I've seen the term *stone ground* used to describe refined flour like *stone ground wheat flour*. Flour described this way is refined. Make certain you pay attention to ingredient lists if you are on the perfect diet.

Triticale Flour: (pronounced trit-a-KA-lee) A whole grain flour that can be used in quick bread recipes calling for whole wheat pastry flour. Use about ¾ as much triticale flour as whole wheat pastry flour. Triticale is a man-made grain, a hybrid of both wheat and rye. It is usually mixed with hard whole wheat flour for kneaded yeast breads but can be made into a flatter 100% triticale bread. Too much kneading is detrimental to its gluten. Triticale flour is not refined; therefore, it does not have to say *whole* in its name.

Unbleached Flour: The word *unbleached* is usually associated with white or refined flour that has not been chemically bleached. Unbleached white flour should be eliminated on the perfect diet. Occasionally whole wheat flour will be bleached and brominated. These processes should be avoided since they destroy nutrients. You are more likely to find whole wheat flour that has been bleached and brominated in the grocery store than in natural foods stores. (Although not normally labeled this way, I have seen ingredients listed as *unbleached stone ground whole wheat flour*. Don't let the word *unbleached* in this instance confuse you. It *is* a whole grain product.)

Wheat Germ: The inner portion of the wheat berry that is removed when whole wheat berries are processed into white flour. Although fresh, raw wheat germ is highly nutritious, it is very perishable because of its polyunsaturated oil. Buy raw wheat germ only if it is stored in the refrigerator. Commercially toasted wheat germ has a longer shelf life than raw wheat germ. Although toasting destroys some of its nutrients, the enzymes that speed rancidity are also destroyed. Buy only enough raw wheat germ to use quickly or toast it in a 300° oven, stirring often. Store all wheat germ in the refrigerator (not the freezer since freezing destroys its vitamin E). A test for freshness is to taste a pinch of the wheat germ. It should be sweet tasting, not bitter. Bitter wheat germ is rancid and should never be eaten. 1 pound = approximately 4 cups.
Percent Calories From Fat: 27
Fat Grams in 2 Tablespoons: 1

White Flour: The starchy white endosperm of the wheat berry with the bran and germ of the whole grain lacking. Eliminate white flour on the **Perfect Whole Foods** diet. Little or none should be used with the liberal diet. Substitute ⅞ cup whole wheat flour for each cup of white flour (⅞ cup = 1 cup minus 2 tablespoons). Select hard whole wheat flour or whole wheat pastry flour according to what you are making.

Whole Wheat Bread Flour: See **Whole Wheat Flour, Hard** below.

Whole Wheat Flour, Hard: Flour made from hard wheat berries which contain sufficient gluten for yeast bread making. Same as whole wheat bread flour.
1 pound = approximately 3½ cups.
1 cup wheat berries = 1⅓ to 1½ cups whole wheat flour.

Whole Wheat Pastry Flour: Flour made from soft wheat berries, having less gluten than hard whole wheat flour. Whole wheat pastry flour is used in making biscuits, cakes, and cookies. Same as *soft* whole wheat flour.

Whole Wheat Flour, Soft: See **Whole Wheat Pastry Flour** above.

Yeast, Baking: A type of living organism used in bread-making to produce carbon dioxide so the bread dough will rise.
1 package dry baking yeast = almost 3 teaspoons.

Whole Grain Bread Recipes

Whole Wheat Bread (Unsweetened, 100% Whole Grain)

Here's a basic recipe for making yeast bread. If you are an inexperienced baker, perfect this recipe before trying other yeast breads. I've explained the words italicized below beginning on page 195.

2 cups *warm water*
2 teaspoons baking yeast
¼ teaspoon *diastatic malt*
¹⁄₁₆ teaspoon *ascorbic acid powder*, optional
1 teaspoon *lecithin granules*, optional
Approximately 5 cups hard whole wheat flour
½ teaspoon salt

In a mixing bowl, add yeast to water and let it sit until dissolved. Add diastatic malt, ascorbic acid powder, lecithin granules, and 2 cups of flour. Stir briskly with a spoon for a couple of minutes to strengthen the *gluten*. Cover and let sit for 1/2 to 1 1/2 hours at room temperature (or overnight in the refrigerator).

Stir mixture down. Add salt and 2 more cups of flour. Mix to form a *soft dough*. Measure 1 cup additional flour. Spread ¼ of it on the counter and turn dough onto floured counter. Set bowl aside. *Knead* dough for 15 minutes, adding a little more flour from your measuring cup when the dough starts to stick to the surface. (Too much flour will make the bread dense and heavy.) You should not need more flour than is in your measuring cup and you may not use all of it. After you have kneaded for 15 minutes, don't add more flour. Knead until dough is no longer floury but has become slightly shiny and a little sticky. Do *Test 1* (p. 196) to determine if you have kneaded the dough enough (hole should fill up).

Oil the mixing bowl. You don't need to wash it first. Put dough into bowl and then turn dough over so that top is oiled and won't dry out. Cover and let *rise* in a warm place (70 to 80°) for 45 minutes to an hour or until double in volume. Do *Test 2* (p. 196) (hole should remain intact). If you have time after the first rising, *punch the dough down* with your fist to let the gas out, cover and let rise again. If you do this several times, texture of the bread will be better. But don't forget to punch the dough down. (If you do forget, bread will develop a sour flavor.)

Oil a 9 x 5-inch bread pan with *Oil-Lecithin Combination* (p. 205). Knead dough a couple of times and *shape* dough into a loaf. Place in pan with smooth side up. Cover with another 9 x 5-inch pan or with a towel and let dough rise until not quite double in volume. The length of time it takes to rise depends upon the temperature of the room as well as the number of risings the dough has had–the more risings, the faster the bread will rise.

Bake in a 350° preheated oven until bread is *done*, about 45 to 60 minutes. Remove from pan and place bread over top of pan crosswise to allow air to circulate while bread is cooling. If you like a soft crust, cover it with a clean cloth while cooling. Slice with serrated knife. Makes 1 loaf. Learn to make one loaf before multiplying ingredients to make 2 or 3 loaves at one time.

Percent Calories From Fat: 5
Total Fat Grams In Recipe: 11

Spelt Yeast Bread (Unsweetened, 100% Whole Grain): Substitute whole spelt flour for the whole wheat flour. Substitute diastatic malt powder made from spelt berries for wheat berry diastatic malt to make this bread 100% Spelt. See *Diastatic Malt Powder* recipe below.

Kamut Yeast Bread (Unsweetened, 100% Whole Grain): When using kamut flour in this recipe, it's necessary to make a few changes. Use only 1½ cups of water. Substitute diastatic malt made from kamut berries for wheat berry diastatic malt to keep this bread wheat-free. See *Diastatic Malt Powder* recipe below.

Whole Wheat Bread (Sweetened, 100% Whole Grain): Use 1 to 2 tablespoons raw honey or molasses in place of diastatic malt, if desired, for a liberal whole foods diet. Also, you may add ¼ cup gluten flour to the 2 cups of flour in Step 1, for a lighter bread.

Whole Wheat & Whole Rye Bread (Unsweetened, 100% Whole Grain): Replace 2 cups whole wheat flour in Step 1 with 2 cups whole rye flour. Dough will be stickier than when you use all whole wheat flour.

Whole Wheat-Bulgur Bread (Unsweetened, 100% Whole Grain): Increase water to 2½ cups. Bring that water to a boil and stir in ⅓ cup raw bulgur. Let sit and cool until slightly warm. Sprinkle in yeast and continue with the basic recipe, adding only 1 more cup of whole wheat flour in Step 2. You will use less than the 5 cups flour total for which the recipe calls.

Whole Wheat-Sprout Bread (Unsweetened, 100% Whole Grain): Stir in ½ cup sprouted wheat berries at the beginning of Step 2.

Whole Wheat-Oatmeal Bread (Unsweetened, 100% Whole Grain): Stir in ½ cup leftover, cooked oatmeal (or any other cooked whole grain) at the beginning of Step 2.

Diastatic Malt Powder

This recipe is very important for making yeast bread for the perfect diet. Although you can find diastataic malt powder commercially, I don't think brands are available currently that contain no refined ingredients. Before buying any commercial diastatic malt, check the ingredients carefully. The brands that I found contain wheat flour and dextrose in addition to the sprouted grain. Making it at home isn't all that difficult, and one recipe will be enough for many loaves of bread.

1 cup hard wheat berries (or any whole grain that sprouts easily like triticale, spelt, or kamut)
Canning ring
Wide-mouth quart canning jar
Netting or plastic strainer

Place wheat berries in clean jar and attach ring over netting or plastic strainer. Cover berries with warm water and soak overnight. Drain, rinse, and drain again, placing jar upside down, tilted so excess water can drain out and air can circulate. Keep in a warm, dark place, rinsing and draining twice a day. When the sprouts are about the same length as the grain, rinse and drain well, then spread the sprouts on 2 ungreased cookie sheets. Dry in a 120° F. oven, no hotter, for about 12 or more hours, or until the sprouts are thoroughly dry and crunchy. If your oven setting doesn't go this low, then try setting the dial to the left of the lowest setting and see if the oven elements turn on. If so, then use an oven thermometer to adjust the dial to get the temperature to around 120°. A hot oven (over 140°) will destroy the enzymes in the diastatic malt. Grind dried sprouts in a blender, seed grinder, or food mill. Remove any pieces that didn't get thoroughly ground. Store in a dry, airtight container at room temperature. Will keep indefinitely. Use in yeast breads in the amount of about ¼ teaspoon to 1 teaspoon diastatic malt powder per loaf of bread. (Read more about **Diastatic Malt Powder** on page 195.)

Whole Wheat Machine Bread (Unsweetened, 100% Whole Grain)

Since bread machines come in an assortment of brands with various sizes and directions, use the following recipe (developed for use in a DAK Auto Bakery/Turbo Baker II) as a guide. If your machine capacity is less than 4 cups of flour, then reduce all ingredients proportionately. Making a 100% whole grain flour will produce a shorter loaf than one with white flour.

½ teaspoon baking yeast
4 cups hard whole wheat flour (don't pack the flour down)
¼ teaspoon diastatic malt (p. 195, 209)
¹⁄₁₆ teaspoon ascorbic acid powder (p. 195)
½ teaspoon salt
1 teaspoon lecithin granules, optional
1¾ cups water (120 to 130°)
Additional flour or water, if necessary

Add ingredients to machine in order recommended by your machine (reduce the amounts for a smaller machine). Turn machine on, observing the mixture carefully. If the dough doesn't form into a ball after a minute or two of kneading, but rather some stays stuck on the bottom of the pan, open the lid and while bread is kneading, sprinkle flour on the dough, just a little at a time until a ball is formed. If the dough clumps together or forms a very rough ball soon after kneading begins, sprinkle warm water on the dough. Don't add so much that the dough loses its shape and become stuck on the bottom of the pan, but if it does, then add just a bit of flour until the dough forms a ball. This procedure insures that the dough is the correct consistency since flour varies in absorbency and packs down easily, making your amount vary from time to time.

100% whole grain breads require more kneading and rising than breads made with refined flour. If your machine isn't programmed for two kneading and two rising cycles, then you can program it yourself by stopping your machine after the first kneading, letting the dough rise for 20 to 45 minutes, and then restarting the machine.

Percent Calories From Fat: 5
Total Fat Grams In Recipe: 9

Spelt Machine Bread (Unsweetened, 100% Whole Grain): Use 3¾ cups spelt flour instead of whole wheat flour. If you are allergic to wheat or want a 100% spelt bread, use diastatic malt made from spelt berries. (See *Diastatic Malt* recipe on page 209.)
Pizza Dough, Rolls, or Hamburger Buns (Unsweetened, 100% Whole Grain): Prepare the dough in the machine, let it rise, then stop the machine before it bakes. Shape the dough by hand and bake it in your regular oven. (See *Whole Grain Pizza* recipe on page 100 for pizza instructions.)
Whole Wheat Raisin-Nut-Cinnamon Machine Bread (Sweetened, 100% Whole Grain): Add 1½ teaspoon ground cinnamon to dry ingredients. Five minutes before kneading is complete, add ½ cup currants or raisins and ¼ to ½ cup nuts (pecans, English walnuts, or black walnuts) that are at room temperature. Omit currants and raisins for perfect diet.
Whole Wheat French Bread (Unsweetened, 100% Whole Grain): If your machine has a French bread setting, use the *Whole Wheat French Bread* ingredients on page 216. Add ingredients to your machine in the order recommended by your machine, reducing the amounts if your machine won't hold 3 cups of flour. Spray the bread with water a couple of times while it is baking.

Whole Wheat Vita Mix Bread (Unsweetened, 100% Whole Grain)

If you have a Vita Mix *appliance, you can grind wheat berries and make your bread dough, all in a few minutes. The following recipe is adapted to the* **Perfect Whole Foods** *diet and calls for no sugar, honey, or fruit juice. If you are familiar with the* Vita Mix Introductory Bread Recipe, *these instructions should make sense.*

2 cups hard wheat berries
¼ teaspoon salt
1 teaspoon baking yeast
⅛ teaspoon diastatic malt (p. 195, 209)
¾ teaspoon lecithin granules, optional
Pinch of ascorbic acid powder, optional
Approximately 1½ cups water at room temperature
1 bread pan: 7¾ x 3⅝-inch size
Whole wheat flour, for adjusting consistency and shaping

Oil bread pan with *Oil-Lecithin Combination* (p. 205). Grind wheat 1 minute, then tap berries from spigot and add salt. Grind 3 minutes longer. Add yeast and diastatic malt plus optional lecithin granules and ascorbic acid powder, mixing *Up, Down, Off.* Add water and mix *Up, Down, Up, Down, Off.* Scrape down sides with spatula and push dough into blades. Knead the bread in the container, using 5 or 6 *Down-Release Action* strokes. Punch down with spatula. Do this knead and punch cycle about 6 or 7 times. If dough is very dry or too moist, adjust the consistency early in the kneading-punching process by adding water or whole wheat flour to the dough (a teaspoon or less at a time). Sprinkle 1 or 2 teaspoons whole wheat flour onto counter. Bring dough above the blades by doing a few kneading strokes. Drop dough onto floured counter. Scrape container to get remaining dough into one corner and add it to dough on counter. Add cold water to container, replace lid, and clean by running machine. Now knead the dough briefly to work in flour and shape into loaf. Place in pan and cover. Preheat oven to 375°. Let rise for about 20 minutes in a warm place. Bake for 35 to 45 minutes or until bread is done.

Percent Calories From Fat: 5
Total Fat Grams In Recipe: 8

Spelt Vita Mix Bread (Unsweetened, 100% Whole Grain): Substitute spelt berries for the wheat berries.
Kamut Vita Mix Bread (Unsweetened, 100% Whole Grain): Substitute kamut berries for the wheat berries, using 1 cup plus 1½ tablespoons water.

Whole Wheat Yeast Biscuits (Unsweetened, 100% Whole Grain)

These biscuits are leavened with both yeast and baking soda. Make them when you have an hour to let them rise. Use triticale, spelt, or kamut flour in place of whole wheat pastry flour if you are allergic to wheat or want to have more variety in your diet (see recipe variations below).

1 tablespoon baking yeast
¼ cup warm water
2½ cups whole wheat pastry flour
¾ teaspoon baking soda
¼ teaspoon salt
¼ cup oil (plus about ½ teaspoon oil to oil cookie sheet)
¾ cup or more buttermilk

Dissolve the yeast in the warm water. Oil cookie sheet with a small amount of oil. Stir the dry ingredients together in a mixing bowl. Add ¼ cup oil, yeast mixture and enough buttermilk to form a soft dough. Turn onto a floured board and gently knead for about 30 seconds before rolling ½-inch thick and cutting with a biscuit cutter. Place biscuits, sides touching, on cookie sheet, cover with a towel, and let stand for at least one hour in a warm place. Bake in a 425° oven for 9 to 11 minutes. Makes 1½ to 2 dozen.

Perfect Whole Foods: Make certain buttermilk does not have whey or starch such as tapioca added. If you like, use approximately ¾ cup skim milk plus 4½ teaspoons vinegar added as the acid ingredient.
Percent Calories From Fat: 30
Total Fat Grams In Recipe: 60 (2 or 3 grams per biscuit depending on number of biscuits you make)

Wheat-Free Yeast Biscuits (Unsweetened, 100% Whole Grain): Substitute 1¾ cups + 2 tablespoons spelt, kamut, or triticale flour for the whole wheat pastry flour.

Let us be of good cheer, remembering that the misfortunes hardest to bear are those that never come.
                                                                    Lowell

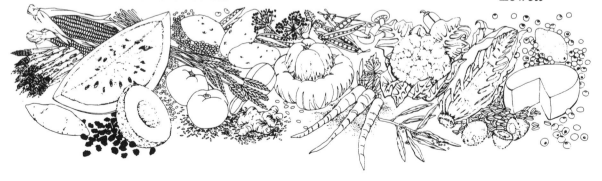

Whole Wheat Sourdough Bread (Unsweetened, 100% Whole Grain)

You can double or triple this recipe when your starter is mature and when you have perfected the techniques. Make sure you feed your starter larger amounts of flour and water so you'll have enough starter for doubling or tripling plus at least 1 cup left over. If you are unfamiliar with bread baking terms, please read the definitions of Done, Knead Dough, Rise, Shape, *and* Test 1, *on pages 195 to 196.*

1½ cups whole wheat sourdough starter (see recipe on page 214), brought to room temperature
  in a large glass bowl
1 cup lukewarm water (spring or purified)
1½ to 3 cups hard whole wheat, plus more for kneading
¾ to 1 teaspoon salt
Clean cotton towel

Add water and salt to starter, mixing gently with a plastic or wooden spoon. Stir in enough flour to make a moist dough. Sprinkle about ¼ cup flour on counter, add dough, and knead for about 10 to 15 minutes, adding as little flour as possible so you have a soft dough that is not sticky. Do *Test 1* (p. 196). Hole should fill up almost immediately. Return dough to original large bowl and cover with a damp cotton towel. Let rise at room temperature for 2 to 4 hours, the time depending on the warmth of the room and the age of the starter. A new starter will take closer to 4 hours; an older starter will take less time, perhaps about 2 hours. The dough should be well-risen, but should not smell sour.

Prepare a 9½ x 5-inch bread pan by oiling with *Oil-Lecithin Combination* (p. 205). Shape dough with damp hands by gently forming it into a loaf. Do not force air out of the dough. If you make more than one loaf, fill each pan about half full of dough. Cover with a damp cotton towel. Let rise at room temperature again, for ½ to 4 hours, until broken air bubbles begin to show on the surface. Bake in a 400° preheated oven for 20 minutes, then lower temperature to 350° and bake 20 to 40 minutes longer or until bread is golden brown and sounds hollow when tapped. Remove from pan and cool on wire rack. Cool thoroughly before slicing. Store either in a paper bag at cool room temperature up to a week, a plastic bag in the refrigerator up to 2 weeks, or longer in the freezer.

Percent Calories From Fat: 5
Total Fat Grams In Recipe: 9

Wheat-Free Sourdough Bread (Unsweetened, 100% Whole Grain): Use spelt, kamut, triticale, or whole rye flour for the starter and bread (see directions that follow for the starter). You'll find that each grain's starter and dough has a different feel to it, yet each makes a delicious bread.

Whole Grain Sourdough Starter (Unsweetened, 100% Whole Grain)

Use this recipe for making a good quality starter. The leavening comes totally from wild yeast in the air. Once you make this starter, you can keep it growing for many years to come. With age, the starter will become more active and your bread will, therefore, rise more quickly. Also, the bread will become better-tasting with time. Don't let the lengthy instructions scare you. I've tried to give complete directions so you won't have to guess about any procedures. It's not as difficult as it appears.

2 cups hard whole wheat, whole rye, spelt, or kamut flour (organically grown and freshly ground, if possible) plus more for daily feeding
Approximately 1½ cups lukewarm water (spring or distilled) plus more for daily feeding
Large glass or earthenware bowl, sterilized
2-quart, wide-mouth jar, sterilized
Cotton cloth for covering jar

Note: To sterilize equipment (including the jar) for making sourdough culture, boil it in water for 10 minutes. This will destroy undesirable bacteria present so that only yeast from the air will be grown. Cool the equipment before proceeding with the recipe. In the instructions that follow, I suggest that you use your clean fingers to mix the flour and water together. It may seem like an inconsistency that I ask you to sterilize the equipment yet use your hands to mix the ingredients. However, clean hands that are free of sores and infections will not contaminate the starter with undesirable bacteria or mold. They may even help innoculate the beneficial yeasts.

In a large glass bowl, mix the flour and about 1½ cups water (using clean fingers or a plastic or wooden spoon, not a metal one) to make a thin dough or a very thick batter. Flours vary in absorbency and textures, so the 1½ cups of water is approximate. The mixture should be a solid, yet pourable mass. Stir to remove all lumps. Transfer the mixture to the sterilized jar and cover with a clean cloth. Set in a cool room, about 65 to 70°.

Daily feedings for the next 6 days: Once a day, for the next 6 days, transfer mixture to the sterilized and cooled bowl. (The transferring from one container to another adds beneficial oxygen to the mixture.) Add ¼ cup water (spring or distilled), mixing with a non-metal spoon. Then mix in approximately ⅓ cup whole grain flour (vary the amount of flour so the mixture will be a solid, yet pourable mass. Each flour is different in its absorbency). Sterilize the jar again before pouring the mixture back into it. Always cover the jar with a clean cloth.

On the 7th day, remove the cloth, cover the jar with a lid (don't feed it this time), and refrigerate the starter for 7 to 10 days. At this point, your starter should be a bubbly, very thick yet pourable batter and smell somewhat fruity yet sour. Feed once more after the 7 to 10 days according to the directions that follow; allow it to sit at room temperature for several hours until starter is bubbly, cover with lid, and refrigerate; the starter will be mature and ready to use the next day.

Feeding the mature starter: Every 7 to 10 days, stir separately into the starter ¾ cup lukewarm water and approximately 1 cup flour, using a plastic or wooden spoon. Add enough flour to make a thick yet pourable batter. You don't need to transfer the mixture to a bowl anymore. Cover the jar with a clean cotton cloth and leave it at room temperature for several hours after feeding, until starter is very bubbly again. Remove cloth, add lid, and then refrigerate it once again.

The starter needs to be fed every 7 to 10 days. Always wait at least 12 hours, preferably 24, after feeding the starter before using it to make bread. If you make bread sooner, you won't have good leavening. Remove from the jar just the amount of starter you plan to use and let it come to room temperature. Refrigerate the remaining starter.

If you won't be baking bread for a while, continue to feed the starter every 7 to 10 days. If you accumulate too much, then give some to a friend or throw some away. If you know you won't be able to feed the starter for longer than 7 to 10 days, then feed the starter less water in proportion to flour (½ cup water to 1 cup whole wheat flour). A thicker starter is less likely to turn sour.

If a grey liquid forms on top of the starter, it is a sign of oxidation and nothing to worry about. You can either stir it back into the starter or pour it off. If, however, the starter turns bright orange, this indicates that the starter has been contaminated by undesirable mold or bacteria. Throw the starter away, sterilize the container, and begin a new starter.

If you don't want to make sourdough bread regularly, then freeze your starter. You can freeze it for several months, thaw it in the refrigerator for 24 hours, remove from the refrigerator, feed it, and leave it at room temperature until it becomes bubbly, refrigerate, and use it the next day to bake bread.

When the starter is older and more active, you can begin feeding it more than 1 cup flour and ¾ cup water each 7 to 10 days. You can then make several loaves of bread at a time.

Whole Wheat French Bread (Unsweetened, 100% Whole Grain)

¾ cup water
½ cup buttermilk or plain, nonfat yogurt
1 teaspoon baking yeast
Approximately 3 cups hard whole wheat flour
½ teaspoon salt
Whole grain cornmeal

Combine water and buttermilk or yogurt. Heat until their temperature is warm but no hotter than 100°. Add yeast; when it has dissolved, stir in 1 cup flour. Beat until the dough is smooth. Add salt and 1 cup more flour, mixing well. Place ¼ cup additional flour on counter and turn dough onto it. Knead for about 10 minutes, adding as much of the remaining ¾ cup flour as needed to make a very stiff dough. Oil bowl, place dough in bowl, turning the dough over so that top is oiled. Cover and let rise in a warm place until doubled in volume; punch down. Oil a cookie sheet and dust with cornmeal. Press the air out of the risen dough and shape it into a long loaf. Place on cookie sheet. Cover and let rise in a warm place until almost doubled again. Preheat oven to 400°. Make diagonal slashes across loaf gently with a very sharp knife. Slashes should be about ¼-inch deep and 2-inches apart. As you put the bread into the oven, spray or gently brush it with water. Spray or brush again in about 20 minutes. The water will produce a chewy, crusted bread. Bake for about 30 to 40 minutes total. Serve hot. Makes 1 loaf.

Perfect Whole Foods: Select buttermilk without starch or whey added.
Percent Calories From Fat: 5
Total Fat Grams In Recipe: 7

Whole Wheat Machine French Bread (Unsweetened, 100% Whole Grain): If your bread machine has a setting for French bread and will hold 3 cups of flour, use this recipe with the machine bread instructions (p. 210).
Wheat-Free French Bread (Unsweetened, 100% Whole Grain): If you have determined that you can tolerate spelt, then substitute whole spelt flour for the whole wheat flour, adjusting the amount of flour to make a stiff dough.

Please Read These Important Notes:
If you have strictly followed the **Perfect Whole Foods** diet for at least two weeks, but you are not feeling dramatically better, see page 35 for additional steps that may be necessary.

If you are allergic to wheat, do not substitute spelt or kamut without first determining that you can tolerate them.

If you are being treated for *Candida*, please see specific guidelines on page 315, Appendix A: If You Have Candidiasis.

Whole Wheat English Muffins (Unsweetened, 100% Whole Grain)

2 cups skim milk
½ teaspoon diastatic malt (p. 195, 209)
1 tablespoon soft butter
½ teaspoon salt
1 tablespoon baking yeast
4 to 4½ cups hard whole wheat flour
Whole grain cornmeal

Combine milk, diastatic malt, butter, and salt in large saucepan. Heat until warm (85 to 100°). Add yeast and let sit for a few minutes until bubbly. Slowly mix in 3½ to 4 cups flour until you have a soft dough. Knead on floured counter for 5 minutes. Let dough rise in covered, oiled saucepan for an hour. Punch down and roll on floured counter to ½-inch thick. Cut into circles about 4-inches in diameter, using an empty bowl or other container. Place on cookie sheets liberally sprinkled with cornmeal. Cover and let rise about 30 minutes. Transfer to a medium-hot, lightly oiled griddle or skillet. Bake about 10 minutes on each side, reducing heat if muffins get brown. Cool on wire rack. To serve, split muffins and toast under broiler. Makes ten 4-inch muffins.

Percent Calories From Fat: 10
Fat Grams In 1 Muffin: 2

Raisin-Whole Wheat English Muffins (Sweetened, 100% Whole Grain): Add ¾ teaspoon cinnamon and ½ cup raisins to the warm milk mixture. Do not use raisins on the perfect diet.
Wheat-Free English Muffins (Unsweetened, 100% Whole Grain): Substitute spelt or kamut flour for the whole wheat flour, varying the amount of flour to make a soft dough. Do not use diastatic malt made from wheat. (Diastatic Malt can be made from any grain that sprouts easily. See recipe on page 209.)   For the liberal diet, you can use 1 teaspoon of barley malt or honey in place of the diastatic malt.

Whole Wheat Bagels (Unsweetened, 100% Whole Grain)

2 cups warm water
2 teaspoons baking yeast
½ teaspoon diastatic malt (p. 195, 209)
2 eggs, beaten
2 teaspoons oil
1 teaspoon salt
7 cups hard whole wheat flour
Poppy or sesame seeds, optional

Dissolve yeast in warm water. Add diastatic malt, eggs, oil, and salt. Stir. Add 3 cups flour and beat well using mixer. Cover and let sit for 15 to 30 minutes. Stir in 3 more cups of flour. Dough will be stiff. Knead in final cup of flour, continuing to knead about 15 minutes. Dough should become very stiff, yet smooth and elastic. Place dough on counter, cover with inverted bowl, and leave alone for 30 minutes. Preheat oven to 400° and heat a large pot of water on stove. Oil 2 cookie sheets. To shape: Cut dough into thirds and each third into 6 pieces. Roll each piece between hands into a 9-inch strip. Overlap 1-inch on each end to form a doughnut shape and seal seam by manipulating dough. Drop bagels into boiling water for about 1 minute, remove, place on cookie sheet, sprinkle with poppy or sesame seeds, and bake for 20 to 25 minutes. Makes 18.

Percent Calories From Fat: 10
Fat Grams In 1 Bagel: 2

Raisin-Whole Wheat Bagels (Sweetened, 100% Whole Grain): Add raisins after beating the first 3 cups of flour into egg mixture. Do not use raisins on the perfect diet.

Wheat-Free Bagels (Unsweetened, 100% Whole Grain): Substitute spelt or kamut flour for the whole wheat flour, varying the amount of flour to make a very stiff dough. Do not use diastatic malt made from wheat. (Diastatic Malt can be made from any grain that sprouts easily. See recipe on page 209.) For the liberal diet, you can use 1 teaspoon of barley malt or honey in place of the diastatic malt.

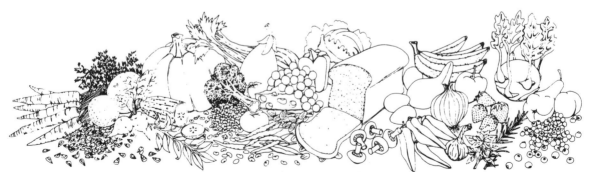

God is the silent partner in all great enterprises.   **Abraham Lincoln**

Melba Toast

If you have homemade or bought bread that's a few days old, make it into Melba Toast.

Preheat oven to 300°. Place slices of day-old unsweetened, 100% whole grain bread on a cookie sheet. Bake 30 to 45 minutes or until crisp. Serve hot or cold.

Whole Wheat-Oatmeal Bread (Sweetened)

I sometimes use this recipe, doubled or tripled, during the holidays to make bread for friends, teachers, and relatives. The gluten flour makes it lighter than most 100% whole grain breads and it pleases even those who don't normally eat whole wheat bread. You can also make it into rolls for a special meal. Don't use this recipe for your daily bread since it has too much honey and butter for everyday eating.

3 cups hot skim milk or boiling water
1½ cups rolled oats
¼ cup raw honey
¼ cup butter
1 teaspoon salt
½ cup warm water
2 tablespoons baking yeast
¼ cup gluten flour, optional
4 to 6 cups hard whole wheat flour

Pour hot or boiling liquid over oatmeal, honey, butter, and salt in a large bowl. Cool to lukewarm. Dissolve yeast in warm water. Add to oat mixture. Beat in gluten flour, if used, and enough whole wheat flour to make a soft dough. Knead approximately 10 minutes, adding flour as necessary. Return dough to mixing bowl that has been oiled. Cover with a towel and let rise in a warm place until double, approximately one hour. Punch down and let rise again for a lighter loaf. Punch down and divide into 2 loaves. Shape and place in two bread pans that have been oiled with *Oil-Lecithin Combination* (p. 205). Let rise until almost double. Bake at 350° for about 45 minutes or until done. Remove from pans and cool on rack. Cover while cooling for a soft crust. Makes 2 loaves.

Perfect Whole Foods: No
Percent Calories From Fat: 19
Total Fat Grams In Recipe: 68 (34 grams per loaf)

Wheat-Free Whole Grain-Oatmeal Bread (Sweetened, 100% Whole Grain): Omit the gluten and substitute spelt flour for the whole wheat flour.

Carrot-Walnut Muffins (Unsweetened, 100% Whole Grain)

These muffins have no refined sweeteners added—only diastatic malt, a whole food that can be used on the perfect diet.

1 egg, slightly beaten
1¾ cups buttermilk or sour milk
2 tablespoons oil
½ cup shredded carrots
2 cups hard whole wheat flour
¾ teaspoon baking soda
1 teaspoon cinnamon
4 tablespoons diastatic malt powder (p. 195, 209)
2 to 4 tablespoons chopped walnuts

Preheat oven to 400°. Oil muffin tins with *Oil-Lecithin Combination* (p. 205). In a bowl, combine buttermilk, beaten egg, oil, and carrots. In a larger mixing bowl, combine dry ingredients and nuts. Add liquid ingredients to dry ingredients, mixing only until flour is wet. Spoon into muffin tins and bake for 10 to 12 minutes. Makes 12 muffins.

Perfect Whole Foods: Use buttermilk with no added starch or whey. Or make sour milk by placing 5¼ teaspoons vinegar in measuring cup and adding enough milk to make 1¾ cups.
Percent Calories From Fat: 27 using 2 tablespoons nuts; 30 using 4 tablespoons
Fat Grams In 1 Muffin: 4 using 2 tablespoons nuts in recipe; 5 using 4 tablespoons

Wheat-Free Carrot-Walnut Muffins (Unsweetened, 100% Whole Grain): Use 1½ cups spelt or triticale, 1 cup + 2 tablespoons kamut flour, or 2 cups whole barley flour in place of the whole wheat flour. Do not use diastatic malt made from wheat. (Diastatic malt can be made from any whole grain that sprouts easily. See recipe for *Diastatic Malt* on page 209.)

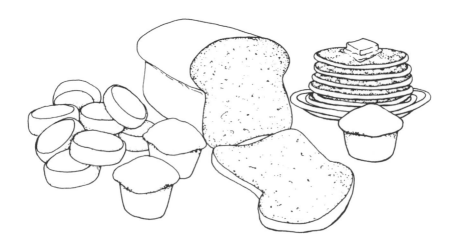

Blueberry Muffins (Unsweetened, 100% Whole Grain)

*These muffins are a treat to eat when you're on the **Perfect Whole Foods** diet. If you are on a liberal diet, you may want to omit the diastatic malt and add a tablespoon or so of honey to the liquid ingredients for sweeter and browner muffins.*

1 cup fresh or frozen blueberries
1 egg, slightly beaten
1¾ cups buttermilk or sour milk
2 tablespoons oil
2 cups hard whole wheat flour
4 tablespoons diastatic malt powder (p. 195, 209)
¾ teaspoon baking soda
1 teaspoon cinnamon

Preheat oven to 400°. Oil muffin tins with *Oil-Lecithin Combination* (p. 205). Combine flour, diastatic malt, soda, and cinnamon in a large bowl, mixing well. Mix together milk, oil, and beaten egg, and stir into dry ingredients, mixing only until flour is wet. Gently mix in the blueberries. Spoon into muffin tins and bake for 15 to 20 minutes. Makes 12 muffins.

Perfect Whole Foods: *Use buttermilk with no added starch or whey. Or make sour milk by placing 5¼ teaspoons vinegar in measuring cup and adding enough milk to make 1¾ cups.*
Percent Calories From Fat: 23
Fat Grams In 1 Muffin: 3

Wheat-Free Blueberry Muffins (Unsweetened, 100% Whole Grain): Substitute 1½ cups spelt or triticale flour, 1¼ cups kamut flour, or 2 cups whole barley flour for the whole wheat flour. Do not use diastatic malt made from wheat. (Diastatic malt can be made from any whole grain that sprouts easily. See recipe for *Diastatic Malt* on page 209.)

Those who have given of themselves to others, live forever within the hearts of those they've touched.
Julie Schaffer

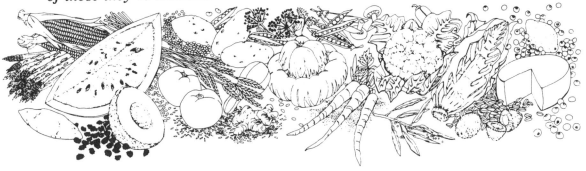

Pumpkin Muffins (Unsweetened, 100% Whole Grain)

If you're on the perfect diet, you'll enjoy these moist muffins.

½ cup cooked, pureed pumpkin, winter squash, carrots, or sweet potatoes
1 egg, slightly beaten
1½ cups + 2 tablespoons buttermilk or sour milk
2 tablespoons oil
2 cups hard whole wheat flour
4 tablespoons diastatic malt powder (p. 195, 209)
¾ teaspoon baking soda
1½ teaspoons ground cinnamon
½ teaspoon ground cloves
2 to 4 tablespoons chopped nuts

Preheat oven to 400°. Oil muffin tins with *Oil-Lecithin Combination* (p. 205). In a bowl, combine flour, diastatic malt, soda, spices, and nuts. Mix together buttermilk, oil, beaten egg, and pumpkin; stir into dry ingredients, mixing only until flour is wet. Spoon into muffin tins and bake for 15 to 20 minutes. Makes 12.

Perfect Whole Foods: Use fresh or frozen vegetables rather than canned; if you use sweet potatoes, do not peel them. Read buttermilk ingredient list carefully and don't buy those with added whey and starches like tapioca. Or make sour milk by placing 4½ teaspoons vinegar in measuring cup and adding enough milk to make 1½ cups + 2 tablespoons.
Percent Calories From Fat: 27 using 2 tablespoons nuts
Fat Grams In 1 Muffin: 5 using 2 tablespoons nuts

Wheat-Free Pumpkin Muffins (Unsweetened, 100% Whole Grain): Use 1½ cups whole spelt or triticale flour, 1¼ cups kamut flour (if you tolerate them), or 2 cups whole barley flour in place of the whole wheat flour. Do not use diastatic malt made from wheat. (Diastatic malt can be made from any whole grain that sprouts easily. See recipe for *Diastatic Malt* on page 209.)

Please Read These Important Notes:
If you have strictly followed the **Perfect Whole Foods** diet for at least two weeks, but you are not feeling dramatically better, see page 35 for additional steps that may be necessary.

If you are allergic to wheat, do not substitute spelt or kamut without first determining that you can tolerate them.

If you are being treated for *Candida*, please see specific guidelines on page 315, Appendix A: If You Have Candidiasis.

Lemon-Poppy Muffins (Unsweetened, 100% Whole Grain)

Even if you must eliminate fruit for a while on the perfect diet, you can eat these muffins since the lemon flavor comes from lemon oil rather than lemon juice. Here's that special treat you've been looking for!.

2 cups hard whole wheat flour
4 tablespoons diastatic malt powder (p. 195, 209)
2 tablespoons poppy seeds
¾ teaspoon baking soda
1 egg, slightly beaten
1¾ cups buttermilk or sour milk
2 tablespoons oil
8 drops lemon oil

Preheat oven to 400°. Oil muffin tins with *Oil-Lecithin Combination* (p. 205). Stir together dry ingredients, including poppy seeds, and mix well. Combine milk, oil, beaten egg, and lemon oil and stir into dry ingredients, mixing only to moisten. Spoon into 12 muffin tins, almost filling them, and bake for 10 to 15 minutes. Makes 12 muffins.

Perfect Whole Foods: Read the buttermilk ingredient list carefully so you won't select a brand with added starch or buttermilk flakes (containing whey). Or make sour milk by adding 5¼ teaspoons vinegar to measuring cup and adding enough milk to make 1¾ cups.
Percent Calories From Fat: 27
Fat Grams In 1 Muffin: 4

Wheat-Free Lemon-Poppy Muffins (Unsweetened, 100% Whole Grain): Substitute 1½ cups spelt or triticale flour, 1¼ cups kamut flour, or 2 cups whole barley flour for the whole wheat flour. Do not use diastatic malt made from wheat. (Diastatic malt can be made from any whole grain that sprouts easily. See recipe for *Diastatic Malt* on page 209.)

Carob-Nut Muffins (Unsweetened, 100% Whole Grain)

1½ cups hard whole wheat flour
½ cup carob powder
4 tablespoons diastatic malt powder (p. 195, 209)
¾ teaspoon baking soda
2 to 4 tablespoons chopped nuts
1 egg, slightly beaten
1¾ cups buttermilk or sour milk (p. 244)
2 tablespoons oil
1 teaspoon vanilla (alcohol-free)

Preheat oven to 400°. Oil muffin tins with *Oil-Lecithin Combination* (p. 205). Sift together dry ingredients and stir in chopped nuts. Combine milk, oil, beaten egg, and vanilla and stir into dry ingredients, mixing only to moisten. Spoon into 12 muffin tins, almost filling them, and bake for 10 to 15 minutes. Makes 12 muffins.

Perfect Whole Foods: Read buttermilk ingredients carefully so you won't select a brand with added starch or buttermilk flakes containing whey.
Percent Calories From Fat: 29
Fat Grams in 1 Muffin: 4

Wheat-Free Carob-Nut Muffins (Unsweetened, 100% Whole Grain): Use 1 cup + 2 tablespoons spelt or triticale flour or 1 cup kamut flour or 1½ cups whole barley flour for the flour. Do not use diastatic malt made from wheat. (Diastatic malt can be made from any whole grain that sprouts easily. See page 209.)

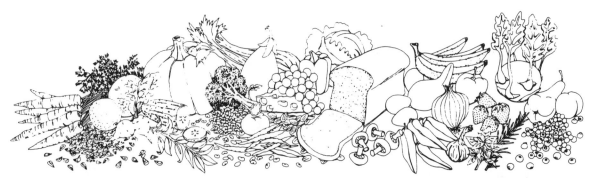

If we fill our hours with regrets over the failures of yesterday, and with worries over the problems of tomorrow, we have no today in which to be thankful.   **Unknown**

Orange-Pecan Muffins (Unsweetened, 100% Whole Grain)

2 cups hard whole wheat flour
4 tablespoons diastatic malt powder (p. 195, 209)
¾ teaspoon baking soda
2 tablespoons grated orange rind
2 to 4 tablespoons chopped pecans
1 egg, slightly beaten
1¾ cups buttermilk or sour milk
2 tablespoons oil
12 drops orange oil

Preheat oven to 400°. Oil muffin tins with *Oil-Lecithin Combination* (p. 205). Stir together dry ingredients, including orange rind and chopped nuts. Mix well. Combine buttermilk, oil, beaten egg, and orange oil and stir into dry ingredients, mixing only to moisten. Spoon into 12 muffin tins, almost filling them, and bake for 12 to 14 minutes. Makes 12 muffins.

Perfect Whole Foods: Read the buttermilk ingredient list carefully so you won't select a brand with added starch or buttermilk flakes (containing whey). Or make sour milk by adding 5¼ teaspoons vinegar to measuring cup and adding enough milk to make 1¾ cups.
Percent Calories From Fat: 29
Fat Grams In 1 Muffin: 4

Wheat-Free Orange Pecan Muffins (Unsweetened, 100% Whole Grain): Substitute 1½ cups spelt or triticale flour, 1¼ cups kamut flour, or 2 cups whole barley flour for the whole wheat flour. Do not use diastatic malt made from wheat. (Diastatic malt can be made from any whole grain that sprouts easily. See recipe for *Diastatic Malt* on page 209.)

Brown Rice Muffins (Unsweetened, 100% Whole Grain)

One of my clients with allergies developed this muffin recipe and Corn Muffins, *the recipe that follows.*

1 cup brown rice flour
½ cup amaranth flour
2 teaspoons cream of tartar
½ teaspoon baking soda
1 cup water
¼ cup oil
1 egg, slightly beaten

Preheat oven to 375°. Oil muffin tins with *Oil-Lecithin Combination* (p. 205). In a mixing bowl, stir together the dry ingredients, mixing well. Combine water, oil, and beaten egg and stir into dry ingredients, mixing only to moisten. Spoon into 12 muffin tins and bake for 20 to 25 minutes.

Percent Calories From Fat: 42
Fat Grams In 1 Muffin: 6

Corn Muffins (Unsweetened, 100% Whole Grain)

½ cup whole grain cornmeal
½ cup brown rice flour
¼ cup amaranth flour
1½ teaspoons cream of tartar
½ teaspoon baking soda
½ cup water
2 tablespoons oil
1 egg

Preheat oven to 450°. Oil muffin tins (6 muffin cups only) with *Oil-Lecithin Combination* (p. 205). In a mixing bowl, stir together the dry ingredients, mixing well. Combine water, oil, and beaten egg and stir into dry ingredients, mixing only to moisten. Spoon into 6 muffin tins that were previously oiled, and add about ½-inch water to the bottom of any empty muffin cups. Bake for 25 to 30 minutes. Makes 6 muffins.

Percent Calories From Fat: 36
Fat Grams In 1 Muffin: 7

Oat Bran Muffins

1 cup oat bran
1½ cups hard whole wheat flour
1 teaspoon baking soda
½ cup chopped nuts, optional
½ cup dried fruit, optional
1⅓ cups buttermilk
1 egg, slightly beaten
2 tablespoons oil
2 tablespoons raw honey

Preheat oven to 425°. Oil muffin pans with *Oil-Lecithin Combination* (p. 205). Mix bran and flour with baking soda and optional nuts and fruit. Combine buttermilk, beaten egg, oil, and honey together in another bowl. Gently add dry ingredients to wet ones, stirring only until combined. Let sit for 5 minutes. Pour into muffin pans, filling almost full and bake 10 to 12 minutes. Makes 12 muffins.

Perfect Whole Foods: Omit dried fruit and honey. Stir 4 tablespoons diastatic malt or 1 teaspoon stevia powder into the dry ingredients. (For information about stevia, see page 297.) Make certain the buttermilk has no starch or whey added. (Or make sour milk by placing 4 teaspoons vinegar in measuring cup and adding enough milk to make 1⅓ cups. Adjust batter consistency by adding extra buttermilk or water.)
Percent Calories From Fat: 23
Fat Grams In 1 Muffin: 4

Wheat-Free Oat Bran Muffins: Use 1 cup + 2 tablespoons spelt or triticale flour, 1 cup kamut flour, or 1½ cups whole barley flour for the whole wheat flour. If you substitute diastatic malt for the honey, use malt made from sprouted spelt, kamut, or triticale. (See the recipe on page 209.)

All people smile in the same language.

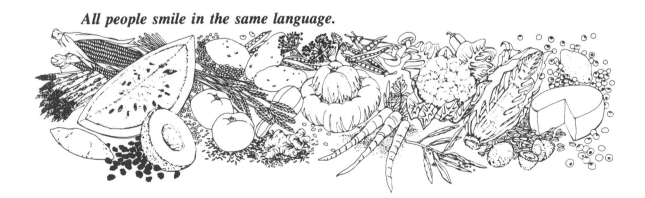

Paula's Super Muffins

Paula King created this recipe for super good muffins. Paula and her husband Ron are proprietors of Great Harvest Bread Company in Lexington, Kentucky, a whole wheat bakery.

2 cups hard whole wheat flour
1 cup wheat bran
1 cup fresh wheat germ
1 teaspoon *Rumford* Baking Powder
1 teaspoon baking soda
2 teaspoons cinnamon
½ cup nonfat milk powder
3 eggs, slightly beaten
1 cup plain nonfat yogurt
½ cup sunflower oil
½ cup raw honey
½ cup skim milk
1½ cups chopped nuts
1 cup raisins, dates, or other dried fruit
1½ cups grated carrots
1½ cups mashed ripe bananas

Preheat oven to 350°. Oil muffin tins with *Oil-Lecithin Combination* (p. 205). Mix dry ingredients together. Combine remaining ingredients in separate bowl. Add to dry ingredients. Mix until moist. Pour into muffin cups and bake about 20 minutes or until toothpick inserted comes out clean. Makes about 24 muffins.

Perfect Whole Foods: No.
Percent Calories From Fat: 46
Fat Grams In 1 Muffin: 11

Paula's Super Pumpkin Muffins: Substitute pumpkin for the bananas.
Paula's Super Applesauce Muffins: Substitute applesauce for the bananas.

Refrigerator Bran Muffins

1 cup boiling or warm water
2½ cups oat or wheat bran
2½ cups whole wheat flour (pastry)
2½ teaspoons baking soda
½ cup fresh wheat germ
½ cup oil
½ cup raw honey
2 eggs, slightly beaten
2 cups buttermilk

Pour boiling water over 1 cup of the bran, if using wheat bran. Pour warm, not boiling, water over 1 cup of the bran if using oat bran. In another bowl, mix flour, soda, wheat germ, and remainder of the bran. Combine oil, honey, beaten eggs, and buttermilk and add to bran and water. Stir to mix and then add to dry ingredients, stirring only to moisten. Cover tightly and store in refrigerator until you are ready for muffins. Add more milk if the batter has thickened. Pour into muffin tins which have been oiled with *Oil-Lecithin Combination* (p. 205). Bake at 400° for 15 to 20 minutes. The batter will keep in refrigerator for several days. Makes about 3 dozen.

Perfect Whole Foods: No, because of the honey.
Percent Calories From Fat: 36
Total Fat Grams In Recipe: 4

Cornbread (Unsweetened, 100% Whole Grain)

1 cup whole grain yellow cornmeal
1 cup whole wheat pastry flour
¼ teaspoon salt
½ teaspoon baking soda
1 tablespoon diastatic malt, optional (p. 195, 209)
1 cup buttermilk or sour milk (p. 244)
2 tablespoons oil
2 eggs, beaten

Preheat oven to 400°. Oil a 8 or 10-inch cast iron skillet with *Oil-Lecithin Combination* (p. 205) and place in oven for a few minutes to get hot just before the batter is ready. Mix dry ingredients thoroughly. Combine buttermilk and oil and add beaten eggs. Pour milk-egg mixture into dry ingredients, stirring just until combined. Do not over mix. Pour into hot skillet and bake for 20 minutes. You can also bake it in an oiled 8-inch square cake pan; however, the crust will not be crisp. (Don't pre-heat the cake pan.) Cut into about 8 pie-shaped pieces.

Percent Calories From Fat: 28
Fat Grams In 1 Piece: 5

Wheat-Free Cornbread (Unsweetened, 100% Whole Grain): Use ¾ cup spelt or triticale flour, ⅝ cup (½ cup + 2 tablespoons) kamut flour, or 1 cup whole barley flour for whole wheat flour.
Egg-Free Cornbread (Unsweetened, 100% Whole Grain): Omit eggs and bake only 15 minutes.

Hoe Cakes (Unsweetened, 100% Whole Grain)

1 cup whole grain cornmeal
½ cup whole wheat pastry flour
¾ teaspoon baking soda
1½ cup buttermilk
1 tablespoon oil, total

Combine dry ingredients. Add milk and mix into dry ingredients, stirring only until dry ingredients are wet. Let batter sit for a few minutes. Oil heavy iron skillet or griddle and heat. Pan fry as you would pancakes, browning on each side. Stir batter gently each time you start to make more cakes. Serve hot. Good with bean soup. Makes eight or nine 4-inch cakes.

Perfect Whole Foods: Read the ingredient list to make certain buttermilk does not have starch or whey added. Or make sour milk by placing 4½ teaspoons vinegar in measuring cup and adding milk to make 1½ cups.
Percent Calories From Fat: 19
Fat Grams In 1 Hoe Cake: 3

Wheat-Free Hoe Cakes (Unsweetened, 100% Whole Grain): Substitute ⅓ cup spelt flour, triticale flour, or oat bran or ½ cup whole barley flour for the whole wheat flour.

Millet Cakes (Unsweetened, 100% Whole Grain)

Prepare this pancake-like bread if you are looking for an unsweetened 100% millet bread. If you are not on the perfect diet, include a teaspoon or so of honey to the batter.

½ cup millet flour
¼ teaspoon baking soda
½ cup buttermilk or sour milk
1 teaspoon oil, total

Combine dry ingredients. Add milk and mix into dry ingredients, stirring only until dry ingredients are wet. Oil heavy iron skillet or griddle and heat. Pan fry as you would pancakes, browning on each side. Makes three 5-inch cakes.

Perfect Whole Foods: Make certain buttermilk does not have starch or whey added. Or make sour milk by placing 1½ teaspoons vinegar in measuring cup and adding enough milk to make ½ cup.
Percent Calories From Fat: 21
Fat Grams In 1 Millet Cake: 2

Oat Bran Snack Bread (Unsweetened, 100% Whole Grain)

1 cup whole wheat pastry flour (plus about ½ teaspoon flour to sprinkle on oiled cookie sheet)
1 cup oat bran
½ teaspoon baking soda
¼ teaspoon salt
1 tablespoon oil (plus about ½ teapoon more to oil cookie sheet)
1 cup + 2 tablespoons buttermilk or sour milk
Shredded low-fat cheese, optional

Preheat oven to 450°. Oil a 9-inch circle on a cookie sheet and sprinkle with a teaspoon flour. Combine dry ingredients. Combine liquid ingredients in another bowl and add to dry ingredients, stirring gently to moisten. Pour onto cookie sheet and, using floured hands, pat into a circle ½-inch thick. Bake for about 10 minutes. Cut into wedges and, while hot, top with shredded low-fat cheese, if desired. Serves 5 or 6.

Perfect Whole Foods: Make certain buttermilk does not have starch or whey added. Or make sour milk by placing 1 tablespoon vinegar in measuring cup and adding enough milk to make 1 cup + 2 tablespoons.
Percent Calories From Fat: 19
Fat Grams In 1 Piece: 4 (without cheese)

Wheat-Free Oat Bran Snack Bread (Unsweetened, 100% Whole Grain): Use ¾ cup spelt or triticale flour, ½ cup + 2 tablespoons kamut flour, or 1 cup whole barley flour for the flour.

Squash Roll-Ups

2 cups whole wheat pastry flour
2½ teaspoons *Rumford* Baking Powder
⅛ teaspoon salt
¼ cup oil
⅔ cup mashed, cooked winter squash (or carrots, pumpkin or sweet potatoes)
1 tablespoon butter, melted

Preheat oven to 450°. Mix together dry ingredients. Add oil and mix until evenly distributed. Add squash and enough water to form a soft ball (about 2 to 4 tablespoons, the amount of water depending on the consistency of the cooked squash). Knead 4 or 5 times. Dust counter with flour and roll ball into a 12-inch circle. Spread with melted butter. Cut circle into 12 wedges. Starting at wide end, roll each wedge, placing point side down on ungreased cookie sheet, 1-inch apart. Bake 10 to 12 minutes. Makes 12.

Perfect Whole Foods: Substitute ⅝ teaspoon (½ + ⅛) baking soda and 1½ teaspoon cream of tartar for the baking powder. Use squash, carrots, or pumpkin rather than peeled sweet potatoes.
Percent Calories From Fat: 38
Fat Grams In 1 Squash Roll-Up: 6

Wheat-Free Squash Roll-Ups: Use 1½ cups spelt or triticale or 2 cups whole barley flour.

Whole Wheat Pancakes (Unsweetened, 100% Whole Grain)

2 cups buttermilk or sour milk (p. 244)
2 eggs, beaten
2 cups whole wheat pastry flour
1 teaspoon baking soda
1 teaspoon oil, total

In large bowl, combine buttermilk and eggs. In another bowl combine soda and flour, mixing well. Add flour mixture to liquids, mixing only until large lumps disappear. Cook on a lightly oiled griddle or skillet over medium heat. Turn when top of pancake is partially set. Makes about twenty-four 3-inch pancakes.

Percent Calories From Fat: 20
Fat Grams In 1 Pancake: 3 when recipe makes 9 pancakes; 4 when recipe makes 8

Wheat-Free Whole Grain Pancakes (Unsweetened, 100% Whole Grain): Substitute 1½ cups spelt or triticale flour, 1¼ cups kamut flour, or 2 cups whole barley for the whole wheat flour.
Dairy-Free Whole Grain Pancakes (Unsweetened, 100% Whole Grain): Substitute 1 cup unsweetened soy milk, or nut milk plus 1 cup water for the 2 cups skim milk.
Whole Grain Blueberry Pancakes (Unsweetened, 100% Whole Grain): Stir 1 cup fresh or frozen blueberries into the batter.
Buckwheat Flapjacks (Unsweetened, 100% Whole Grain): Substitute ⅝ cup (½ cup + 2 tablespoons) buckwheat flour for 1 cup whole wheat flour.

Overnight Blender Pancakes (Unsweetened, 100% Whole Grain)

By soaking whole grains overnight in water in the blender container, you'll just have to add the other ingredients in the morning, blend, let the mixture sit for 30 minutes while you're getting dressed, and then bake on an oiled griddle. You'll have scrumptious-tasting pancakes with very little work.

1 cup whole grains (soft wheat, spelt, triticale, or kamut berries, oat groats, or hulled barley)
2 eggs
½ cup nonfat milk powder
½ teaspoon baking soda
1 tablespoon cider vinegar (or add 1 teaspoon cream of tartar to dry ingredients)
1 tablespoon oil, total

Soak whole grains in 1¾ cups of water in the blender container overnight at room temperature. Next morning, add eggs and blend until smooth, stopping occasionally to scrape down the sides to make certain all grains are ground. Mix together the dry milk and soda. Stir them in along with vinegar and blend to thoroughly mix. Let sit about 30 minutes and then bake on an oiled griddle. Turn over when tops have bubbled and are partially set. Makes about fifteen 3-inch pancakes.

Percent Calories From Fat: 24
Fat Grams In 1 Pancake: 2

Dairy-Free Overnight Blender Pancakes: Add 2 tablespoons more whole grains and omit milk.

Vita Mix Pancakes (Unsweetened, 100% Whole Grain)

If you have a Vita Mix *appliance, you can grind the grain, add remaining ingredients, and have pancake batter in just a few minutes.*

1½ cups soft whole wheat, spelt, kamut, or triticale berries or hulled barley
½ teaspoons baking soda
2 eggs
2 cups skim milk
1 tablespoon apple cider vinegar (or add 1 teaspoon cream of tartar with the soda)
1 tablespoon oil, total
Extra skim milk or whole grain flour, if necessary

Grind whole grains in Vita Mix for 1 minute. Remove container and tap against counter top so that kernels stuck in spigot will drop into container. Add baking soda and grind for 1 minute longer. Add eggs and milk mixed with vinegar; blend until mixed. Adjust consistency, if necessary, by adding a little flour or more skim milk and mixing. Cook on a lightly oiled griddle, pouring from the container. Turn pancakes when they are slightly set on top. Makes about twenty-four 3-inch pancakes.

Percent Calories From Fat: 19
Fat Grams In 1 Pancake: 1

Chickpea Pancakes (Unsweetened, 100% Whole Grain)

For those with multiple food allergies, here's a pancake recipe made without wheat, eggs, or milk. Beat in an egg if your diet allows it or use milk in place of the water.

¾ cup brown rice flour or millet flour
¼ cup chickpea flour
¼ teaspoon baking soda
½ teaspoon cream of tartar
1 cup water (or milk, if tolerated)
2 tablespoons oil, divided

Mix dry ingredients together. Combine wet ingredients, using only 1 tablespoon oil and reserving the other tablespoon for oiling the griddle. Using a mixer, beat the wet and dry ingredients together just until lumps disappear. Drop by ¼ cupfuls on hot, lightly-oiled griddle or skillet. Turn over when tops are almost set. Stir batter each time you start to prepare a pancake since flour tends to settle to the bottom. Makes about eight 4-inch pancakes.

Percent Calories From Fat: 40
Fat Grams In 1 Pancake: 8

Silver Dollar Pancakes (Unsweetened, 100% Whole Grain)

Here's a recipe I developed especially for those with grain allergies. Spread these tiny pancakes with airy butter, nut butter, or natural fruit jam, according to your preferences and diet. Use ¼ cup flour the first time you prepare it and then double the recipe next time if you like that particular flour and want more than 6 or 7 tiny pancakes. If you find you don't like the pancakes made from one flour, don't hesitate to try another one since they are all quite different. Some are better than others, but allergies often limit the ones you can use.

¼ cup of the flour of your choice: amaranth, whole barley, buckwheat (dark or white), corn (probably is refined), oat bran, whole oat flour, quinoa, whole rye, spelt, teff, triticale, or whole wheat (whole wheat pastry or soft rather than hard)
¼ cup or more carbonated mineral water
Pinch of salt, optional

Combine flour and salt. Stir in the carbonated water until you have a smooth, pourable batter with a consistency of very thick cream or thin gravy. Begin with the ¼ cup water and add about 1 teaspoon at a time until you have the right consistency. Heat a *SilverStone* skillet or griddle until medium hot and pour 2-inch rounds, turning over when tops are almost set. If you don't have a *SilverStone* skillet or griddle, you can use an oiled skillet. Cook until lightly browned. Makes six or seven 2-inch pancakes.

Perfect Whole Foods: Make certain the carbonated mineral water does not have sugar added. Do not use corn flour since it is refined.
Percent Calories From Fat: 4 using whole wheat flour
Total Fat Grams In Recipe: Less than 1 using whole wheat flour

Soda-Leavened Silver Dollar Pancakes (Unsweetened, 100% Whole Grain): Stir a pinch (about ¹⁄₁₆ teaspoon) of baking soda into ¼ cup whole grain flour, mixing very well. Add ½ teaspoon lemon juice, lime juice, or vinegar to ¼ cup water (not carbonated) or milk. If, after stirring in this liquid, the batter is too thick, add more of the same plain water or milk. Cook in *SilverStone* skillet or griddle as instructed above. Do not use the lemon or lime juice if you are on the perfect diet.

Sweetened Silver Dollar Pancakes: If you are on a liberal diet, add ½ to 1 teaspoon sweetener such as honey, maple syrup, molasses, or date sugar to the batter. This will make the pancakes brown better and give them a slightly sweet taste.

Whole Wheat Waffles

When my family and I visit my parents in Tennessee, my mother, Ann Oakes, usually serves these waffles for a hearty breakfast or brunch. She has them prepared ahead of time, stored in the freezer and pops the frozen waffles into the toaster to heat them up. Served with eggs, whole grain corn grits, and fruit that's in season, we have breakfast on the table in no time.

2 cups whole wheat pastry flour
4 teaspoons *Rumford* Baking Powder
1¾ cups skim milk
2 eggs, well beaten
2 tablespoons oil

Combine the flour and baking powder. Combine the milk, eggs, and oil in another bowl. Add the liquid ingredients to the dry ingredients, stirring until dry ingredients are moistened. Batter will be slightly lumpy. Bake in preheated waffle iron, using about ¾ cup batter for a 4-section waffle. Bake approximately 5 minutes or until waffles no longer steam. Makes four 4-section waffles.

Perfect Whole Wheat: Use 1 teaspoon baking soda instead of the baking powder; place 2 tablespoons cider vinegar in your measuring cup and add enough skim milk to equal 1¾ cups.
Percent Calories From Fat: 25
Fat Grams In One 4-Section Waffle: 11

Wheat-Free Whole Grain Waffles: Use 1½ cups spelt or triticale flour, 1 cup minus 1 tablespoon kamut flour, or 2 cups whole barley flour for the whole wheat flour.
Dairy-Free Whole Wheat Waffles: Substitute ¾ cup unsweetened soy, nut, or zucchini milk and 1 cup water for the 1¾ cups of skim milk.

Seasoned Wheat Chips

Whole Wheat Chapatis or Whole Wheat Flat Bread (homemade or bought)
Granulated garlic
Granulated onion
Chili powder

Preheat oven to 350°. Cut each chapati into 6 or 8 pie-shaped pieces. Sprinkle with seasonings. Place on ungreased cookie sheet and bake for about 4 minutes. Turn them over and bake about 4 minutes longer. Watch carefully since they burn easily.

Perfect Whole Foods: Pay close attention to the ingredient list so you won't buy flat breads with baking powder or white flour added.
Percent Calories From Fat: 27
Fat Grams In Chips From 1 Chapati: 5

Taco Corn Chips: Use soft corn tortillas (whole grain corn tortillas if you're on the perfect diet). Bake at 400° for 4 or 5 minutes, turn chips over, and bake 4 or 5 minutes longer. Since corn tortillas vary in thickness, you may need to adjust the cooking time for your favorite brand.

Basic Crackers (Unsweetened, 100% Whole Grain)

This recipe should be especially helpful if you must eliminate traditional yeast breads because of allergies. Simply choose from the flours, oils, and optional flavorings that you can use. The amount of water is approximate—enough to make the mixture stick together without being too sticky to knead and roll out.

1 cup flour of your choice: amaranth, whole barley, buckwheat (dark or white), garbanzo or chick pea, kamut, corn (probably is refined), quinoa, whole rye, spelt, teff, triticale, whole wheat pastry
2 tablespoons oil of your choice: almond, apricot, avocado, canola, corn, olive, peanut, pumpkin seed, safflower, sesame, soy, sunflower, or walnut
1 or 2 flavorings, to taste (optional): sea salt or mineral salt, caraway seeds, chia seeds, cinnamon powder, dill seeds, nutmeg powder, poppy seeds, or sesame seeds

Preheat oven to 375°. Oil a cookie sheet (without sides) using same oil you are using in the crackers. If you are using seeds, place them in a cup and press them with the back of a spoon to bruise them and intensify their flavor. Mix the flour and flavorings together. Add the oil, mixing until crumbly. Next, add about ¼ cup water or enough to make the mixture stick together. Knead briefly and flatten slightly on cookie sheet. Cover with a piece of wax paper and roll on cookie sheet until dough is thin, about ⅛-inch thick. Using a pizza cutter or a table knife, cut into crackers. Sprinkle with salt, if desired. Place in preheated oven and, after 6 or 8 minutes of baking, remove those crackers which are browned to a wire rack and continue baking the others. Check them every 1 or 2 minutes, removing crackers as they are done.

Perfect Whole Foods: *Do not use corn flour since it is refined.*
Percent Calories From Fat: 38 using whole wheat flour
Total Fat Grams In Recipe: 27 using whole wheat flour

Think positively, act positively, pray positively and believe positively, and powerful results will be yours.   *Norman Vincent Peale*

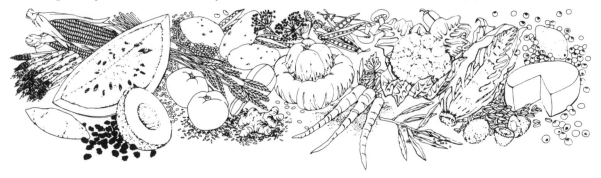

Toasted Pitas

Toasted commercial pita bread can be used in a variety of ways. Toasted lightly, you can stuffed it with Tofu Salad (p. 118) plus plenty of veggies for a delicious sandwich. Toast it until it's crisp, cut it into pie-shaped pieces, and serve it with dips like Eggplant Dip *or guacamole. (See dip recipes on pages 260 to 262.)*

100% Whole Wheat Pita Bread (unsweetened)

Cut pita bread in half and toast, using a toaster or oven broiler.

Percent Calories From Fat: 5
Fat Grams In 1 Pita: Less than 1

Chapatis (Unsweetened, 100% Whole Grain)

These flat breads are often available at natural food stores and food co-ops, but if you want to make your own, here's the recipe. If you buy whole wheat chapatis, make certain they do not have baking powder in them if you are on the perfect diet.

1 cup hard whole wheat flour
¼ teaspoon salt
1 tablespoon oil
Approximately ¼ cup water

Mix flour and salt in bowl. Work in oil with fork or fingers. Add water, mixing and kneading until it all sticks together. If it remains crumbly, add more water, a teaspoon at a time. Knead on an oiled surface for 10 minutes. Dough will become smooth and elastic. Invert bowl over dough and let it sit for 30 minutes to make rolling easier. Divide into 6 portions. Shape each into a ball and cover to prevent drying. Roll each ball starting from the center into a 6-inch circle. Keep the rolled chapatis covered. Heat a large, heavy, ungreased griddle or skillet. Place a chapati on the griddle and cook until it puffs up a little and bottom is brown in spots. Turn and cook on other side. As each chapati is cooked, wrap in towel or napkin to keep warm. Serve them warm or cool or store. Makes 6.

Percent Calories From Fat: 27
Fat Grams In 1 Chapati: 5

Whole Grain Flat Bread (Unsweetened, 100% Whole Grain)

These tortilla or chapati-type flat breads can be used for sandwiches by wrapping them around sliced meat and shredded vegetables or by spreading nut butters on them and rolling them up. Reheat them in the oven or toaster. They freeze well.

1 cup flour of your choice: amaranth, whole barley, buckwheat (dark or white), corn (probably is refined), garbanzo or chickpea, kamut, oat, quinoa, whole rye, spelt, teff, triticale, or hard whole wheat
¼ teaspoon salt
1 flavoring, if desired: ½ teaspoon ground cinnamon or a pinch of ground allspice, cloves, ginger, nutmeg, caraway seeds, dried chives, dill seeds, or garlic powder

Combine flour, salt and optional flavorings in a bowl. Add ¼ cup water and mix. If it remains crumbly, add more water, a teaspoon at a time, until it all sticks together. Since some flours absorb more water than others, you may need to use up to ½ cup. Knead in the bowl for 5 to 10 minutes or until dough becomes smooth and elastic, adding more flour to bowl if necessary to keep dough from being sticky. If you have the time, cover bowl and let dough sit for 15 to 30 minutes to make rolling easier. Divide dough into about 6 golf-ball size portions. Shape each into a ball and cover to prevent drying. Sprinkle a little flour on wax paper, place one portion on floured paper, sprinkle more flour on top and cover with another piece of wax paper. Flatten dough slightly and roll, starting at the center, into a 5 to 6-inch circle, about ⅛-inch thick. Lift the wax paper off dough frequently to prevent it from sticking. Sprinkle on a little more flour if there is the tendency to stick. Turn wax paper covered dough over and, as with top of dough, lift paper off other side of dough. Use as little flour as possible, but enough to prevent sticking. If at any time dough sticks on the wax paper and tears, you can scrape it off, reshape into a ball, and roll again.

As you get one rolled, place it in a large, heavy medium-hot griddle or skillet (not greased). While continuing to roll out more dough, cook the first bread until it puffs up a little and the bottom is brown in spots. Turn and cook on the other side. As each flat bread is cooked, wrap it in a towel or napkin to keep it warm. Or use an airtight container and freeze. Makes approximately 6.

Perfect Whole Foods: Do not use corn flour since it is refined.
Percent Calories From Fat: 4 using whole wheat flour
Total Fat Grams In Recipe: 1 using whole wheat flour

Fruited Flat Bread: Add ½ cup of mashed or pureed fresh fruit or dried fruit puree* and decrease the amount of water. Add a teaspoon of water at a time until the flour and fruit mixture will form a ball. Follow instructions above for kneading, shaping, and cooking.
*Dried fruit purée: Soak dried fruit in water overnight. Drain and puree in food processor. Do not use dried fruit purée on the perfect diet.

Whole Grain Pie Crust

I have tried, without success, to find a way to make pie crust low in fat. It takes fat to make a tender, flaky crust rather than crunchy like crackers. My best advice is to use this recipe with discretion.

1 cup rolled oats, blended in food processor until fine
1 cup whole wheat pastry flour
3 tablespoons oil
Approximately ⅓ to ½ cup ice water

Preheat oven to 375°. Combine dry ingredients. Add oil and mix with food processor, fork, or fingers. Add ice water slowly while mixing until ingredients form a ball. Roll between 2 sheets of wax paper and place in pie pan, being careful not to stretch the crust. Finish edge by pressing with fork tines or fluting with fingers. For pre-baked crust, prick with a fork and bake until nicely browned, about 10 to 15 minutes. Filled crust will make 5 to 6 servings.

Percent Calories From Fat: 35
Total Fat Grams In Recipe: 50

Wheat-Free Whole Grain Pie Crust: Use 1 cup whole barley flour or ¾ cup spelt, triticale or kamut flour in place of the whole wheat pastry flour.

Whole Wheat Crepes (Unsweetened, 100% Whole Grain)

These crepes may be used with a variety of fillings and sauces. Add scrambled eggs, roll, and top with Creole Sauce *(p. 269) for a special brunch. Or stuff with steamed vegetables and drizzle with* Cheese Sauce *(p. 267). Serve these or create your own crepe fillings for elegant whole foods cooking.*

¾ cup skim milk
1 tablespoon oil
1 egg
¾ cup whole wheat pastry flour

Place all ingredients in blender in the order listed. Cover and blend on high speed until smooth. Refrigerate for at least an hour before cooking. Batter should be thin. If it is thick after sitting in refrigerator, add a tablespoon or so of water and stir. Cook on an electric crepe-maker according to directions. Or, using a seasoned 6 to 8-inch crepe pan, oil and heat over medium-high heat, add 2 to 3 tablespoons batter, lift and tilt pan to spread batter, return to heat, and cook until brown on one side. Top should be dry. Invert pan so that crepe is removed onto a paper towel. Repeat until all crepes are cooked. Stack crepes with paper towels between them. You may store them in an airtight container and refrigerate them several days before using. Makes about 10 crepes.

Percent Calories From Fat: 30
Fat Grams In 1 Crepe Without Filling: 2

Wheat-Free Whole Grain Crepes: Substitute ½ cup plus 1 tablespoon spelt or triticale flour, ½ cup kamut flour, or ¾ cup whole barley flour for the whole wheat flour.

Sprout Bread (Unsweetened, 100% Whole Grain)

Sprout Bread, sometimes called Essene *Bread or* Manna, *is one of the first varieties of bread ever made. It was originally baked in the sun. The following recipe calls for hard wheat berries; other grains such as soft wheat berries, spelt berries, triticale berries, kamut berries, rye berries, oat groats, and millet can be used instead. Also, grains can be combined. Sprout Bread has a slightly sweet taste since grains become sweet when sprouted. Just as with diastatic malt, Sprout Bread can be used on the* **Perfect Whole Foods** *diet because it is a whole food. The grain has not been refined or processed. If you are on a liberal diet, try soaking dried fruit and nuts and adding them to the dough before shaping.*

- Sprout at least ½ cup hard wheat berries for 2 or 3 days or until sprouts are the same length as the grain. Do not rinse on the morning of making the bread. (See recipe for *Diastatic Malt* on page 209 for instructions on sprouting wheat.)
- Using a food processor with metal blade attachment, grind about 2 or 3 cups of sprouts at a time for 1 or 2 minutes, scraping down sides occasionally. This mass is your bread dough.
- Oil cookie sheet and sprinkle with whole grain corn meal.
- Shape the dough with wet hands into round loaves with flattened tops. You don't have to knead. Just work with the dough to press out air pockets and make a fairly smooth surface.
- Bake on cookie sheet at 150 to 275° for several hours (2 to 8) or until bread is somewhat firm on the outside but still moist inside but not really sticky. With a low baking temperature, few nutrients will be lost. The higher baking temperature will produce a more crusty loaf. Baking time will be determined by the amount of moisture in sprouts, the size and shape of loaf, and oven temperature. If you underbake it, you can always bake it longer even after you've cut into it.
- Cool on wire rack and store in plastic bag at room temperature if it is to be eaten within a few days; or store in the refrigerator where it will keep for several weeks.

Percent Calories From Fat: 5
Total Fat Grams In Recipe: 2

Seeded Sprout Bread (Unsweetened, 100% Whole Grain): Knead sunflower seeds, flax seeds, and sesame seeds into ground wheat sprouts, using 1 tablespoon raw sunflower seeds and 1 teaspoon each flax and sesame seeds per ½ cup wheat (or other grain) berries. (Measure grain before sprouting.)

I can do all things through Christ Who strengthens me.   Philippians 4:13

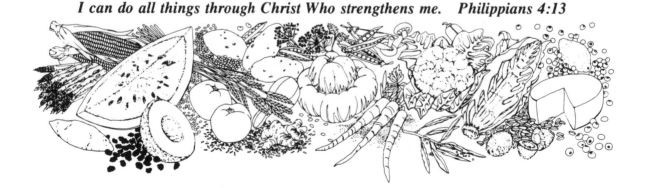

DAIRY PRODUCTS

Choose nonfat and low-fat dairy products most of the time when you buy dairy foods. Although many of the high-fat products are free of refined carbohydrates, eating them regularly or in quantity will provide too much total fat and saturated fat for a healthy diet. (Read about cheese and cottage cheese, under **Main Dishes** on pages 67, 68, and 75.)

I've included recipes in this section for making three cultured products: buttermilk, yogurt, and kefir. Each is simple to make and is less expensive to make than buy. If you take the time to sterilize the jars in which you will make cultured dairy products, you won't grow undesirable bacteria along with the desirable ones. Your product will have a better flavor and you will be able to use it over and over as a starter for the next batch.

Nonfat yogurt makes an excellent substitute for high-fat dairy products like sour cream. When drained of its whey, yogurt can also take the place of cream cheese (see recipe for *Yogurt Cheese*, page 246).

Ways to Use Plain Yogurt

- In place of sour cream on baked potatoes or on brown rice. Add a little salt and garlic powder, prepared mustard, nutritional yeast, or herbs to complement the food you are serving. (See *Herbed Tater Toppers* on page 270 for more ideas.)

- Mixed with homemade or commercial mayonnaise to avoid so much fat from mayonnaise. Use this combination in making egg salad, potato salad, slaw, and other foods using mayonnaise.

- As a topping for cooked vegetables instead of butter. Add a dollop of plain yogurt (room temperature) to beets, broccoli, or green beans.

- As a topping for pancakes or waffles. First stir a little vanilla extract into the yogurt. Then add some fresh fruit, if desired.

- As a treat by itself with 2 tablespoons pecan meal or chopped pecans sprinkled over yogurt.

Perfect Whole Foods: Use only alcohol-free vanilla (commercial or homemade) or omit vanilla.
Percent Calories From Fat: 0 from plain, nonfat yogurt; 22 from plain, low-fat
Fat Grams In 1 Cup: Less than 0.5 in plain, nonfat yogurt; 4 in plain, low-fat

Dairy Facts

Butter: Butter is used rather than margarine on the *Perfect Whole Foods* diet since it is a natural product with no hydrogenated fat added. Because it is a saturated fat, butter should be used sparingly. (See complete information about fats beginning on page 44.)
Percent Calories From Fat: 100
Fat Grams In 1 Teaspoon: 4

Buttermilk: A cultured milk product, buttermilk varies in fat content depending on the kind of milk used in its preparation. Commercial buttermilk often contains a starch stabilizer. Don't use these on the perfect diet. Gelatin stabilizers are okay. When flakes are added, the flakes are made of whey, a source of refined carbohydrates. Select buttermilk with the lowest fat content, as long as other ingredients are okay. If you cannot find buttermilk without refined carbohydrates added, you can substitute sour milk in baked goods. For instructions on making this buttermilk substitution, see **Sour Milk** on page 244. Don't use buttermilk powder on the perfect diet since the brands I have found contain added whey.
Percent Calories From Fat: 10 in buttermilk with ½% butterfat
Fat Grams In 1 Cup: 1 in buttermilk with ½% butterfat

Cheese: See pages 67, 68, and 75 for a complete discussion of aged cheeses and cottage cheese.

Cream, Half and Half: A cream that's made with half milk and half heavy cream. Because it is rich in saturated fat, half and half should not be used often.
Percent Calories From Fat: 77
Fat Grams In 1 Tablespoon: 2

Cream, Sour: A high-fat dairy product that should not be used often. Read the ingredient list carefully since some sour cream products have sweeteners and starches added. (Plain, nonfat yogurt makes a good substitute for sour cream.)
Percent Calories From Fat: 87
Fat Grams In 1 Tablespoon: 3

Cream, Light Sour: Most light sour cream products contain sweeteners and starches and should be eliminated on the perfect diet. However, *Alta-Dena* does make a good light sour cream that contains no refined carbohydrates and may be used on the perfect diet.

Cream, Whipping: A dairy product that should be used only occasionally because almost all of its calories come from fat.
Percent Calories From Fat: 97
Fat Grams In 1 Tablespoon: 6

Goat's Milk: If you are allergic to the whey protein of cow's milk (lactalbumin and lactoglobulin), you might be able to tolerate milk and cheese from other animals such as goats and sheep since the whey proteins in these milks are different from those of cow's milk. Carefully check the ingredients of goat cheeses made in the U.S. since they are sometimes made with partial cow's milk for a milder-flavored cheese.

Kefir: (pronounced KEY-fur) A liquid, milder-than-yogurt, cultured milk product that is made from kefir grains or pellets. These grains settle to the bottom of the liquid and can be reused over and over. Kefir can also be made with a starter from a previous batch, just like making buttermilk and yogurt. Commercial kefir products usually have sweeteners added. Kefir grains are available, so those on **Perfect Whole Foods** can make plain, unsweetened kefir. Grains and instructions may be ordered from R.A.J.-Jungreis, 35 Park Avenue, Blue Point, NY 11715.

Lactose: Milk sugar that naturally occurs in dairy products. The perfect diet allows dairy products in moderate amounts since the trace nutrients needed for the metabolism of lactose is present in the milk. However, products with lactose added as an ingredient should be eliminated since pure lactose is a refined sugar.

Lactose Intolerant: Those individuals who do not produce the enzyme lactase that is needed for the digestion of lactose or milk sugar. Symptoms of lactose intolerance include indigestion, bloating, cramping, diarrhea, or gas after consuming milk and some milk products. Some who are lactose intolerant can tolerate a little milk, others none. Many, however, are able to eat cultured milk products. (See **Milk, Cultured**, below.)

Lactose-Reduced Milk: Milk to which the enzyme lactase has been added, resulting in 70% less lactose. If you are lactose intolerant, you may or may not be able to digest this product. It all depends on how sensitive you are to lactose. Lactose-reduced milk is usually a low-fat product. Read the label of lactose-reduced milk carefully if you are on the perfect diet.

Milk, Cultured: Milk to which a beneficial bacteria culture has been added and allowed to grow. These bacteria are beneficial to the body because they establish themselves in the intestinal tract where they help with protein digestion and manufacture some of the B vitamins. They also help prevent the overgrowth of harmful yeast like *Candida albicans* which also resides in the intestinal tract. The use of antibiotics destroys the beneficial bacteria in the intestines and harmful bacteria. If cultured products with active culture (as well as supplements providing active Acidophilus and Bifidus culture) are used during and following antibiotic therapy, they can help replenish the beneficial bacteria and prevent yeast overgrowth. Various strains of bacteria are used to produce cultured milk, with each strain producing a different product. Yogurt is the most commonly known cultured milk product. Others are buttermilk, acidophilus milk, kefir, piima, and viilia.

Milk, Low-Fat: Commercial milks that are called *low-fat* include ½, 1, and 2 percent fat by weight. Notice that the percent calories from fat is not the same as the percent fat by weight.
Percent Calories From Fat: 10, 23, and 35, respectively
Fat Grams In 1 Cup: 1, 3, 5, respectively

Milk, Powder, Instant Nonfat: Dried skim milk powder that has been processed so that it dissolves easily in water. When reconstituting instant nonfat milk powder with water, use ⅓ cup milk powder to 1 cup water. Use either *instant* or *non-instant nonfat milk powder* in recipes that simply call for *nonfat milk powder*. See also **Non-Instant Nonfat Milk Powder** that follows.

Milk Powder, Non-Instant Nonfat: Dried skim milk powder that has not been instantized. It is less processed than instant nonfat milk powder. It is also harder to mix with water. The *non-

instant milk powder is preferred over the instant variety for making cultured milk products. When using non-instant milk powder in baked goods, add the powder along with the other dry ingredients and then use water in place of the liquid milk. When reconstituting into liquid milk, add ¼ cup non-instant nonfat milk powder to 1 cup water. Use either *instant* or *non-instant nonfat milk powder* in recipes that simply call for *nonfat milk powder*.

Milk, Skim: Commercial milk that is called *skim milk* has less than ½ percent fat by weight.
Percent Calories From Fat: 4 or less
Fat Grams In 1 cup: Less than 0.5

Milk, Sweet Acidophilus: Milk to which the bacteria culture, *lactobacillus acidophilus*, has been added. While refrigerated the mixture is not held at a temperature that allows the culture to predigest the lactose in the milk. However, once it is drunk and in the gastrointestinal tract, the culture will digest the lactose, so those intolerant to lactose can usually tolerate this milk. The milk cannot be used in cooking, heated, or added to hot liquids without destroying the bacteria culture. Sweet acidophilus milk is usually available as a low fat product and does *not*, as the name suggests, have sugar added. Read the ingredient list carefully if you are on the perfect diet.

Milk, Whole: 3.5% fat by weight. A lower fat milk is preferable since the percent calories from fat is much too high to be used often. Don't confused the percent fat by weight (used in meats and dairy products) with the percent calories from fat since the two are totally differnt. Since milk is mostly water, the percent of fat by weight is low, but not the percent calories from fat.
Percent Calories From Fat: 48
Fat Grams In 1 Cup: 8

Sour Milk: If you're on the perfect diet and can't find buttermilk made without whey or tapioca starch added, you can substitute sour milk for buttermilk in baked goods. To make one cup sour milk, place one tablespoon vinegar or lemon juice in a measuring cup. Fill the cup with milk (skim, 1%, or 2%, whichever you use) and let it sit for a minute or so. Don't use lemon juice if you're on the perfect diet. You may need to add extra flour to baked goods since sour milk is thinner than buttermilk.

Sterilize: To sterilize equipment for making cultured milk products or a sourdough starter, boil it in water for 10 minutes. This will destroy any undesirable bacteria that are present in the jar so that only the desirable ones from the starter will be grown during the incubation period.

Yogurt: A dairy product that has been cultured with beneficial bacteria. Those bacteria are allowed to grow and multiply. The resulting product is thick and slightly tangy. If you're on the perfect diet, buy plain yogurt rather than vanilla or fruit-flavored. Read ingredient lists carefully to eliminate the tapioca, whey, and whey protein concentrate that are sometimes added. Also select yogurt with *live*, *active* or *viable* bacteria culture since these friendly bacteria are beneficial to the intestinal tract. Don't buy those pasteurized or heat-treated after culturing. (See page 241 for **Ways to Use Plain Yogurt**.) Low-fat yogurt is generally 1.5% fat by weight. Nonfat yogurt is the preferred type of yogurt to use rather than low-fat or whole milk yogurt.
Percent Calories From Fat: 48 in whole milk yogurt; 22 in low-fat; 0 in nonfat
Fat Grams In 1 Cup: 7 in whole milk yogurt; 4 in low-fat; less than 0.5 in nonfat

Dairy Recipes

Carob Yogurt

*If you have just started the perfect diet and you had been eating lots of sugar, you may not like this recipe. Wait a couple of weeks to try it—after your tastebuds have adjusted to the diet. (See **Stevia** on page 297 for an explanation about this herbal sweetener.)*

1 cup plain, nonfat yogurt
2 teaspoons carob powder
⅛ teaspoon powdered stevia

Mix ingredients together and serve. Makes one 1-cup or two ½-cup servings.

Carob-Mint Yogurt: Add 1 drop peppermint oil to Carob Yogurt. Use a dropper since you will get more than one drop if you pour it and the mint flavor will be too strong.

Percent Calories From Fat: 2
Total Fat Grams In Recipe: Less than 0.5

Super Yogurt Treat

This delicious treat for the perfect diet was developed by Ann Kirtley. It's also good without the fruit, but if you want a super treat, add a piece of fresh fruit!

¾ cup nonfat yogurt
1 to 3 teaspoons natural peanut butter, almond butter, or cashew butter
1 fresh fruit such as banana, apple, peach, or pear, chopped or sliced (optional)

Mix yogurt and nut butter in a bowl. Stir in optional fresh fruit. Serves 1 or 2.

Percent Calories From Fat: 22 using 1 teaspoon peanut butter, 27 using 3 teaspoons
Total Fat Grams In Recipe: 6 using 1 teaspoon peanut butter, 9 using 3 teaspoons

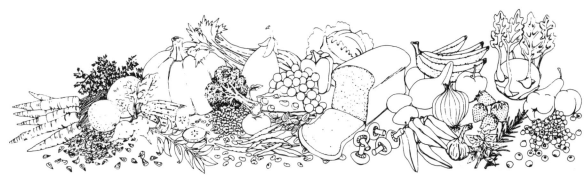

Stand still and consider the wondrous works of God.   **Job 37:14**

Lemon Yogurt

Why not liven up plain, nonfat yogurt with a drop of lemon oil!

1 cup plain, nonfat yogurt
1 or 2 drops pure lemon oil

Mix ingredients together and serve. Makes one 1-cup or two ½-cup servings.

Orange Yogurt: Use 1 or 2 drops of pure orange oil.

Percent Calories From Fat: 2
Total Fat Grams In Recipe: Less than 0.5

Spiced Yogurt

1 cup plain, nonfat yogurt
¼ teaspoon *Cinnamon Spice Blend* (p. 256), or more, to taste

Mix *Spice Blend* into yogurt and serve. Makes one 1-cup or two ½-cup servings.

Percent Calories From Fat: 2
Total Fat Grams In Recipe: Less than 0.5

Yogurt Cream Cheese

Here's a nonfat, cream cheese-type spread that you can make by draining the whey from either homemade or commercial plain, nonfat yogurt. (Don't use yogurt with gelatin as an ingredient since it keeps the whey from separating out.) Special yogurt cheese funnels are available in kitchen specialty shops. Or, you can use cheesecloth to make yogurt cheese.

2 cups plain, nonfat yogurt (without gelatin)

If you are using cheesecloth, you'll need a couple of layers of 12-inch squares. Place yogurt in the center of the two-ply square and pull ends together, fastening with a rubber band. Place yogurt bundle, rubber band end up, in a large funnel sitting in a tall glass. Place it in the refrigerator to drain for about 14 hours for cream cheese consistency. You can drain the yogurt up to 24 hours or as little as 6 hours for a thicker or thinner cheese. Remove cheese from the cloth and refrigerate in an airtight container. (Wash cheesecloth thoroughly and it can be re-used. 2 cups yogurt makes approximately 1 cup yogurt cream cheese.

Percent Calories From Fat: 1
Total Fat Grams In Recipe: 1

Homemade Yogurt

Through trial and error, I have found that my best homemade yogurt is made using non-instant nonfat milk powder, water, and a heating pad. Using the instant variety of milk powder or skim milk has not been successful for me. If, for some reason, your yogurt does not thicken, all is not lost. Use the liquid yogurt-milk in cooking.

¼ cup fresh nonfat, plain yogurt (homemade or fresh commercial with active yogurt cultures and no stabilizers like gelatin or tapioca added)
1 cup non-instant nonfat milk powder (should be fresh)
1 quart jar with lid, both sterilized in boiling water and cooled
Metal slotted spoon and measuring cups, sterilized
Blender with blender container sterilized
3½ cups warm water (100° F.)
A heating pad
Large, clean, heavy towel

- Turn heating pad on medium heat in a protected area. Cover with a large towel folded in half.
- Pour 1 cup of the warm water into the blender and the remainder into the jar. Turn blender on low and add the milk powder and yogurt. As soon as the mixture is smooth, turn it off and pour the mixture into the jar of water. If foam has formed, skim it off with a slotted spoon. Stir to combine liquids.
- Place jar on heating pad, between towel halves so that both jar and heating pad are completely covered.
- Check yogurt after 3 hours. If the yogurt is finished, it will be slightly set or firm. If it is not set, cover and check again every 30 minutes. When it is ready, gently move it to the refrigerator without disturbing it and without adding a lid. Even a bump before it has cooled could make the whey or liquid separate out. Make certain there is room all around the jar so that cold air can circulate.
- When cool, add lid to jar. Makes 1 quart.

Percent Calories From Fat: 2
Total Fat Grams In Recipe: 1

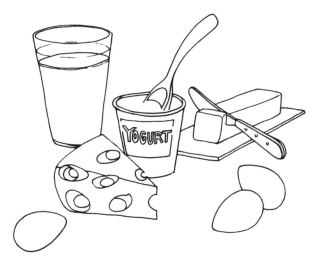

Buttermilk

½ cup cultured buttermilk (homemade or commercial with no stabilizers like gelatin or tapioca added)
1 cup non-instant nonfat milk powder
1-quart jar with lid, sterilized in boiling water
Almost 3½ cups water, slightly above room temperature (about 80°)
Metal slotted spoon and measuring cup, sterilized in boiling water
Blender with blender container sterilized in boiling water

Pour 1 cup of the water into the blender container. Add remaining water to the quart jar. Turn blender on low and add the milk powder and buttermilk. As soon as the mixture is smooth, turn blender off and pour the milk-mixture into the jar of water, stirring to combine. If there is foam on top, skim it off with a slotted spoon. Add lid to jar and let sit in a warm spot for 6 to 8 hours or until slightly thickened. Refrigerate. Use some of this buttermilk to start your next batch.

Perfect Whole Foods: Read commercial buttermilk labels carefully so you won't buy those with starch or buttermilk flakes (containing whey) added.
Percent Calories From Fat: 3
Total Fat Grams In Recipe: 2

Variation: Use warmed (about 80°) commercial skim or ½-percent milk in place of the milk powder and water. You do not need to use a blender if you use liquid milk. Simply mix starter and milk together.

Kefir from Starter

3 tablespoons fresh, plain, low-fat kefir (commercial or homemade)
Almost 1 quart skim milk
1-quart jar, sterilized in boiling water
Metal slotted spoon, measuring cup and pan, all sterilized

Heat milk to room temperature (70 to 80°). Add kefir to milk. Stir with sterilized spoon. Cover and let sit, undisturbed, for 24 hours at room temperature. Refrigerate.

Perfect Whole Foods: Do not use commercial kefir that has a sweetener added.
Percent Calories From Fat: 6
Total Fat Grams In Recipe: 2

Variation: To use non-instant nonfat milk powder, reconstitute 1 cup in 1 cup water (room temperature) in a blender and add kefir starter. As soon as the mixture is smooth, turn it off and add it to almost 3 cups of water. If foam has formed, skim it off with a sterilized slotted spoon. Cover and let sit, as directed above.

TOPPINGS

In this section, I've grouped together several foods that don't belong in other categories yet don't need their own section. If a food doesn't fit into the category of **Main Dishes, Whole Grains, Vegetables, Whole Grain Breads, Dairy, Beverages, Fruits**, or **Desserts**, then you'll probably find it in this section. I've included discussions or recipes for seasonings, salt, dressings, syrups, sauces, gravies, dips, nuts, nut butters, and nut milks.

So many everyday sauces, dips, gravies, and dressings that we Americans typically eat add undesirable salt, sugar, white flour, or fat. While many recipes in this section are not totally lacking in fat and salt, they contain no sugar or white flour. The amount of salt used is much less than in comparable processed foods. Omit the salt entirely if you wish.

Check the **Quick Reference for Name Brand Products** beginning on page 360 for brands of commercial spaghetti sauce, pizza sauce, salad dressing, mayonnaise, peanut butter, and nut butter prepared without refined carbohydrates. Always read the ingredient lists before purchasing these products to make certain the ingredients have not been changed since this book was published.

Remember that homemade dressings and sauces are much less expensive than commercial ones. When you make them yourself, you can also control the amount and kind of oils and salt. I like to store homemade dressings in empty, thoroughly cleaned commercial dressing bottles. The bottles with plastic lids are best because acid ingredients like vinegar or lemon juice will not react with plastic as they do with metal.

Topping Facts

Almond Butter: A good-tasting nut butter made from either raw or roasted almonds.
Percent Calories From Fat: 81
Fat Grams In 1 Tablespoon: 9

Arrowroot: A starchy thickening agent derived from a tropical tuber. Because arrowroot is refined like cornstarch, eliminate it from the *Perfect Whole Foods* diet. Instead, use a whole grain flour for thickening. For a liberal diet, you may use arrowroot or cornstarch; use the same amount of arrowroot as you would cornstarch. Don't, however, bring the arrowroot liquid to a boil as you would cornstarch. Stop cooking it as soon as it thickens or the boiled arrowroot will thin back down.

Bouillon Cubes and Broth Powders: Most of these products have sugar or starch added and should not be used on the perfect diet. They also usually contain MSG or hydrolyzed protein of which MSG is a component. I have found a product suitable for the perfect diet and without MSG. *Gayelord Hauser's All Natural Vegetable Broth* powder is excellent used as a broth (1 rounded teaspoon to a cup of hot water) or as a tasty seasoning blend. Before using it on the perfect diet, since products can change, read the ingredient list carefully to make certain undesirable ingredients have not been added.

Cashew Butter: A good-tasting nut butter spread made from cashews. It is available commercially made from raw or roasted cashews. If oil has separated out, store the jar upside down for a few days before opening it and shake it occasionally to mix the oil with the cashew butter. After opening, store cashew butter (and all high-fat products) in the refrigerator.
Percent Calories From Fat: 74
Fat Grams In 1 Tablespoon: 8

Cornstarch: A highly refined corn product. It should not be used on the *Perfect Whole Foods* diet. Thicken sauces and gravies with whole grain flour, substituting three times as much whole wheat flour if a recipe calls for cornstarch.

Crushed Red Pepper: A hot spice also known as *pizza pepper* and used in Mexican and Italian foods.

Diastatic Malt Powder: A whole foods sweetener made from sprouted, dried, and ground grains. It may be used on the perfect diet since it is a whole food that has not been refined.
You can prepare diastatic malt using the recipe on page 209. Do not use other malt products while on *Perfect Whole Foods* since they are concentrated sweeteners.

Flaxseed Oil: In its fresh form, flax oil is an excellent source of the Omega-3 fatty acid. Since the essential polyunsaturated fatty acids are fragile, do not cook flax oil; use it raw. You can also buy whole flaxseeds and grind them in a nut/seed grinder as an Omega-3 source. To release the oil, you must grind the seeds rather than eat them whole.
Percent Calories From Fat: 100
Total Fat Grams In 1 Teaspoon: 5

Gelatin: An incomplete animal protein product which when dissolved in a liquid and refrigerated forms a gel. 1 envelope = 2¼ teaspoons.

Ghee: Ghee, or clarified butter, is butter in which the water-soluble milk solids are removed. When butter is used for frying or sautéing, it is the milk solids that can burn and turn black. The milk solids are the most perishable part of butter. Ghee is traditionally used in Indian and French cooking. See page 259 for instructions for making ghee.

Ginger: Fresh ginger root should be firm when bought and then stored in a plastic bag in the refrigerator to keep it from drying out. Use it as a seasoning by thinly slicing, grating, or mincing the root. It's not necessary to remove the thin outer skin before using. When recipes call for *fresh ginger*, you'll have better results if you use the fresh rather than substituting *powdered ginger*.

Guar Gum: A natural fiber from the legume *guar*. Use guar gum as a thickener in foods that do not need to be cooked as in dressings. You may use it on the **Perfect Whole Foods** diet.

Herbs: ⅓ to ½ teaspoon dried herbs = 1 teaspoon fresh herbs.
½ teaspoon powdered herbs = 1 teaspoon leaf herbs.

Kelp: A sea vegetable that contains many trace minerals. Use the powdered form as a seasoning.

Kuzu (also spelled kudzu): (pronounced KOO-zoo) A tasteless and easily digested Japanese thickening agent. Dissolve kuzu in a cool liquid before boiling it to thicken. When adding the dissolved kuzu to a hot liquid, add it slowly while stirring constantly to prevent lumping. If it is purchased in chunks too large to measure easily, pound kuzu into smaller pieces before measuring. Eliminate kuzu from the **Perfect Whole Foods** diet. Use the following proportions to determine the amount of kuzu you should use for a liberal diet:
1 tablespoon kuzu per cup liquid = thin sauce for stir-fried vegetables.
2 tablespoons kuzu per cup liquid = gravy consistency.

Mayonnaise: Two brands of sugar-free mayonnaise, *Duke's* and *Mrs. Clark's*, are available. Make certain you buy the *regular*, not *light* varieties which contain sugar and starch. I've included a recipe for *Egg-Free Soy Mayonnaise* (p. 266) in case you can't find the commercial sugar-free mayonnaises. Although recipes are available for making mayonnaise with eggs, I don't recommend them since the eggs are not cooked. (Raw eggs can have been linked to salmonella poisoning.)

Miso: (pronounced MEE-so) A flavorful, fermented soybean paste, with or without added grains, that is used in soups and stews and sometimes used in sauces, dips, and spreads. In general, milder misos are lighter in color and are combined with a grain. Do not use *white miso* if you are on the perfect diet since it is made from refined rice. Some other grains added to miso can be refined also. If the label does not make it clear that the grain is whole, then buy the miso made without grains for the perfect diet. Buy miso that is unpasteurized and keep it in the refrigerator. Unpasteurized miso is a *live* food, rich in beneficial bacteria and enzymes. To add to soups, blend a little broth with the miso and stir the broth back into the soup. Do not boil

after the miso is added or the live components will be destroyed. To make a tasty broth, dissolve a small amount of miso in hot water. Since miso is salty, you will likely not need to add more salt to foods you prepare with miso.
Percent Calories From Fat: 11
Fat Grams In 1 Tablespoon: Less than 0.5

Miso, Natto: A chunky miso used as a condiment. Since one of its ingredients is barley malt, do not use natto miso on the **Perfect Whole Foods** diet.

Mustard: Most commercially prepared mustard is made without sugar or refined starch. Occasionally, however, sugars and starches are included, so check the ingredient list carefully before buying mustard if you are on the perfect diet.

Nutritional Yeast: This is a good tasting, non-leavening yeast that can be used for flavoring popcorn or vegetables and is a good source of B vitamins, including vitamin B-12. Nutritional yeast has a cheesy taste. Don't substitute brewer's yeast or torula yeast in recipes that call for nutritional yeast since the flavor is not the same. (All types are okay for the perfect diet.)

Olive Oil, Pure: Is usually extracted from the olives with chemical solvents. Virgin olive oil is a better choice.

Olive Oil, Virgin: Virgin olive oil is the term that denotes a high quality, low heat, no solvent product. *Extra virgin* is unrefined oil that comes from the first pressing (most delicate flavor and most expensive), *fine virgin* from the second pressing, and *virgin* from the third pressing (more acidic and least expensive of the virgin oils).
Percent Calories From Fat: 100
Total Fat Grams In 1 Teaspoon: 5

Peanut Butter, Natural: Natural peanut butter is simply peanuts ground into a spread. Salt is sometimes added. Keep all nut butters (and nuts) refrigerated and stir the oil, if it separates, back into the nut butter before using. Most commercial peanut butter has sugar, hydrogenated fat, and salt added.
Percent Calories From Fat: 77
Fat Grams In 1 Tablespoon: 8

Pecan Butter: A delicious nut butter that can easily be made in your food processor (see recipe on page 259).
Percent Calories From Fat: 94
Fat Grams In 1 Tablespoon: 8

Pecan Meal: Finely ground pecans that are used for topping cooked cereals as well as using in desserts. Make certain commercial pecan meal is fresh, not rancid. (Do not eat any fats that are rancid.)
Percent Calories From Fat: 94
Fat Grams In 1 Tablespoon: 4

Pine Nuts: Also called pignolias. These are small, buttery, and sweet-tasting nuts.
Percent Calories From Fat: 87
Fat Grams In 1 Tablespoon: 5

Potato Flour: A highly refined potato product. Do not use it on the perfect diet.

Potato Starch: A highly refined potato product. Do not use it on the perfect diet.

Safflower Oil: Safflower oil is available in a number of forms. Regular or polyunsaturated safflower oil (preferably unrefined) can be used raw as a source of essential fatty acids. High-oleic or monounsaturated safflower oil is available in expeller-pressed (refined) form and is sometimes used for moderately-high-temperature cooking, as in stir-frying. For more information about oils, see page 44.
Percent Calories From Fat: 100
Total Fat Grams In 1 Teaspoon: 5

Salt: Be selective when choosing salt. Iodized table salt has sugar added, usually dextrose, to stabilize the iodine. Both iodized and non-iodized commercial salts are heated to very high temperatures (1200-1500° F.) to remove moisture and combine the salt with the additives. Other additives include sodium bicarbonate (a bleaching agent) and an aluminum compound (an anti-caking agent). Some medical scientists believe that the extremely high heat as well as additives make salt a greater health risk than it need be. Rather than commercial table salt, use modest amounts of unrefined, unheated (solar-dried rather than kiln-dried) mineral, sea, or rock salt. These salts contain trace amounts of natural minerals (including iodine) in addition to sodium and chloride.

Salt in Processed Foods for the *Perfect Whole Foods* Diet: In general, it's safe to assume that the salt added to processed food does not have sugar added since manufacturers purchase the least expensive form of salt—non-iodized. Products made by natural foods companies often use sea salt and will list it with the ingredients.

Salt, Mineral: Mineral salt is a natural source of minerals in addition to sodium chloride. Also, it has no sugar or dextrose added as table salt often does. True mineral salt, very difficult to obtain, is approximately 13% trace minerals, 80% sodium chloride, and 7% moisture. *Lima* Sea Salt, available in some food co-ops and health food stores, is probably one of the best unrefined mineral salts sold today. Its sodium chloride content is almost 94%, higher than true mineral salt but lower than other salts available in natural food stores. *Lima* Sea Salt has not been chemically treated and is solar evaporated.

Salt, Rock: Another salt that is not refined nor subjected to heat. Pure rock salt also has a natural balance of minerals in addition to sodium and chloride.

Salt, Sea: Sea salt has no sugar added unless it is iodized. The degree of processing greatly varies from one product to another. Sea salt generally has 2 to 3% minerals in addition to sodium and chloride. Select solar-dried rather than kiln-dried sea salt.

Sesame Butter: A sesame seed butter made from *roasted, unhulled* sesame seeds. (Sesame butter made using *raw unhulled* seeds is very bitter.) *Tahini* (sometimes called *sesame tahini*), another type of sesame seed butter, is made from raw or roasted, *hulled* sesame seeds. Sesame butter is richest in flavor, tahini made from roasted seeds is milder than sesame butter, and tahini made from raw seeds is the mildest of the three. Since they are interchangeable, select the one whose flavor you enjoy the most.
Percent Calories From Fat: 84 for sesame butter and tahini
Fat Grams In 1 Tablespoon: 10 for sesame butter and tahini

Sesame Oil, Unrefined: A monounsaturated oil that is suitable for cooking. For more information on oils, see page 44.
Percent Calories From Fat: 100
Fat Grams In 1 Teaspoon: 5

Sesame Seeds, Hulled: Tiny, creamy-white seeds with the hull or husk removed. They are used with the perfect diet. Although hulled sesame seeds have less calcium than unhulled ones, the calcium in the hull is not available to the body since it is combined with oxalic acid (p.162).
Percent Calories From Fat: 84
Fat Grams In 1 Tablespoon: 4

Sesame Seeds, Unhulled: Tiny, light brown seeds with hull or husk intact. They are used with **Perfect Whole Foods**.

Shoyu Sauce: (pronounced shoy-U) A naturally-fermented soy sauce that is used on the perfect diet if alcohol is not added as a preservative. Read the ingredient list carefully.

Sodium Restriction: If you need to restrict the sodium in your diet, then restrict the following high sodium foods and ingredients that are typically used on the **Perfect Whole Foods** diet: sea, mineral, and rock salt, shoyu and tamari soy sauces, miso, baking soda, canned tuna and salmon, cheese, olives, many canned tomato products like *V-8 Juice* and tomato sauce, prepared mustard, salad dressings, and some whole grain crackers, breads, salted peanut butter, and salted nuts. (*Rumford* Baking Powder, while a preferred product due to its being without the aluminum in most baking powders, is still a high-sodium ingredient. It is used only with a liberal whole foods diet.)

Soy Sauce: See **Shoyu Sauce** and **Tamari Soy Sauce** in this list.

Sunflower Butter: A nut butter made from sunflower seeds.

Sunflower Seeds: Make certain you buy fresh sunflower seeds since they become rancid when stored improperly or too long. Sometimes the rancid flavor of roasted seeds is concealed with a heavy dose of salt. Raw sunflower seeds are more likely to be fresh if they are even-colored and unbroken.
Percent Calories From Fat: 76
Fat Grams In 1 Tablespoon: 9

Tahini: (pronounced ta-HEE-ne) Sesame seed butter made from raw or roasted hulled seeds. See **Sesame Butter** on page 254 for a comparison of *sesame butter* and *tahini*.
Percent Calories From Fat: 84
Fat Grams In 1 Tablespoon: 10

Tabasco Sauce: A product made from peppers which can be used with the perfect diet.

Tamari Soy Sauce: This is a naturally-fermented soy sauce that is made from soybeans, water, salt, and sometimes wheat and alcohol. Naturally fermented soy sauce is sometimes called shoyu. For the **Perfect Whole Foods** diet, select a brand of tamari or shoyu soy sauce with no alcohol added as a preservative. Use sparingly since soy sauce is very high in sodium. Most brands of soy sauce from the grocery store are made of soy flakes or defatted soybean meal plus sugar, chemicals, and alcohol.

Tapioca: A refined starchy thickener prepared from the cassava root. Don't use on perfect diet.

Thickeners: Don't use cornstarch, potato starch, potato flour, arrowroot, tapioca, and kuzu while on **Perfect Whole Foods**, and use whole wheat flour or other whole grain flour as a thickener. Read about these specific thickeners in this section.

Vanilla Extract: Use alcohol-free vanilla extract (commercial or homemade) while on the perfect diet. You can also use the vanilla bean. Do not use artificial vanilla called vanillin.

Vinegar: A product, usually made from fruit juice, that results from fermentation of the fruit sugar into alcohol. The alcohol is then converted into an acid by bacteria. Vinegar can be used on the **Perfect Whole Foods** diet. Buy raw (unpasteurized) vinegars, either apple cider, wine, or malt, with sediment in the bottles. Shake the bottles well before using. This sediment, called the *mother*, is a mixture of beneficial bacteria and enzymes. Avoid distilled vinegar.

Vinegar, Balsamic: A variety of aged Italian vinegar that is deep reddish brown. It has a slightly sweet taste and is good sprinkled over a vegetable salad for a zero fat, zero calorie dressing. It can be used with the perfect diet.

Walnuts, Black and English: Good-tasting nuts and good sources of essential fatty acids. Store shelled nuts in the refrigerator or freezer.
Percent Calories From Fat: 85 and 88, respectively
Fat Grams In 1 Tablespoon: 5

Whole Wheat Flour for Thickening: Refined white flour is often used for thickening sauces and gravies. Since white flour is not used on the perfect diet, whole wheat flour can be used as a thickener instead. Whole wheat flour has less thickening ability than white flour since whole grains are made up of the germ and bran as well as starch, the thickening agent. White flour contains a greater percentage of starch and, therefore, more thickening ability. When substituting whole wheat flour for white flour in a recipe for sauces and gravies, use one-half more whole wheat flour than white flour. For example, if your recipe calls for 2 tablespoons white flour, use 3 tablespoons whole wheat or other whole grain flour.

Topping Recipes

Cereal or Yogurt Toppers

If you are new to whole foods and find oatmeal and other cooked whole grains rather bland, especially without sugar, remember that your taste for whole foods will change. Your taste for foods will become enhanced so that, rather than being bland, grains will each have a unique flavor. In the meantime, try adding two or three of these toppings to your cooked cereals. All except two are allowed on the perfect diet. Serve with or without milk, unsweetened soy milk, or nut milk (see recipe below), as desired. You can also add these toppings to plain yogurt for a delicious breakfast.

Raw seed mixture (sunflower, pumpkin, sesame, etc.), soaked in water at least overnight in the refrigerator - a jar full will stay fresh almost a week
Freshly ground flaxseeds
Fresh nut pieces (pecans, almonds, etc.)
Fresh or frozen fruit (frozen berries are delicious, convenient, and very nutritious!)

Cinnamon Spice Blend (see below)
Dried fruit (raisins, apricot pieces, etc.)
Unsweetened coconut
Diastatic Malt Powder (p. 209)
Dash of cinnamon or nutmeg
Alcohol-free vanilla (commercial or homemade)
Pinch of stevia (p. 296)

Perfect Whole Foods: Omit dried fruit and coconut.

Nut Milk

Use this dairy-free nut milk over cereals, in quick breads, or in sauces in place of milk. Dilute nut milks with water for less fat and a milder flavor.

¼ cup raw nuts or seeds (such as almonds, cashew nuts, sunflower seeds, or sesame seeds)

Soak nuts or seeds in 2 cups of water overnight in the refrigerator. Place in blender and process about 2 or 3 minutes. Strain, if desired, and use the residue in cooked cereals and breads. Makes about 2 cups.

Percent Calories From Fat: 81 (using almonds and not straining)
Fat Grams In 1 Cup: 8 (using almonds and not straining)

Cinnamon Spice Blend

Use a dash of this spice blend to top cooked cereals, plain yogurt, or a baked sweet potato. It will add a unique taste.

1 teaspoon finely grated orange or lemon peel (if using fresh peel, let stand uncovered for an hour or so to dry out)
1 teaspoon each of ground nutmeg, ground cloves, and ground ginger
2 teaspoons ground cinnamon

Mix ingredients together and store in an airtight container.

Homemade Alcohol-Free Vanilla

For the perfect diet, either use this recipe or buy the commercial variety made with glycerine.

4 to 8 vanilla beans
⅔ cup warm water
2 teaspoons liquid lecithin

Soak beans in water for several hours, then blend in blender on high speed until beans are very fine. Bring mixture to a boil in a covered pan. Pour into jar and cover tightly. Let it sit overnight. Strain, put back into blender, add lecithin while blending on low speed, and pour into a bottle with a tight-fitting lid. Store in the refrigerator.

Percent Calories From Fat: 100 for lecithin only (Figures are not available for vanilla beans.)
Total Fat Gram In Recipe: 9 from lecithin

Apple Butter

1 cup dried apple pieces
1 cup apple juice or water
⅛ teaspoon ground cinnamon
Pinch ground cloves

Combine ingredients and let sit at room temperature until apples absorb juice. Blend in food processor or blender until smooth.   Place in a covered jar and store in the refrigerator. Makes 1½ cups.

Perfect Whole Foods: No
Percent Calories From Fat: 2
Total Fat Grams In Recipe: 1

Apricot Preserves

My friend Rita Hardman makes this recipe regularly and serves it at breakfast on whole grain toast.

1 cup very finely diced dried apricots (cut with scissors)
1 cup apple juice or water

Combine ingredients in a pint jar with a lid and let sit at room temperature until apricots absorb the juice. Refrigerate and serve on whole grain toast. Makes 1½ cups.

Perfect Whole Foods: No, because of dried fruit and juice.
Percent Calories From Fat: 2
Total Fat Grams In Recipe: 1

Malted Syrup

One of my clients, while on the perfect diet, developed this simple recipe for syrup.

1 teaspoon butter
2 tablespoons skim milk or water
¼ cup diastatic malt powder (p. 209 and 195)

Melt butter in a small saucepan. Add liquid and diastatic malt powder, stirring over low heat only until ingredients are mixed well.

Percent Calories From Fat: 27
Total Fat Grams In Recipe: 5

Orange-Banana Syrup

1 large ripe banana
⅓ cup orange juice

Blend ingredients in food processor or blender, and serve immediately. Good served over pancakes. Makes about ¾ cup.

Perfect Whole Foods: No, because of the orange juice.
Percent Calories From Fat: 5
Total Fat Grams In Recipe: 1

Strawberry-Banana Syrup: Add a few fresh or frozen and partially-thawed unsweetened strawberries.

Sunshine Butter

Here's a recipe for a delicious butter spread that provides beneficial essential fatty acids from flax seed oil. Don't use it if you must restrict your saturated fats because of high blood cholesterol.

1 stick butter (½ cup), softened
½ cup fresh flaxseed oil

Blend ingredients together in a blender or food processor or with a hand blender. Store in the refrigerator in an airtight, opaque container that excludes light. Return to the refrigerator immediately after using it. Makes 1 cup.

Percent Calories From Fat: 100
Fat Grams In 1 Teaspoon: 4

Ghee

Ghee, or clarified butter as it is sometimes called, can be used for frying or sautéing. It won't scorch and turn black as will butter since the milk solids have been removed. Butterfat is more stable to high temperature cooking than many other fat and is a wonderful flavor-enhancer of foods.

1 pound unsalted butter

Melt butter in a heavy pan and bring it to a boil, immediately reducing the heat to simmer. Skim off the white foam as it accumulates on top and thickens. Do not stir; leave the bottom milk-solid layer and middle oily layer alone. The oily layer will become clear and the bottom layer will become golden brown. However, don't let the bottom layer actually burn. Continue to simmer until all of the water is evaporated, about 20 minutes. You'll know that the water is evaporated when the bubbling stops and the sound changes to a hissing frying sound. Remove from heat quickly and cool. Pour the ghee or oil into a covered opaque container such as a crock. Use the browned sediment for seasoning vegetables or adding to breads. Ghee can be stored at room temperature or in the refrigerator. Makes about 1¾ cups.

Percent Calories From Fat: 100
Fat Grams In 1 Teaspoon: 5

Roasted Nuts

Raw nuts or seeds, shelled or unshelled (select from almonds, peanuts, sunflower seeds, etc.)

Preheat oven to 300°. In a shallow pan, roast nuts in a single layer, stirring occasionally. Shelled nuts should be cooked for 15 to 25 minutes and unshelled for 20 to 40, the exact time depending upon the thickness of the nuts. Cool and store in an airtight container in the refrigerator.

Percent Calories From Fat: Most vary from 70 to 85. (Chestnuts are about 10 percent fat.)
Fat Grams In 1 Tablespoon: 4 to 5 (Chestnuts, less than 0.5)

Pecan Butter

It doesn't take much of this scrumptious nut butter to add a welcome bit of flavor to toast or crackers.

2 cups raw pecan pieces

In blender or food processor with blade attachment, process pecans until they become creamy. You may need to stop the machine occasionally and stir nuts with a spatula to make certain they all become processed. Makes 1 scant cup.

Percent Calories From Fat: 94
Fat Grams In 1 Tablespoon: 8

Raw Walnut Butter: Use English or black walnuts in place of pecans.
Raw Pumpkin Seed Butter: Use pumpkin seeds (shelled) in place of pecans.

Creamy Spinach Dip

Anita Courtney, community nutritionist at the Lexington-Fayette County Health Department, developed this reduced-fat version of spinach dip. Serve it with fresh, crunchy vegetables such as carrots, celery, broccoli, and cauliflower.

10-ounce package frozen chopped spinach, thawed
2 cups plain, nonfat yogurt
1 tablespoon mayonnaise
½ cup finely chopped green onions
½ cup finely chopped fresh parsley
¼ teaspoon salt
⅛ teaspoon black pepper

Place thawed spinach in a colander and drain well, squeezing out excess moisture. Combine ingredients in food processor bowl and, using blade attachment, mix until spinach is finely chopped. Makes 3½ cups.

Perfect Whole Foods: Make certain mayonnaise is unsweetened.
Percent Calories From Fat 26
Fat Grams In ¼ Cup: 1

Claire's Famous Yogurt Dip

This is great for dipping carrots, celery, broccoli, cauliflower, or whole wheat pita strips. Makes a tasty salad dressing, too!

1 cup plain, nonfat yogurt
1 small onion, finely minced
¼ teaspoon chili powder
¼ teaspoon dill weed
Few drops of *Tabasco Sauce*
¼ teaspoon raw cider vinegar

Mix ingredients and refrigerate for at least two hours. Makes about 1½ cups.

Percent Calories From Fat: 1
Total Fat Grams In Recipe: Less than 0.5

Eggplant Dip

Try this Middle Eastern dip (sometimes called Baba Ghanouj) with toasted pita bread that has been cut into wedges and with fresh vegetables. If you take it to a party or picnic, be sure to take a copy of the recipe along with you. You'll get requests!

1 medium eggplant
½ teaspoon salt
1 to 2 cloves garlic, minced
¼ cup lemon juice
3 tablespoons tahini
1 tablespoon olive oil
¼ teaspoon cumin or chili powder
1 tablespoon fresh parsley, snipped with scissors into tiny pieces

Preheat oven to 375°. Bake eggplant on a cookie sheet for about 45 minutes or until tender. Cool slightly and remove peel. Place pulp in food processor bowl with blade attachment. Add salt, garlic, lemon juice, tahini, oil, and cumin or chili powder, processing until smooth. Pour into serving bowl and let sit about 30 minutes at room temperature. Garnish with parsley just before serving. Makes 2 or 3 cups.

Perfect Whole Foods: Substitute ¼ cup water plus 2 or 3 drops of lemon oil for the lemon juice.
Percent Calories From Fat: 62
Total Fat Grams In Recipe: 31

Loretta's Tofu Guacamole

For a small party or family, make one-third of this recipe. I sometimes make this guacamole without the tofu by mixing 1 pureed avocado with about ¼ jar Pace Mild Picante Sauce. Whether you use the tofu or not, serve guacamole with baked corn chips, fresh veggies, or taco salad.

⅓ pound tofu
16-ounce jar medium *Pace* Picante Sauce (use mild or hot if you like)
3 medium avocados
2 large cloves garlic, minced optional
Juice from 1 lemon, optional

Pureé the tofu and avocados in a food processor or mash with fork. Combine with the Picante Sauce and optional garlic and lemon juice. Makes 4 or 5 cups.

Perfect Whole Foods: Omit baked chips unless the package says they are made from whole grain corn. Omit lemon juice or substitute 2 tablespoons water plus 1 drop of lemon oil.
Percent Calories From Fat: 72
Fat Grams In 2 Tablespoons: 3

Amy's Guacamole

The employees at Good Foods Co-op prepare this recipe for sampling in the store. Each employee who makes it adds his or her special touch. It's never exactly the same, but always delicious! Here's Amy Brown's version. Reduce the amounts if you're making it for a small group.

4 avocados
1 large tomato, cut into cubes
3 cloves garlic, minced
1 red onion, chopped
Juice of ½ lime or lemon
1 teaspoon or more cumin
Dash of cayenne

Mash avocados and stir in remaining ingredients. Serve immediately with baked corn chips or raw vegetables. Makes about 6 cups.

Perfect Whole Foods: Don't use baked chips unless the package says they are whole grain. Substitute 1 tablespoon water plus 1 drop lemon oil for the lime or lemon juice.
Percent Calories From Fat: 74
Fat Grams In ¼ Cup: 5

Homemade Catsup

Since most commercial catsup is about one-third sugar, you may want to try this recipe even if you're not on the perfect diet. (Or try Westbrae's Un-ketchup, *a delicious unsweetened commercial product.)*

6-ounce can tomato paste
2 tablespoons raw cider vinegar
3 tablespoons water
¼ teaspoon salt
½ teaspoon dried oregano
¼ teaspoon granulated garlic
Pinch of cumin, nutmeg, and black pepper
Pinch of stevia extract, optional (see page 297)
¼ teaspoon prepared mustard

Mix ingredients together and refrigerate in a covered jar. Makes slightly more than 1 cup.

Percent Calories From Fat: 5
Total Fat Grams In Recipe: 9

Herbed Buttermilk Dressing

1 cup buttermilk; plain, nonfat yogurt; or plain kefir
½ teaspoon granulated onion
1 garlic clove, minced
¼ teaspoon paprika
1 teaspoon raw cider vinegar
2 tablespoons lemon or lime juice
Pinch of crushed red pepper
Dashes of cinnamon, coriander, and cumin
¾ teaspoon guar gum, optional (don't use with yogurt)

Place buttermilk or kefir in a jar with tight-fitting lid or place yogurt in mixing bowl. Combine dry ingredients together and add to buttermilk, kefir, or yogurt. Cover jar with lid and shake until dry ingredients are mixed in and buttermilk or kefir is slightly thickened. With yogurt in bowl, use a spoon to mix ingredients. If guar gum is not used, the buttermilk or kefir will not thicken, but the dressing will taste the same. Allow dressing to sit in the refrigerator for at least an hour for flavors to blend. Shake or stir before serving. Makes 1⅛ cups.

Perfect Whole Foods: Substitute 1 drop of lemon oil for the lemon or lime juice.
Percent Calories From Fat: 16 using 1% fat buttermilk
Total Fat Grams In Recipe: 2 using 1% fat buttermilk

Zero Dressing

1 cup tomato juice
1 tablespoon raw cider vinegar or lemon juice
⅛ teaspoon pepper
⅛ teaspoon garlic powder
¼ teaspoon dried oregano leaf
1 tablespoon finely chopped fresh onion or 1 teaspoon dried onion flakes
1 teaspoon fresh parsley, snipped with scissors into tiny pieces or ¼ teaspoon dried
½ teaspoon guar gum, optional

Place juice and vinegar in a jar. Combine dry ingredients together and add to jar. Cover with lid and shake until dry ingredients are mixed in and juice is slightly thickened. If guar gum is not used, juice will not thicken, but dressing will taste the same. Allow to sit in refrigerator for at least an hour for flavors to blend. Shake again before serving. Makes 1⅛ cups.

Perfect Whole Foods: Use vinegar, not lemon juice.
Percent Calories From Fat: 3
Total Fat Grams In Recipe: Less than 0.5

Thousand Island Dressing

My husband Jim has always liked Thousand Island Dressing. Here's my reduced-fat, no-sugar version.

¼ cup unsweetened catsup (homemade–*Homemade Catsup*, page 262 or
   commercial–*WestBrae's* Un-Ketchup)
¼ cup plain, nonfat yogurt
1 tablespoon mayonnaise (*Duke's* or *Mrs. Clark's*) or *Egg-Free Soy Mayonnaise* (p. 266)
2 teaspoons unsweetened dill pickle relish
2 teaspoons fresh parsley, snipped with scissors into tiny pieces

Combine ingredients together and store in the refrigerator in an airtight glass container. Makes
a little more than ½ cup.

Fat-Free Thousand Island Dressing: Omit the mayonnaise.

Percent Calories From Fat: 55
Fat Grams In 1 Tablespoon: 1

Blue Cheese-Yogurt Dressing

*This recipe uses yogurt instead of traditional mayonnaise and sour cream and, therefore, has much less
fat than most blue cheese dressings.*

1 cup plain, nonfat yogurt
¼ cup crumbled blue cheese
1 small clove garlic, pressed with garlic press or crushed with flat part of knife.

If garlic has large pieces remaining, finely mince them with knife. Mix ingredients together and
refrigerate in a non-metalic, airtight container at least an hour to blend flavors. Makes 1¼ cups.

Percent Calories From Fat: 53
Fat Grams In 1 Tablespoon: 1

Creamy Coleslaw Dressing

¼ cup unsweetened mayonnaise
½ cup plain nonfat yogurt
¼ cup raw cider vinegar
Salt and pepper, optional

Combine ingredients in bowl. Vary the amount of ingredients according to the quantity of
coleslaw you are preparing, but keep these proportions. Makes 1 cup. Stir this into your choice
of shredded or chopped cabbage, carrots, green peppers, and onions for a delicious slaw.

Percent Calories From Fat: 86
Fat Grams In 1 Tablespoon: 3

Herb Dressing

¼ cup water
¼ cup raw cider vinegar
½ cup oil
1 teaspoon dried onion flakes
½ teaspoon salt
⅛ teaspoon black pepper
½ teaspoon each: granulated garlic, dried oregano, dried parsley flakes, dried basil, and dried mustard powder

Measure ingredients into a glass bottle or jar. Cover, shake, and allow to sit in the refrigerator for at least an hour. Shake again before using. Makes about 1 cup.

Percent Calories From Fat: 98
Fat Grams In 1 Tablespoon: 7

Creamy Italian Dressing: Place above ingredients in a blender along with 1 teaspoon liquid lecithin. Whip until smooth and creamy. Store in bottle or jar in the refrigerator.

Anne-Sophie's Vinaigrette Dressing

One summer we had a French exchange student stay with us for a month. Anne-Sophie made an excellent salad dressing but measured none of the ingredients. I watched her closely several times so I could write the recipe down. Here are my instructions for making her dressing.

⅛ teaspoon salt
Dash pepper
1 to 2 teaspoons Dijon or mild yellow prepared mustard
4 tablespoons wine vinegar
8 tablespoons olive oil (or part olive plus part milder-tasting oil)

In a shallow bowl (Anne-Sophie used a cereal bowl), mix together the salt, pepper, mustard and vinegar. Slowly add the oil, drizzling a tablespoon at a time, while beating the mixture constantly with a tablespoon. Store in the refrigerator in a small jar and shake well before using. Makes ¾ cup.

Perfect Whole Foods: Use mustard without wine or sweetener.
Percent Calories From Fat: 95
Fat Grams In 1 Tablespoon: 9

Egg-Free Soy Mayonnaise

½ cup liquid soy milk (unsweetened)
½ cup oil
1 tablespoon raw cider vinegar
¼ teaspoon each salt, granulated onion, and paprika

Combine soy milk and half the oil in blender or food processor for a minute at high speed. Slowly drizzle the remaining oil. Add vinegar, salt, granulated onions, and paprika and blend until mixture thickens. Transfer into a glass jar, cover tightly, and refrigerate. Makes 1 cup.

Percent Calories From Fat: 99
Fat Grams In 1 Tablespoon: 7

Miso Dressing

The following recipe is delicious on vegetable salads and over steamed potatoes or brown rice. If you have very traditional taste, you may not like its earthy flavor.

1½ tablespoons miso (made with whole grains or no grains for perfect diet)
1 tablespoon grated fresh ginger
2 tablespoons raw apple cider vinegar
1 tablespoon tahini
⅜ cup oil (¼ cup + 2 tablespoons)

Using a blender, combine miso, ginger, vinegar, and tahini. Slowly add the oil while blender is going, as in making mayonnaise. Slowly add the ⅜ cup water (¼ cup + 2 tablespoons) and blend until thick and creamy. If ginger root is not blended until almost a liquid, then strain the dressing. Store in jar in the refrigerator. Makes over 1 cup.

Percent Calories From Fat: 87
Fat Grams In 1 Tablespoon: 5

Creamy Tahini

This non-dairy sauce is good as a mayonnaise-like spread for sandwiches. Or you can thin it with water and drizzled it cold over a vegetable salad, or warmed over cooked veggies, grains, or potatoes.

4 tablespoons tahini
½ teaspoon tamari or shoyu soy sauce (alcohol-free)
½ teaspoon granulated onion

Mix ingredients together with 4 tablespoons water in a small bowl or cup. Store in an airtight glass container in the refrigerator. Makes ½ cup.

Percent Calories From Fat: 69
Fat Grams in 1 Tablespoon: 4

Whole Grain Creamy Sauce

1 cup skim milk, divided
3 tablespoons whole grain flour (hard or soft wheat, triticale, whole barley, brown rice, spelt, etc.)
¼ teaspoon salt or herbs to taste

Begin heating ¾ cup milk in a small saucepan. In a measruing cup or bowl, blend the flour with the ¼ cup cold milk, stirring until free of lumps. Add flour-milk mixture to the warmed milk, stirring constantly. Stir and cook until uniformly thickened. Add salt or herbs. Makes slightly over 1 cup.

Percent Calories From Fat: 4
Total Fat Grams In Recipe: Less than 1

Thin Creamy Sauce: Use 1½ tablespoons whole grain flour.
Thick Creamy Sauce: Use 6 tablespoons whole grain flour.
Cheese Sauce: Stir into thickened sauce ½ cup shredded low-fat cheese, ¼ teaspoon paprika and ¼ teaspoon dry mustard.
Mushroom-Onion Sauce: Sauté ¼ cup chopped mushrooms and ¼ cup chopped onions in ½ teaspoon oil before adding the milk and flour as directed above.
Onion Sauce: Sauté ⅓ cup finely chopped onions in ½ teaspoon oil before adding the milk and flour as directed above.

Cheesy-Tamari Sauce

This sauce, used in French Style Rice *(p. 140), is also good served over steamed cauliflower or broccoli.*

4 tablespoons whole grain flour (wheat, barley, triticale, spelt, etc.)
¼ cup skim milk
¾ cup shredded low-fat cheese
1 to 2 teaspoons tamari or shoyu soy sauce (alcohol-free)

Begin by heating ¾ cup water in a small saucepan. In a cup or bowl, blend the flour with the skim milk, stirring until free of lumps. Add flour-milk mixture to the warm water, stirring constantly. Stir and cook until uniformly thickened. Add the cheese and tamari sauce, stirring until blended. Makes 1⅓ cups sauce.

Percent Calories From Fat: 38
Total Fat Grams In Recipe: 16

Quick Pasta Sauce

This recipe is almost as simple as opening a jar of spaghetti sauce. It does not, however, have added sugar as do most commercial brands. It is also much lower in salt and fat.

28 or 29-ounce can tomato pureé
1 tablespoon dried onion flakes
1 tablespoon dried parsley flakes
½ teaspoon granulated garlic
2 teaspoons dried basil
1 teaspoon dried oregano leaves
½ teaspoon dried thyme
½ teaspoon dried marjoram
⅛ teaspoon black pepper
1 bay leaf
½ to ¾ teaspoon salt, optional (don't use if tomato purée is salted)
1 to 3 teaspoons olive oil, optional

Combine ingredients in a quart jar along with 2 tablespoons water, stirring with a long spoon. Refrigerate for several hours, preferably all day. If you need the sauce immediately, simmer it for about 20 minutes. If the sauce is stored for several days, you will need to add additional water to make the right consistency. Makes about 1 quart sauce.

Percent Calories From Fat: 2 without oil; 10 using 1 teaspoon oil
Total Fat Grams In Recipe: 1 without oil; 5 using 1 teaspoon oil

Chunky Quick Pasta Sauce: Use canned crushed tomatoes in place of tomato pureé. Don't add salt if crushed tomatoes are salted.

Barbecue Sauce

This is good with leftover turkey or chicken. Simply cut leftovers into fine pieces and heat in some of the sauce. Use sauce also in preparing Barbecued Tempeh *on page 93.*

1 onion, chopped
1 green pepper, chopped
½ cup diced celery
3 cups tomato juice
6-ounce can tomato paste
2 tablespoons raw cider vinegar
⅛ teaspoon cayenne pepper
1 teaspoon tamari or shoyu soy sauce (alcohol-free)

Combine all ingredients in pan, bring to a boil, reduce heat, cover and simmer for 45 to 60 minutes. Makes 5 to 6 cups sauce.

Percent Calories From Fat: 2
Total Fat Grams In Recipe: 2

Creole Sauce

Serve this over cooked whole grains, beans, poultry or fish for a colorful, as well as flavorful, addition.

1 teaspoon oil
1 small onion, chopped
¼ cup chopped green pepper
1 cup sliced mushrooms
1 clove garlic, minced
1 rib celery, thinly sliced
1 tomato, chopped
1 cup tomato sauce (sugar-free and starch-free)

Sauté all vegetables, except tomato, in oil for about 5 minutes. Add chopped tomato and tomato sauce, bring to a gentle boil, and cook another 2 or 3 minutes. Makes about 3 cups.

Percent Calories From Fat: 26
Total Fat Grams In Recipe: 6

Seasoned Onions

These liven up any sandwich!

1 giant yellow onion, thinly sliced and separated into rings
2 teaspoons dried oregano leaves (do not use oregano powder)

In a plastic bag add onions and oregano. Add twist-tie to bag and then mix onions and oregano together. Refrigerate at least 24 hours before using.

Percent Calories From Fat: 5
Total Fat Grams In Recipe: 1

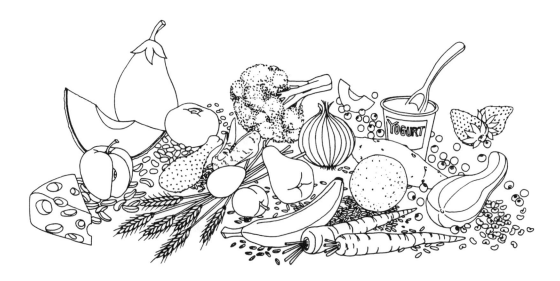

Onion Butter

Cook this in the oven while baking your potatoes or rice and use it as a delicious topping.

2 tablespoons ghee (p. 259) or butter
1 onion, chopped
1 clove garlic, minced

Preheat oven to 350 to 375°. The exact temperature depends on the temperature at which you're baking other food. Place all ingredients in small casserole, cover, and bake for approximately 1 hour.

Percent Calories From Fat: 85
Total Fat Grams In Recipe: 25

Sour Cream Substitutes

To avoid the fat of sour cream, use light sour cream if the ingredients are okay. Or use one of these substitutes.

• Plain, nonfat yogurt
• Low fat (1%) cottage cheese whipped in food processor with water, skim milk, broth, or lemon juice to the consistency of sour cream

Perfect Whole Foods: Do not use lemon juice.
Percent Calories From Fat: 4, yogurt; 13, cottage cheese
Total Fat Grams In Recipe: 1 in 2 cups of yogurt; 2 in 1 cup of cottage cheese

Herbed Tater Topper

For a baked potato topping, use one of the Sour Cream Substitutes *listed above and stir in one or two of these seasonings.*

Basil
Celery seed
Chopped chives
Dash of salt
Dill
Granulated garlic powder
Miso Dressing (p. 266)
Salsa

Creamy Tahini (p. 266)
Nutritional yeast
Granulated onion powder
Other herbs as desired
Paprika
Parsley
Prepared mustard

Another idea for a steaming hot baked potato topping is to sprinkle it with flaxseeds. The warm seeds give the potato an almost buttery taste.

FRUITS

Ripe, fresh, and whole are the most nutritious forms of fruits to eat. If you're on the **Perfect Whole Foods** diet, you'll quickly learn to appreciate the delicious flavor of naturally sweet fruit when you eliminate all other forms of sugar from your diet. If you're being treated for *Candida*, you will develop an even greater appreciation since you must omit fruit for a few months.

Fruit juice is not included on the **Perfect Whole Foods** diet because the fiber has been removed; what is left is concentrated fruit sugars. Without fiber, the fruit sugar is absorbed too quickly.

Although you should not use lemon and lime juice while on the perfect diet, you can use several products with fruit flavoring since they contain no concentrated fruit sugar. Even if you must eliminate fruit (on the *Candida* diet), you can use pure lemon, lime, and orange oil. These oils are good for flavoring plain yogurt. Don't use too much though; you only need a drop or two per cup of yogurt. You can also use the oil to make delicious muffins. See the *Lemon-Poppy Muffins* on page 223 and the *Orange-Pecan Muffins* on page 225. These muffins are a special treat if you're on the *Candida* diet.

You can also use lemon, lime, and orange peel, as long as they are not sweetened or candied, on the perfect diet and on the *Candida* diet. Citrus peels are particularly good in baked goods. Do not use lemon juice powder since it contains corn syrup solids as well as lemon solids and lemon oil.

The terms *natural lemon flavoring* and *natural lime flavoring* are used on ingredient lists when either lemon or lime juice or lemon or lime oil is used. Since there's no way to know which is used, eliminate all products with natural lemon or lime flavoring listed on the ingredient list unless you call the company and find that oil rather than juice is used. For example, *Perrier Water with Natural Lemon Flavoring* is flavored with a small amount of lemon juice and, therefore, should not be used on the perfect diet.

Fruit Products That May Be Used on the Perfect Whole Foods Diet

Whole, fresh fruit (not juiced or dried)
Frozen fruit (not juiced)
Lemon, lime, and orange oil
Lemon, lime, and orange peel

If you are being treated for Candida, *eliminate fresh and frozen fruit until your doctor tells you to resume it.*

Fruits are usually very low in fat. Because cooking destroys many of the nutrients in fruit and often involves adding undesirable fats and sugars, eat most of your fruit raw. If occasionally you want something a little different, then check the recipes that follow to find that treat. Some of these recipes are for raw fruit desserts and others require some cooking.

Fruit Facts

Apples: Considered to be the all-American fruit. Select apples that are firm and well-colored with no soft or bruised spots. Store them in the refrigerator. Sliced apples won't turn brown if the cut pieces are dipped in lemon juice diluted with water (1 part lemon juice to 3 parts water). Do not do this if you are on the perfect diet.
1 pound = 3 medium, fresh apples = 3 cups sliced or diced.

Apricots: Ripen at room temperature (see **Ripening Fruit** on page 274) and store in the refrigerator. 1 pound fresh = 8 to 12 fresh apricots.

Bananas: To slow the ripening process of bananas, store them in an opaque plastic bag in the refrigerator. Remove all of the air you can and close the bag with a twist tie before refrigerating.
1 pound = 3 medium bananas.
4 medium-sized bananas = 1¾ cups mashed bananas.

Blueberries: Choose full, well-colored berries. Avoid those with juice stains on the bottom of the container. This indicates that the berries are very soft or starting to rot. Store blueberries in the refrigerator and use in a day or so or freeze in airtight containers.

Cantaloupes: Should be slightly springy but not too soft. The stem end should have a depressed scar, not a jagged stem. When ripe, the cantaloupe's stem end will be slightly soft. Store ripe cantaloupes in the refrigerator and use in a day or so.

Cherries: Look for full, shiny fruit and avoid dark stems. Store in the refrigerator and use in a few days. 1 pound = 2 cups pitted, fresh cherries.

Citrus Fruits: Oranges, grapefruit, lemons, limes, tangerines, tangelos, and kumquats.

Coconut: A fatty fruit or nut. Most dried coconut from grocery stores has sugar added, but unsweetened dried coconut is available at natural foods stores. It is usually cut fine or coarsely shredded. Use it sparingly because of the high fat content, most of which is saturated fat. Do not use unsweetened dried coconut while on the perfect diet; you may use fresh.
Percent Calories From Fat: 90
Fat Grams In 1 Tablespoon: 3

Cranberries: Available from September to December, cranberries will keep for several weeks in the refrigerator and longer in the freezer. Discard any cranberries that are shriveled, soft, or yellow. Wash cranberries just before using. 1 pound = 1 quart fresh cranberries.

Dates: 1 pound dried = 2 to 2½ cups pitted or about 1¾ cup cut-up. Do not use dried dates on the perfect diet.

Dried Fruit: Fruit from which water has been removed either by the sun or very low temperature ovens or food dryers. Sometimes sweeteners are added before the drying process. All dried fruit is very concentrated in fruit sugar and should be eliminated on the *Perfect Whole Foods* diet.

Grapefruit: Select pink or ruby red grapefruit varieties for a naturally sweeter taste than white grapefruit. Store grapefruit in the refrigerator.

Grapes: Buy grapes that are plump, firm, free of wrinkles, and firmly attached to green stems. Store them in the refrigerator. Wash grapes just before eating to preserve their dusty natural protective coating, called the *bloom*. 1 pound = 1 quart fresh grapes.

Kiwis: Kiwis are ripe when they yield to gentle palm pressure, but are not actually soft. Store ripe kiwis in the refrigerator. Halve a kiwi and eat it with a spoon out of the shell. Or slice it (peeled or unpeeled, whichever you prefer) for salads, fruit mixtures, or a cereal topping.

Lemons: should be fine-textured, plump, and heavy for their size. Do not use lemon juice on the perfect diet; use the juice with all of the pulp.
1 medium = 2 to 3 tablespoons juice.

Limes: should be bright green and heavy for their size. Do not use lime juice on the perfect diet; use the juice with all of the pulp.
1 medium = 1½ to 2 tablespoons juice.

Natural Fruit Flavor: The term *natural fruit flavor*, when used on an ingredient list, can denote a variety of ingredients including fruit juice or the oil of fruit (such as lemon oil). The only way to know the specific ingredient is to ask the manufacturer.

Nectarines: are similar to peaches, only smoother and slightly sweeter. Since nectarines do not get sweeter if they are picked immature, avoid buying very hard, immature ones. They should be firm, but have a slight softening along the seam. Ripen them at home in a paper bag (see **Ripening Fruit** on page 274). When they are ripe, store nectarines in the refrigerator.

Oranges: are good sources of vitamin C. Most U.S. oranges are grown in either Florida, California, Arizona, or Texas. Thin-skinned oranges are juicier than thick, loose-skinned ones. Whichever variety you select, oranges should be firm and heavy for their size. Color does not indicate ripeness. Store all oranges in the refrigerator.

Peaches: Since peaches don't get sweeter if they are picked immature, avoid buying very hard, immature fruit. Ripen peaches at home by the paper-bag method (see **Ripening Fruits**, page 274). Peach varieties are either freestone or clingstone. 1 pound = 4 medium, fresh peaches.

Pears: Pears are always harvested green and should be ripened at home. See the discussion on **Ripening Fruits** that follows. Pears are ripe when they will yield to gentle pressure with the palm of your hand, not your fingertips. Refrigerate when ripe and use within a few days.
1 pound = 4 medium, fresh pears.

Plums: Select plump, firm plums and ripen at home (see instructions that follow on **Ripening Fruit**). Ripe plums will yield to gentle pressure with the palm of your hand. Always wash plums just before eating to preserve the dusty natural protective coating called the *bloom*.
1 pound = 8 to 20 fresh plums.

Prunes: Prunes are especially rich in fiber, potassium, and iron. They shouldn't be used on the perfect diet since they're concentrated in natural sugar. 2 pounds = 2½ cups dried prunes.

Raisins and Dried Currants: 1 pound = 2½ to 3 cups. Do not use dried fruits while on the perfect diet.

Ripening Fruits: Fruits release a gas during the ripening process. This gas promotes further ripening. Therefore, fruits like pears, plums, peaches, and nectarines can be ripened by placing them in a paper bag, closing the bag loosely, and storing at room temperature for a few days. The bag collects the gas which helps the fruit ripen. Check the fruit daily and use immediately or refrigerate when the fruit is ripe.

Strawberries: A fragile fruit that should be eaten soon after purchase. Select firm, dry berries with good color and with the caps attached. Check the box for strawberry stains which may indicate that the berries are soft and starting to rot.

Tangerines: should be heavy for their size, somewhat puffy but with no soft spots. Since they are very perishable, tangerines should be refrigerated and used as soon as possible.

Temperate Fruits: Fruits grown in temperate climates, including apples, pears, peaches, plums, nectarines, figs, cherries, apricots, grapes, all kinds of berries, melons, and kiwis.

Tropical Fruits: Fruits grown only in tropical areas including bananas, pineapples, mangos, papayas, coconuts, and dates (sub-tropical).

Watermelons: It's very hard, even for the experienced buyer, to determine the quality of an uncut watermelon. It's important that the melon be picked mature, but not over-ripe. Skin should be smooth, but not shiny. The ground spot should be yellow or amber, not green or white.

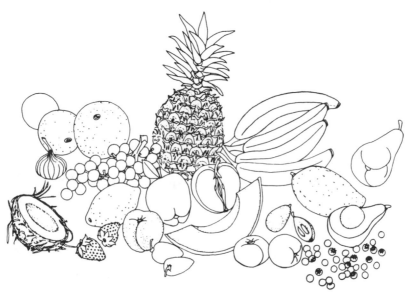

Fruit Recipes

Fried Apples

1 medium apple per person
¼ teaspoon butter per person
Cinnamon, optional

Core apples and slice, leaving on skin. Sauté apple slices in butter for a few minutes. Sprinkle with cinnamon, if desired.

Percent Calories From Fat: 15
Total Fat Grams In Recipe: 2, using 1 apple

Homemade Applesauce

Cooking apples (Jonathan or McIntosh are good)
Heavy pan or skillet with lid

Core and dice unpeeled apples. Place apples in a heavy pan or skillet with a small amount of water to prevent sticking. Cook, covered, until apples are tender, and purée using a food processor, blender, hand blender, or food mill. If too thin, cook slowly, uncovered until thickened. Two pounds makes 2 cups of applesauce.

Percent Calories From Fat: 6
Total Fat Grams In Recipe: 3 (using 2 pounds of apples)

Apple Float

Because of the serious problem of salmonella poisoning from raw egg whites, I use reconstituted NOW Brand Eggwhite Powder in place of the raw egg white in this recipe. To reconstitute, stir 2 teaspoons powder into 2 tablespoons water and let sit for a several minutes. You may need to mix agina and let sit for a few minutes longer.

2 cups unsweetened applesauce, chilled
1 egg white or reconstituted egg white powder equivalent to 1 egg white
1 teaspoon alcohol-free vanilla

Beat egg white until stiff using glass or metal bowl (not plastic since they often have an oily residue on them which prevents the egg white from beating properly). Fold in applesauce and vanilla. Chill before serving. Makes 3 cups.

Perfect Whole Foods*: Use Homemade Applesauce. Don't buy brands of egg white powders that are meant for cake decorating and confections since they contain sugar and starch.*
Percent Calories From Fat: 5
Total Fat Grams In Recipe: 2

Carob-Peanut Applesauce

1 cup unsweetened applesauce
¼ cup natural peanut butter
1 tablespoon carob powder

Mix ingredients until smooth. Serves 2.

Perfect Whole Foods: Use Homemade Applesauce.
Percent Calories From Fat: 56
Total Fat Grams In Recipe: 28

Variation: In place of the peanut butter, use another nut butter such as almond, cashew, pecan, or walnut butter.

Waldorf Apples

Here's a low-fat variation of Waldorf salad that makes a delicious, light dessert.

1 fresh apple, cored and cut into ½-inch chunks
1 fresh orange, cut in half, sections removed
⅓ cup seedless grapes, each halved
2 tablespoons English walnuts
2 tablespoons raisins or currants
⅛ teaspoon cinnamon
⅛ teaspoon nutmeg

Mash 2 or 3 orange sections to create juice. Mix apples, orange sections, orange juice, walnuts, and raisins together. Sprinkle cinnamon and nutmeg on top and stir gently. Cover and refrigerate for several hours for flavors to blend. Makes about 2 cups.

Perfect Whole Foods: Eliminate raisins and currants.
Percent Calories From Fat: 23
Total Fat Grams In Recipe: 9

Almond-Banana-Strawberry Shake

¼ cup raw almonds
1 large banana, peeled and frozen in a plastic bag
½ cup fresh strawberries

Purée almonds and ¾ cup water in a blender. Add frozen banana and strawberries, reserving 2 for garnish. Blend again. Pour into two glasses and top each glass with a fresh strawberry.

Variations: Use other combinations of fruits such as banana and blueberries
Percent Calories From Fat: 51
Total Fat Grams In 1 Serving: 9

Frozen Bananas

2 to 4 ripe bananas, peeled

Place bananas in an airtight, plastic freezer bag and freeze until firm. Eat while frozen, using a small baggie to hold a banana. Use within a week or so or before the bananas turn dark.

Banana Ice Cream: Use a *Champion* Juicer (with the blank attachment rather than the strainer) to homogenize the frozen bananas. Or, using a food processor with steel blades, cut 4 bananas in chunks and pulse until chopped. Then process until smooth and creamy. Serve immediately in individual bowls that have been placed in freezer to get cold.
Grape Sorbet: Use a *Champion* Juicer (with blank, not strainer attachment) to homogenize several pounds of frozen seedless grapes. Freeze in a airtight container and soften slightly before serving.

Percent Calories From Fat: 5
Total Fat Grams In Recipe: 1 (using 2 bananas)

Cranberry Relish

This has become a traditional dish in my home at the holidays. After you try it, you'll never want to eat the jellied cranberries that come in a can.

12-ounce package fresh cranberries
20-ounce can unsweetened, crushed pineapple with juice, or
    1 fresh pineapple, cut into small chunks
1 orange (preferably organically grown), cut into eighths and seeds removed
1 firm, red apple, quartered and cored
¼ cup chopped pecans, optional

One at a time and using food processor with blade, chop until fine the cranberries, orange, and apple. Combine all ingredients and refrigerate for several hours or overnight before serving. Makes about 6 cups.

Perfect Whole foods: *Use 1 fresh pineapple, cut into chunks and then chopped in food processor.*
Percent Calories From Fat: 5 without pecans, 24 with pecans
Total Fat Grams In Recipe: 4 without pecans, 25 with pecans

Orange Sherbet

2 to 4 fresh oranges

Cut oranges into eighths, remove the seeds, and freeze in an airtight container until firm. Eat while frozen, removing peel while eating. It tastes like orange sherbet.

Percent Calories From Fat: 6
Total Fat Grams In Recipe: 1 using 2 oranges

Pineapple Popsicle

Fresh pineapple, peeled and cored
Popsicle sticks

Cut pineapple into wedge-shaped pieces. Insert sticks into wedges and stand in a jar. Freeze and serve.

Percent Calories From Fat: 9
Fat Grams In 1 Cup Of Pineapple: 1

Pineapple Frost

20-ounce can crushed pineapple in unsweetened pineapple juice
¼-½ cup orange or pineapple juice, optional

Freeze the unopened can of pineapple. About 30 minutes before preparing, remove can from the freezer and sit at room temperature to slightly defrost. Or hold can under hot running water for a minute or two. To prepare, add frozen pineapple to food processor bowl, using the blade attachment. Begin processing and add some juice through the processor opening if pineapple is still too frozen to blend. Or let pineapple defrost a few minutes longer if juice is not available. Continue processing until pineapple is smooth and creamy. Serve immediately. Makes 2½ cups.

Perfect Whole Foods: No, since pineapple is canned; also, fruit juice is not allowed. You can freeze fresh pineapple chunks and homogenize them using a Champion Juicer.
Percent Calories From Fat: 1
Total Fat Grams In Recipe: Less than 0.5

Pina Colada

Here's a recipe my chiropractor, Dr. Robert Barnes of Winchester, Kentucky, gave me.

½ cup plain, nonfat yogurt
¼ teaspoon vanilla extract (alcohol-free)
3 tablespoons unsweetened, canned crushed pineapple in juice
1 tablespoon unsweetened, flaked coconut
3 to 4 toasted cashews, broken into pieces

Mix yogurt and vanilla in serving bowl. Top with pineapple, coconut, and cashews. Serve immediately. Makes ¾ cup

Perfect Whole foods: Use fresh pineapple. Use fresh coconut rather than dried.
Percent Calories From Fat: 46
Total Fat Grams In Recipe: 10

Strawberries 'n "Cream"

You'll like this simple yet delicious low-fat dessert whether you're on the **Perfect Whole Foods** *diet or a more liberal diet.*

1 pint fresh strawberries, washed, capped, and sliced
½ cup plain, nonfat yogurt
1 tablespoon diastatic malt powder (p. 209 and 195)
¼ teaspoon alcohol-free vanilla

Arrange strawberry slices in 2 or 3 serving bowls. Combine yogurt with diastatic malt and vanilla. Drizzle yogurt mixture over the strawberries. Serves 2 or 3.

Percent Calories From Fat: 7
Total Fat Grams In Recipe: 1

Peaches 'n "Cream": Substitute 2 or 3 ripe peaches for the strawberries.

Strawberry Milk Shake

½ cup fresh ripe strawberries, cleaned and hulled
1 cup skim milk
1 tablespoon oat bran
1 tablespoon fresh wheat germ
½ teaspoon alcohol-free vanilla
½ cup ice cubes

Reserve and slice 1 strawberry for garnish. Place remaining strawberries, milk, oat bran, wheat germ, and vanilla into blender container and process until smooth. While still blending, add ice gradually and blend until ice is finely cracked. Pour immediately into glasses and garnish with strawberry slices. Makes about 2 cups.

Percent Calories From Fat: 12
Total Fat Grams In Recipe: 1

You are more than you think!   *Walt Stoll, M.D.*

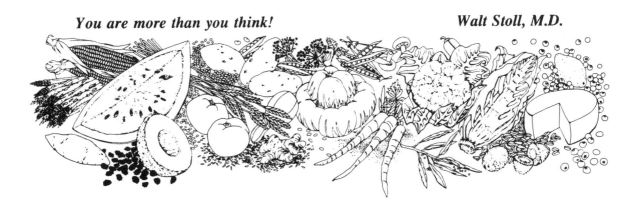

Orange Fruit Smoothie

¾ cup plain, nonfat yogurt
1 fresh orange, cut into halves and then each half into fourths, and peeled
1 ripe banana, peeled and frozen

Place ingredients in blender and puree until almost smooth.   Makes about 2 to 2½ cups.

Percent Calories From Fat: 1
Total Fat Grams In Recipe: Less than 0.5

Kiwi Fruit Smoothie: In place of orange, use 1 fresh kiwi, peeled and cut into chunks.

Watermelon Pops

In a food processor or blender, blend chunks of watermelon (seeds removed) until it becomes a liquid. Pour into plastic popsicle molds, add lids, and freeze until solid. Children loves these.

Percent Calories From Fat: 13
Fat Grams In 1½ Cups: 1

Lemon-Glazed Fruit Ambrosia

Here's a luscious dessert—great for taking to potlucks and picnics. Use just a few different fruits or many, whatever is available.

A variety of fresh fruit in season: strawberries, pineapple, oranges, apples, peaches, blueberries, cantaloupe, watermelon, kiwi, bananas, seedless grapes
½ cup plain, nonfat yogurt
1 drop lemon oil (use a dropper!)

Cut fruit into about 1-inch size pieces. Mix gently. Stir lemon oil into yogurt, mixing well. Add just enough of the yogurt mixture to glaze the fruit, again stirring very gently. Unless you have a large bowl of fruit, you won't use all of the yogurt. Refrigerate until ready to serve.

Percent Calories From Fat: 2
Total Fat Grams In Recipe: Less than 0.5

Easy Stewed Fruit

3 cups dried fruit, one kind only or assorted mixture
1 quart canning jar with lid
Warm, not boiling, water

Cut large pieces of fruit so that all fruits are of similar size. Place fruit in jar and fill with warm water. Refrigerate overnight or longer.

Perfect Whole Foods: *No: dried fruits are not allowed.*
Percent Calories From Fat: 2
Total Fat Grams In Recipe: 3

Banana-Carob Candy

*The recipe for this treat was developed by a friend while she was following the **Perfect Whole Foods** diet. Carol Elkins of King's Mountain, Kentucky makes this and gives samples to her friends. If they like it, she then takes them more, along with the recipe.*

1 cup natural peanut butter
1 cup mashed, ripe bananas (approximately 2 bananas)
2 cups carob powder, divided
1 teaspoon alcohol-free vanilla
1 teaspoon stevia powder (see page 297)

Combine peanut butter and bananas, mixing thoroughly. Sift together 1½ cups of the carob powder and the powdered stevia. Gradually combine the carob powder mixture with the peanut butter-banana mixture and form into ¾-inch balls. Roll in additional carob powder. Refrigerate in an air-tight container. Makes approximately 5 dozen candies.

Percent Calories From Fat: 42
Total Fat Grams In Recipe: 113 (about 2 grams per each ¾-inch piece)

Variations: Add a pinch of cinnamon to the carob powder in which you roll the balls.
Add cream cheese to the peanut butter-banana mixture.

Real Fruit Gelatin

1 envelope (2¼ teaspoons) unflavored gelatin
1½ cups unsweetened fruit juice (any flavor such as orange, grape or apple)

Sprinkle gelatin over ½ cup cold water in a saucepan. Let it sit for a few minutes while gelatin absorbs water. Place over low heat, stirring constantly until gelatin dissolves. Remove from heat. Stir in fruit juice and pour into bowl. Chill until firm. Makes 2 cups.

Perfect Whole Foods: No
Percent Calories From Fat: 3
Total Fat Grams In Recipe: 1

Variation: When gelatin is slightly thickened, add cut up fruit or vegetables and stir. Do *not* use fresh pineapple since it contains an enzyme which will prevent a gel from forming. Chill until firm.

Fruit Kanten

1 cup fruit juice (any flavor such as apple or orange)
1 to 2 cups fresh fruit pieces such as sliced peaches, bananas, strawberries, or apples
1 cup water
2 tablespoons agar flakes

Combine water and agar flakes. Bring to a boil and simmer for 2 minutes. Pour into a bowl, slowly add juice while stirring, and cool for about 10 minutes. Add fresh fruit and let mixture sit to gel. At room temperature it will take about 45 minutes. In the refrigerator, it will gel faster. Makes 3 to 4 cups.

Perfect Whole Foods: No
Percent Calories From Fat: 3
Total Fat Grams In Recipe: 1

Fruit Sherbet

Use these guidelines to prepare any combination of Fruit Sherbet, *using bananas and yogurt as the base.*

1 pound of very ripe fruit such as strawberries, peaches, or blueberries, washed, sliced (not the blueberries), placed on cookie sheet, frozen, transferred to plastic bag, and stored in freezer
1½ pound very ripe bananas, peeled, frozen on cookie sheet, transferred to plastic bag and stored in freezer
½ cup plain, nonfat yogurt

Chill bowl of food processor. Add fruit and process until smooth. Add yogurt and process until blended. Pour into air-tight container and freeze. Let soften briefly before serving. Serves 6.

Percent Calories From Fat: 6, using strawberries
Total Fat Grams In Recipe: 5, using strawberries

BEVERAGES

One question newcomers to whole foods frequently ask me is, *What do you drink?* They are often surprised at my reply, *Water.* There are other acceptable beverages, but pure water is mainly what you should drink to quench your thirst and replace much of the water lost from the body through elimination, exhalation, and perspiration. (Some is replaced by the water in food.)

The fact that water should be both clean and pure makes us suspect tap water, underground wells, and springs. Although the public water systems meet legal standards for water, these standards are not necessarily what we need for optimal health. Although public systems do disinfect water to prevent water-borne diseases, chlorine added to the public water supply can combine with harmless organic particles in water to form cancer-causing trihalomethanes (THMs). Some underground wells and springs are contaminated by industrial pollutants such as pesticides, cleaning solvents, or heavy metals which chlorine cannot help.

If you question the importance of using bottled or purified water rather than tap, then drink bottled water for a while, at least a month, then go back to tap water, and notice the taste difference. The unpleasant taste is, more than likely, caused by undesirable pollutants or additives. Know the water you drink; make certain it is safe.

Bottled spring water is usually the best choice. Select only spring water whose company is reputable and will supply an analysis of its water. Also, make certain the word *spring* is not just part of the brand name. In this case, unless the label also states that it is from a spring, it could be purified tap or well water.

Use private well and spring waters only if you have them analyzed regularly by a laboratory that is certified for testing drinking water. Have the water tested about every three to six months.

Purifying your water at home with a reverse osmosis unit is another good option. Don't use distilled and softened waters. Distilled water is highly refined; all beneficial minerals as well as harmful substances are removed. Don't use artificially softened water since it has harmful minerals like sodium and possibly cadmium and lead added.

If you do use water from the tap for drinking or cooking, take the following precautions. If there has been no water used lately, flush the cold water pipes for a minute or longer. Modern plumbing is made of copper pipes that are assembled using lead-containing solder. By flushing the pipes, any lead concentration in the tap water will be reduced. Use only the cold water since hot water is more likely to have impurities dissolved in it.

There is a variety of fruit-flavored sparkling water beverages on the market, many of which are sources of sugar. Even if you're not on the perfect diet, read the ingredient lists carefully to avoid those with sugar since no one should be drinking water with sugar added! If you are on the perfect diet and want a no-sugar-added, fruit-flavored sparkling water, check with the company to determine if the natural fruit flavor added is from juice, oil, or peel. (Each specific flavor may vary.) If the flavor comes from juice, don't use it while on the perfect diet. Natural flavor derived from the oil or peel of the fruit is okay. One client told me that she adds a small pinch of stevia extract to fruit-flavored sparkling water for a bit of sweetness. You can add a touch of flavor to any water by squeezing a lemon or lime slice (not on the perfect diet, but later) or adding crushed fresh mint to water. A pinch of stevia extract, again, will add a sweet taste.

Plain sparkling waters, club soda, and seltzer are all sugar-free. Club soda is a source of sodium while sparkling water and seltzer are sodium-free. Don't use tonic water since it contains sugar.

With caffeine-containing coffee and black and green teas eliminated from the **Perfect Whole Foods** diet, many people are eager to find substitutes for these. (See page 31 for a complete list of caffeine sources, many of which are found in beverages.) Because decaffeinated coffee and decaffeinated tea contain small amounts of caffeine, they should both be eliminated from the perfect diet.

If you're looking for a hot or cold beverage, you might want to try some of the many herbal teas available. Be aware that certain herbs, in quantity, have a medicinal effect on the body, so select mild teas such as those sold by *Celestial Seasonings*. Don't use the same herb tea over and over, day after day. Even mild teas may have a medicinal effect if overused. Read the ingredient lists carefully since some herbal tea blends have varieties that include barley malt, dried fruit, natural flavor (which can be a refined product), and caffeine-containing green and black teas as ingredients. For example, *Celestial Seasonings'* After Dinner Tea Blend contains caffeine-containing tea. It's easy to pick up a package of the wrong tea if you're in a hurry and don't read the ingredient list.

If you're giving up coffee and are looking for an alternate, beware of grain-based coffee substitutes. Most are made from roasted, ground refined cereals like barley and wheat and contain sweeteners like figs, malt, and molasses. *Postum*, *Pero*, *Roma*, *Cafix*, *Coffree*, and *Bambu* all contain refined ingredients. If you find a coffee substitute made of *whole* grains with no fruit, malt, or other sugar, it may be okay on the perfect diet. Check the ingredients carefully. Although I've seen recipes for making coffee substitutes from whole grains and soybeans, I've not found any that I thought were satisfactory substitutes. Actually, true coffee lovers usually don't care for cereal-based products. The full body and taste are never the same. Remember that decaffeinated coffees can be used by those on a liberal whole foods diet, but should be eliminated from the **Perfect Whole Foods** diet because of the small amount of caffeine.

The subject of diet soda usually comes up when beverages are being discussed. Although some don't actually contain refined carbohydrates, they all contain the artificial sweetener aspartame. Because aspartame or *NutraSweet* causes some people to react with headaches, dizziness, skin problems, stomach pains, constipation, memory loss, and even seizures and other people to crave sweets after using them, I cannot recommend it. Why take the risk of using a substance known to cause serious problems? Besides, if aspartame can also cause sugar cravings, it will only make following a whole foods diet, whether perfect or liberal, more difficult. Instead of drinking diet sodas, try iced herb teas sweetened with stevia instead. (If on the **Perfect Whole Foods** diet, use the green powder or white extract rather than liquid products with alcohol.)

Beverage Facts

Black Tea: Contains caffeine; do not use on the perfect diet.

Club Soda: Carbonated water which has sodium additives. Read about **Seltzer Water** below.

Decaffeinated Coffee: Due to the small amount of caffeine remaining in decaffeinated coffee, do not use *Sanka* and other decaffeinated coffees on the perfect diet.

Decaffeinated Tea: Due to the small amount of caffeine remaining in decaffeinated tea, do not use it on the perfect diet.

Distilled Water: Pure, refined water with no minerals. It's best to drink other kinds of purified water or spring water.

Green Tea: Contains caffeine; do not use on the perfect diet.

Herb Tea: See page 284 for discussion of herb teas.

Mineral Water: Natural mineral water is spring water that has more minerals than most spring water. Natural mineral water can be either still (no gas bubbles) or sparkling (with carbon dioxide gas bubbles). Mineral water with natural bubbles usually has additional carbonation added since most gas usually escapes when the spring water emerges from the underground.

Natural flavors: In some products, the exact ingredients in natural flavors are trade secrets of the company that makes them. Since they may contain very small amounts of sucrose, maltodextrins, and corn syrup solids, products with natural flavors must be eliminated from the perfect diet if the manufacturer cannot disclose the source.

Pau D'Arco: An herb with antifungal properties. It is sometimes made into tea and used as part of the *Candida* treatment program. Also called *Taheebo*. (See page 290 for tea recipe.)

Seltzer Water: Carbonated water with no sodium added.

Smoothie: A refreshing drink, usually dairy-based, with blended fruit (fresh or frozen).

Sparkling Water: Carbonated water to which fruit flavors and sugar may be added. Check the ingredients. If a specific brand has no sugar added but includes natural fruit flavors, check with the manufacturer to determine if the fruit flavor comes from juice, oil, or peel. Citrus oil and peel may be used on the perfect diet as well as the diet during *Candida* treatment, but not juice.

Spring Water: When you buy spring water, make certain that it comes from a source that is analyzed regularly. Also, check the label to determine that it is, indeed, spring water. The word *spring* as part of the company name doesn't indicate its source. It must be labeled spring water.

Spritzers: A mixture of fruit juice and sparkling water. Spritzers are available commercially or can be made at home. Do not use them on the perfect diet.

Taheebo: See **Pau D'Arco** above.

Tea: The term tea usually denotes caffeine-containing products and should be omitted on the perfect diet. You may use herb teas on the perfect diet as long as they contain no caffeine or concentrated fruits (citrus peels are okay) or sugars (like malts).   Also, use a variety of herb teas rather than the same ones over and over since most herbs have medicinal properties.

Tonic Water: Carbonated water which includes sugar and should not be used on the perfect diet.

Water: Make certain the water you drink is pure. Avoid tap water when possible.

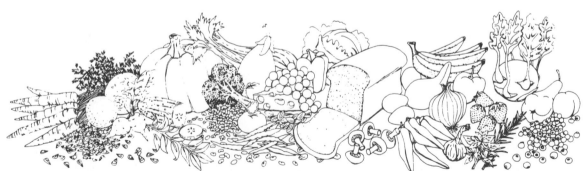

People who stand still may avoid stubbing their toes, but they won't make much progress!
                                 Unknown

Beverage Recipes

Hot Herb Tea

1 tea bag or 1 to 1½ teaspoon loose herb tea per cup
Almost-boiling water

Steep tea bag or loose tea in water in a cup or teapot. After 4 to 6 minutes, remove bag or strain loose tea and serve.

Perfect Whole Foods: Read the ingredient list of herb tea bags and tea blends to make certain tea has no caffeine and no sweeteners such as barley malt or dried fruit are added to tea ingredients.

Sunshine Iced Herb Tea

1 quart water
4 to 6 herb tea bags or 3 tablespoons loose herb tea

Place tea and water in a covered glass jar and place it in the sunshine for 2 to 4 hours. Serve over ice with or without lemon wedges. Makes 4 cups.

Perfect Whole Foods: Read package and label of herb tea bags to make certain tea has no caffeine and no sweeteners such as barley malt are added to the tea ingredients. Do not use lemon.

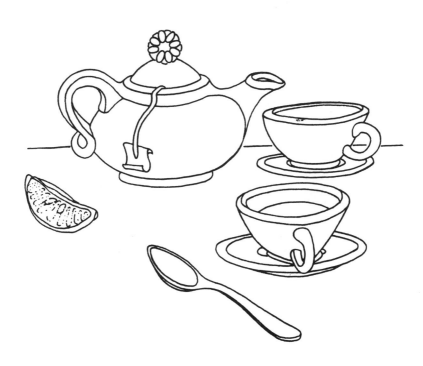

Party Tea

My Co-op friend Mildred Lovins gave me this recipe. We named it Party Tea *since she recently gave the recipe to a friend who served it at a party. This tea is free of caffeine, sugar, alcohol, fat, and sodium! There's no artificial sweetener, coloring, or flavoring either. It's refreshing and delicious!*

4 cups almost-boiling water
¼ cup dried peppermint leaves
2-inch piece cinnamon stick
¼ vanilla bean, split lengthwise

Steep ingredients, either in a cloth tea bag or loose, 5 minutes if you're serving the tea hot and 10 for iced tea. Remove tea bag or strain and serve. Garnish iced tea with a sprig of fresh mint or lemon slice. Makes 4 cups.

Perfect Whole Foods: Do not use lemon.

Ginger Tea

Here's a very refreshing tea. Some say it helps with their digestion.

1 thin slice of fresh ginger root
1 cup almost-boiling water

Steep ginger root in water for a few minutes. Remove ginger root before drinking. Makes 1 cup.

Lemon Tea

Even if you must temporarily eliminate fruits due to their simple sugars, you can enjoy this simple tea. The lemon flavor comes from the oil, and you don't miss the sugar.

1 cup boiling water
2 to 3 drops lemon oil

Drop oil in water. Stir occasionally while drinking. Makes 1 cup.

Pau D'Arco Tea (or Taheebo Tea)

If your doctor has recommended that you drink Pau d'Arco or Taheebo tea as part of your Candida treatment, use the following instructions for preparing it. (Pau D'arco or Taheebo is an herb with anti-fungal properties.) If you find commercial tea bags filled with these herbs, read the ingredient list on the label carefully before using them as they sometimes have lemon, lime, or other fruit added to them. Fruit oil and citrus peel are okay, but not dehydrated fruit juice.

1 teaspoon loose pau d'arco or taheebo tea
3 cups water

Boil the tea and water together for 5 minutes. Remove from heat, cover, and let sit for 20 minutes before straining and drinking. Store unused tea in the refrigerator. Makes about 3 cups.

Herbal Tea with Juice

Use any herb tea and juice combination you prefer. It's excellent with rosehips or Tia Sangria (a blend of hibiscus, cinnamon and rosehips) and 1 quart each of grape-cranberry cocktail and apple-strawberry juice.

Scant ½ cup loose herb tea or about 16 tea bags
7 cups almost-boiling water
2 tablespoons lemon juice
2 quarts unsweetened fruit juice
1 gallon container
Ice water to fill container

Steep tea in almost-boiling water until the water cools to lukewarm or at least 20 minutes. Strain and cool tea. Place in gallon container along with remaining ingredients. Serve chilled or over ice. Makes 1 gallon.

Perfect Whole Foods: No, because of fruit juices.
Percent Calories From Fat: 2
Total Fat Grams In Recipe: 2

Hot Spiced Apple Cider

2 quarts unsweetened apple cider
½ teaspoon whole cloves
2 sticks cinnamon
½ teaspoon allspice

Heat the cider and spices for about 20 minutes. Strain or dip out the spices before serving.
Makes 8 cups.

Perfect Whole Foods: No, because of apple cider.
Percent Calories From Fat: 3
Total Fat Grams In Recipe: 3

Granny's Tea

Here's a refreshing caffeine-free beverage to substitute for iced tea. Several years ago, my mother, Ann Oakes, served it to me. I knew my children, then about 6 and 8 years old, wouldn't drink it if they knew it was made of prune juice. So we called it Granny's Tea and didn't tell them what Granny's magic ingredient was for a while. When they discovered what it was, it didn't matter. They liked it!

By the pitcher: Combine ¼ cup prune juice with 2 quarts water.
By the glass: Combine 1½ teaspoon prune juice with 1 cup water.

Serve over ice.

Perfect Whole Foods: No, because of prune juice.
Percent Calories From Fat: Less than 0.5%
Total Fat Grams In Recipes: Less than 0.5 in 1 gallon

Fruit Spritzer

¾ cup cold fruit juice
¼ cup cold seltzer

Mix and pour over ice. Strong-flavored juices like grape juice can be mixed half juice and half
seltzer. Makes 1 cup.

Perfect Whole Foods: No, because of fruit juice.
Percent Calories From Fat: 1-3, depending on juice used
Total Fat Grams In Recipe: Less than 0.5

Fruit Punch Slush

This makes a perfect punch for entertaining. Serve it from a punch bowl or in individual cups.

3 cups water
2 cups raw honey
6-ounce can frozen orange juice, reconstituted
2 whole oranges, cut into 8ths and then sliced into bite size pieces (peel skin if color added)
5 or 6 ripe bananas, thinly sliced
1 lemon, juiced with pulp added
2 20-ounce cans unsweetened crushed pineapple in juice
Cold seltzer (some prefer to use diet gingerale)

Heat water and honey until honey is dissolved. Do not boil. Add remaining ingredients except seltzer. Freeze in large, flat, non-metallic container (9 x 13-inch heavy plastic container with lid is good).

To serve, either cut into chunks, place in punch bowl and add seltzer or cut into cubes, place in cups and add seltzer. If fruit is frozen solid, let it sit out for a few minutes before cutting. You may use as much or as little seltzer as you like. Frozen fruit yields approximately 20 cups. Using 4 quarts of seltzer will yield 36 cups.

Perfect Whole Foods: No, because of honey, fruit juice, and canned pineapple.
Percent Calories From Fat: 10
Total Fat Grams In Recipe: 5

Hot Carob Cocoa

When my children were little, they'd have this hot carob cocoa as a special treat when they came in from playing in the snow. They learned to prepare it for themselves as they got old enough.

3 tablespoons carob powder
¼ cup water
1 to 3 teaspoon raw honey
2 cups skim milk, heated
½ teaspoon vanilla extract

In a jar, stir carob, water, honey, and vanilla together. Add tight-fitting lid and shake until well blended. Add carob syrup to hot milk, reheat, and stir until mixed. Serves 2.
For young children under 2: Use whole milk. Do not give raw honey to infants under 1 year.

Perfect Whole Foods: No, because of honey.
Percent Calories From Fat: 4
Total Fat Grams In Recipe: 1

DESSERTS

When I first became interested in whole foods, I spent a lot of time developing dessert recipes that I thought were much healthier than the recipes I had been using. I switched from white flour to whole wheat, from white and brown sugars to honey, maple syrup, molasses, and fruit juices, and from chocolate to carob. I had already stopped using shortening, but switched from margarine to butter. I gradually came to the realization that these desserts are high in fat and high in sugar just as traditional desserts made of white flour and white sugar. I now use these recipes only at holiday times or other really special occasions, not regularly as I had been doing.

If you're on a liberal whole foods diet, I hope you, too, will save my dessert recipe collection for special times, not as an end to your meals each day. Many people have the mistaken notion that if a little is okay, a lot is too. Use recipes in this section only if you can tolerate them. Some people who have followed the perfect diet are able to liberalize and use these recipes occasionally; others are not.

If you're presently on the **Perfect Whole Foods** diet, you will be unable to use all recipes in this section. Instead, why not try some special treats like muffins made using diastatic malt (p. 220 to 227) or flavored yogurts (p. 245 and 246).

Only Sweeteners Used on the Perfect Diet

Diastatic malt (See pages 195 and 209.)
Stevia (See "Stevia" on page 296.)

Avoid artificial sweeteners! If you absolutely must use them, use only those with no refined carbohydrates added and use them only occasionally (also read pages 284, 294, 328, and 362).

Many of these recipes, although they contain honey or molasses, are not nearly so sweet-tasting as popular white sugar, white flour desserts. If you serve them to those who consume mostly processed foods, they very likely will not appreciate them as will those who eat whole foods almost exclusively. I've included several cake and cupcake recipes that do not have frostings to go with them. Many people expect cakes to have frosting, but they taste good without and are much healthier that way.

When baking cakes and bar cookies, if you use pans that are slightly different in size from the size I recommend, make certain that you adjust your baking time accordingly. Pans that are smaller in diameter will require longer baking than times I suggest since the batter will be thicker. If you bake something in a larger pan, it will take less time for baking.

Dessert Facts

Amasake: A Japanese rice sweetener that is sometimes used with a liberal whole foods diet. It is a fermented food that's more slowly absorbed than many sweeteners.

Artificial Sweeteners: Although a few people continue to use artificial sweeteners along with whole foods in an attempt to have sweet-tasting foods without actually eating sugar, I highly discourage their use because of the adverse reactions some people experience. If you absolutely must, then use the liquid artificial sweeteners, but only occasionally. Don't use granules and most tablets since they usually include sources of sugar such as dextrose, lactose, and maltodextrin. Those who use artificial sweeteners have a more difficult time totally eliminating sweets since artificial sweeteners can result in cravings for sugar. When you totally eliminate sweets and artificial sweeteners, you'll taste and enjoy the natural flavors of whole grains, vegetables, nuts, and fruits. (See **Stevia**, an alternative to artificial sweeteners, on page 296 and **Aspartame** on page 328.)

Babies and Honey: *Never* give *raw* honey to babies under one year of age. Raw honey, which can carry botulism spores, has been associated with fatal botulism in infants. If present in the honey, these spores do not affect older children or adults, just infants. Babies, actually, should not be given any sweeteners, so this should present no problem.

Barley Malt: A complex carbohydrate grain sweetener that gets its sweet flavor from maltose. It is more slowly absorbed than many other sweeteners. Barley malt is sometimes used on a liberal whole foods diet. It is not used on the perfect diet since the sprouted whole barley is treated with barley enzymes to convert the starch to maltose sugar.

Brown Rice Syrup: A complex carbohydrate grain sweetener that gets its sweetness from maltose. It is more slowly absorbed than many sweeteners. It is sometimes used on the liberal diet. Brown rice syrup is not used on the perfect diet since brown rice is treated with barley enzymes to convert the rice starch to maltose sugar.

Candy: At holiday times as well as throughout the year, natural foods stores often sell a large assortment of candies. Many unsuspecting customers pay several times more than they would have to pay at a grocery store for candy, thinking it must be healthy. Sometimes the first ingredient is sugar. Usually highly saturated fats are also main ingredients. A few ingredients such as carob, sesame seeds, almonds, peanuts, or oatmeal are included which make the products appear healthy. Before you spend a top price for candy for a liberal whole foods diet, make certain it doesn't include ingredients you'd rather not be eating. Read the ingredient lists!

Carob Chips: If you're following a liberal whole foods diet, there are a variety of carob chips and carob candies available, often at health food stores, co-ops, as well as grocery stores. But don't equate carob with *health*. Don't think *If it's made of carob, it must be okay.* Carob powder is a good, wholesome ingredient. However, carob chips, as well as other carob candies, more often than not have highly saturated fats (usually partially-hydrogenated palm kernel oil which is more saturated than the fat in red meat) and sweeteners (often sucrose or fructose if from the grocery store and malted grain sweetener if from a natural food store).

Carob Flour: Same as **Carob Powder**, below.

Carob Powder: Is ground from the carob pod which comes from a tree of the locust family. Carob resembles chocolate but is lower in fat and richer in minerals and natural sugars. Carob, also, has no caffeine-like substances as does chocolate. Roasted carob powder has a flavor more similar to chocolate than raw carob powder. Carob powder may be used on the *Perfect Whole Foods* diet. However, most recipes using carob powder also use sweeteners. To use carob in place of cocoa, use the same amount. One square chocolate can be replaced with 3 tablespoons carob powder plus 2 tablespoons water in a recipe. 1 pound = 4 cups.
Percent Calories From Fat: 4
Fat Grams In 8 Tablespoons: 1

Honey: Although not allowed on the perfect diet, honey is sometimes used on a liberal whole foods diet. Do not, however, get into the habit of using honey, or any sweetener, often or in large amounts. Because honey is sweeter than most other sugars, you can use less for equal sweetness. To substitute honey for 1 cup white sugar, use ½ cup and either decrease a liquid ingredient by approximately ¼ cup or increase a dry ingredient by about ¼ cup. When honey becomes granular, simply sit the jar in a pan of hot water to liquify it. 1 pound honey = 1⅓ cups.

Honey, Buying: When buying honey, select 100% pure, raw, unfiltered honey. The label will probably not say all of this since there are no laws to define these descriptions. If the source is reputable, it will be 100% pure when sold as honey. Most honey is heated some, but should not be actually cooked. If honey is slightly cloudy rather than golden clear, it is probably unfiltered or minimally screened.

Honey, Measuring: When measuring honey, first oil the measuring cup to prevent the honey from clinging. Or, if the recipe calls for oil, just measure the oil first in the same cup that you will use for measuring the honey.

Malt: The concentrated sweet extract, either in powdered or syrup form, of a sprouted grain such as barley, rice, or wheat. Unless the malt is diastatic malt (sometimes called *wheat malt*: sprouted grain, dried, and ground, not concentrated), it should be eliminated from the *Perfect Whole Foods* diet.

***Rumford* Baking Powder**: A baking powder that's aluminum-free. Baking powder is not used on the perfect diet because of the cornstarch (or potato starch in some other brands). Do not use any baking powder regularly on a liberal whole foods diet because of the phosphates they contain.

Shortening: If a recipe calls for shortening or margarine, use butter or oil instead. Replace either margarine or shortening with an equal amount of butter. If you want to use an oil instead of butter, use ⅞ cup for each one cup of butter called for, and either increase the amount of dry ingredients or decrease other liquids. Remember that both butter and oil should not be used in large quantities since they are high fat foods.

Sorghum: A cereal grain that can be eaten whole, cooked like rice, or ground into flour. A sweet syrup is made from the stalks of a certain variety of sorghum. Eliminate sorghum syrup from the perfect diet.

Stevia: An herb that, in its dried form, is about 10 to 15 times sweeter than white sugar. As a white extract, stevia is over 200 times sweeter than sugar! Note that the green powdered herb does not dissolve in liquids whereas the pure white extract does. Read stevia labels very carefully since many brands of white stevia extracts also contain refined ingredients such as maltodextrin and FOS (fructo-oligosaccharides) that should be omitted on the perfect diet. (While FOS has beneficial properties, like serving as food for "friendly" bacteria in the colon, it consists of small chains of fructose molecules which are refined.) You can use pure stevia in a variety of ways to make foods taste sweet without adding refined carbohydrate to the diet. If you're on the perfect diet, you might want to experiment with using either the green or the pure white stevia. One to two tablespoons of the finely ground green herb and about ¼ teaspoon of the white extract are each equal in sweetness to approximately one cup of white sugar. Stevia is also available in liquid forms. Avoid liquid stevia products that are alcohol-based on the perfect diet; glycerin-based stevia is okay. Stevia can be successfully used in puddings, custards, dressings, and fruit and dairy smoothies. When you substitute stevia for white sugar or honey in baking, it's important to adjust other ingredients so the texture of the baked goods will be correct. Adding fruits like applesauce or mashed bananas (unless you're omitting fruit temporarily during *Candida* treatment) will help compensate for the loss of the bulk of sugar and, of course, will add some flavor.

Vanilla Extract: Buy pure vanilla extract and other pure flavorings. Always select real vanilla rather than the artificial vanilla flavoring called *vanillin*. Don't use alcohol-containing extracts while on the perfect diet. It was once thought that alcohol in foods and recipes would evaporate during cooking, but tests have shown that all of the alcohol does not leave the food. Therefore, if you are on the perfect diet, use either alcohol-free commercial vanilla that is glycerin based, alcohol-free vanilla that you make yourself (see recipe on page 257), or vanilla beans.

Please Read These Important Notes:
If you have strictly followed the **Perfect Whole Foods** diet for at least two weeks, but you are not feeling dramatically better, see page 35 for additional steps that may be necessary.

If you are allergic to wheat, do not substitute spelt or kamut without first determining that you can tolerate them.

If you are being treated for *Candida*, please see specific guidelines on page 315, Appendix A: If You Have Candidiasis.

Dessert Recipes

Carob Brownies

My daughter Heather converted a white flour-white sugar brownie recipe into this one when she was 13 years old.

2 eggs
½ cup raw honey
½ cup oil
1 teaspoon pure vanilla extract
1¼ cups whole wheat pastry flour
½ cup carob powder
¼ cup nuts, chopped

Preheat oven to 350°. Oil a 9-inch square pan with *Oil-Lecithin Combination* (p. 205). In a small bowl beat eggs, honey, oil, and vanilla for 1 minute with a mixer. Stir in flour and carob. Spread evenly in pan and sprinkle with nuts. Bake for 20 to 25 minutes. Makes 16 pieces.

Perfect Whole Foods: No, because of honey.
Percent Calories From Fat: 49
Fat Grams In 1 Piece: 9

Wheat-Free Carob Brownies: Substitute 1¼ cups whole barley flour, 1 cup spelt, triticale or millet flour, or ¾ cup for the whole wheat flour.

Granola Bars

¾ cup rolled oats
¾ cup whole wheat pastry flour
¼ cup fresh wheat germ
¼ cup chopped nuts (pecans are good)
¼ cup butter, melted
¼ cup raw honey
1 teaspoon pure vanilla extract

Preheat oven to 325°. Oil a 9-inch square on a cookie sheet with *Oil-Lecithin Combination* (p. 205). Combine the dry ingredients in one bowl and liquid ingredients in another. Add liquids to dry ingredients and mix well. Pat onto the oiled area of the cookie sheet in a 6 x 8-inch rectangle. Cut in center lengthwise and then every inch crosswise, making 16 bars. Bake 20 to 25 minutes or until golden brown. Remove from oven and let them sit 5 minutes, then loosen bars from cookie sheet with a spatula. Slide onto wire rack to cool. Break apart into granola bars when cool.

Perfect Whole Foods: No, because of honey.
Percent Calories From Fat: 47
Fat Grams In 1 Bar: 5

Louis's Favorite Wheat-Free Granola Bars: Use ¾ cup whole barley flour in place of the whole wheat pastry flour and ¼ cup oat bran in place of the wheat germ.

Golden Bars

¼ cup oil
½ cup raw honey
1 tablespoon molasses
1 egg
1 cup + 2 tablespoons whole wheat pastry flour
1 teaspoon *Rumford* baking powder
¼ cup chopped nuts (walnuts are good)

Preheat oven to 350°. Oil a 9-inch square cake pan with *Oil-Lecithin Combination* (p. 205). Combine oil, honey, molasses and egg. Beat together and stir in the flour and baking powder. Pour into cake pan, sprinkle with nuts, and bake for about 15 to 20 minutes. Do not overcook. Edges should be brown with center not browned. Cool on wire rack in pan and cut into 2¼-inch squares. If bars tear when cut, dip knife into water and then cut. Makes 16 pieces.

Perfect Whole Foods: No, because of honey, molasses, and baking powder.
Percent Calories From Fat: 40
Fat Grams In 1 Piece: 5

Wheat-Free Golden Bars: Substitute 1 cup + 2 tablespoons whole barley flour, ⅞ cup (1 cup minus 2 tablespoons) triticale or spelt flour, or 1¼ cups brown rice flour for the pastry flour.

Banana Bread

2 eggs
3 ripe bananas
¼ cup oil
¼ cup raw honey
1 tablespoon lemon juice
2 cups whole wheat pastry flour
1 teaspoon baking soda
¼ cup chopped nuts

Preheat oven to 350°. Oil a 9 x 5-inch loaf pan with *Oil-Lecithin Combination* (p. 205). Process eggs and bananas in blender or food processor until well mixed. Add oil, honey, and lemon juice; mix. Combine dry ingredients in a bowl, mixing soda in very well. Add liquid ingredients and combine just until dry ingredients are moistened. Do not overmix. Stir in nuts. Pour into pan and bake for 40 to 50 minutes. Let cool in pan 10 minutes before turning out onto rack to cool. Best if sliced next day. Makes eighteen ½-inch thick pieces.

Perfect Whole Foods: No, because of honey and lemon juice.
Percent Calories From Fat: 35
Fat Grams In 1 Piece: 5

Wheat-Free Banana Bread: Substitute 2 cups whole barley flour, 1½ cups triticale, spelt, or millet flour, or 1¼ cups kamut flour for the whole wheat flour.

Apple Pudding Cake

¾ cup oil
½ cup raw honey
2 eggs
3 cups chopped, unpeeled apples
2 cups whole wheat pastry flour
1 tablespoon *Rumford* Baking Powder
2 teaspoons ground cinnamon

Preheat oven to 325°. Oil a 9 x 13-inch pan with *Oil-Lecithin Combination* (p. 205). Cream oil and honey. Add eggs and beat. Combine dry ingredients and stir into egg mixture. Add apples, mixing lightly. Pour into pan and bake 25 to 30 minutes. Serve from pan. Makes twelve 3 x 3⅓-inch pieces.

Perfect Whole Foods: No, because of honey and baking powder.
Percent Calories From Fat: 49
Fat Grams In 1 Piece: 15

Wheat-Free Apple Pudding Cake: Substitute 2 cups whole barley flour, 1½ cups triticale or spelt flour, or 1¼ cups kamut for the whole wheat flour.
Peach Pudding Cake: Substitute 3 cups chopped, unpeeled fresh peaches for the apples.

Crazy Carob Cake

This crazy *cake is mixed and baked in the pan. It has* no eggs, no milk, *and when made without wheat flour,* no wheat. *It's great for those who are allergic to these foods.*

2 cups whole wheat pastry flour
1¼ teaspoons baking soda
½ cup carob powder
½ cup oil
⅓ cup raw honey
1⅓ cups water
1¼ teaspoons vanilla
1¼ teaspoons cider vinegar

Preheat oven to 350°. Combine dry ingredients in a 9-inch square cake pan (do not oil). Mix well, especially the baking soda. Combine liquid ingredients together and add to dry ingredients. Blend well, using a fork and scraping the sides so that all the dry ingredinets are mixed. Bake for 20 to 30 minutes. Cool on wire rack and serve from pan. No frosting needed. Makes twelve pieces.

Perfect Whole Foods: No, because of honey.
Percent Calories From Fat: 41
Fat Grams In 1 Piece: 13

Wheat-Free Crazy Carob Cake: Substitute 2 cups whole barley flour, 1½ cups triticale or spelt flour, or 1¼ cups kamut flour for the whole wheat pastry flour.
Applesauce Crazy Cake: Omit carob powder and decrease water to ½ cup. Add to dry ingredients: 1¼ teaspoons cinnamon, ¼ teaspoon cloves, and ¼ teaspoon nutmeg. Add to wet ingredients: 1¼ cups unsweetened applesauce. If desired, stir in ⅓ cup chopped nuts and ½ cup raisins or currants just before baking.

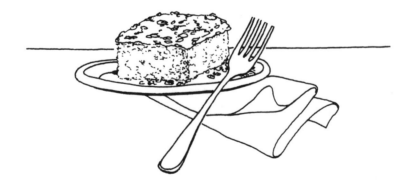

Capricorn Cake

Sonia and Lee Carter developed this recipe to use fruit and vegetable pulp leftover from making fresh juices. It's a moist and tasty cake!

3 cups whole wheat pastry flour
2 teaspoons baking soda
2 tablespoons cinnamon
½ teaspoon nutmeg
½ teaspoon cloves
1 cup oil
1 cup orange blossom honey or other raw honey
2 eggs
2 tablespoons pure vanilla extract
1 cup *Granny Smith* apple pulp
2 mashed bananas or 1 cup carrot pulp
1 cup chopped raw almonds or walnuts or combination
½ cup *each* currants & raisins or 1 cup golden raisins

Preheat oven to 350°. Butter and flour angel food tube cake pan. Mix dry ingredients. In a separate bowl, blend oil, honey, eggs and vanilla. Add to dry ingredients (folding motion with spatula, several times). Dust raisins and currants with a little flour. Add remaining ingredients to batter and mix well. Bake for 1 hour. Cool slightly and unmold. Makes about 24 pieces.

Perfect Whole Foods: No, because of honey and currants or raisins.
Percent Calories From Fat: 45
Fat Grams In 1 Piece: 13

Carrot Cake

If you don't have access to pulp for the Capricorn Cake, *then try this one. It makes a good dessert at Thanksgiving time.*

4 eggs
⅝ cup raw honey
1½ cup oil
3¼ cups whole wheat pastry flour
2 teaspoons *Rumford* Baking Powder
2 teaspoons baking soda
1 teaspoon cinnamon
8-ounce can crushed pineapple in juice, drained
2 cups shredded carrots (about 4 large)
1 cup chopped pecans
1 cup chopped dates
¼ cup additional whole wheat pastry flour

Preheat oven to 350°. Oil Bundt pan or tube pan with *Oil-Lecithin Combination* (p. 205). Beat eggs in a large mixing bowl. Beat in honey and oil. In another bowl, combine 3¼ cups flour, baking powder, baking soda, and cinnamon. Stir into egg mixture. Add drained pineapple and carrots. Mix well. Toss pecans and dates with the additional ¼ cup flour; stir into batter. Pour into pan and bake for about 40 to 55 minutes or until top of cake springs back when lightly pressed. Cool cake for about 15 minutes in pan. Remove from pan and cool on wire rack. Store in an airtight container when cooled. Makes about 24 pieces.

Perfect Whole Foods: No, because of honey, baking powder, canned pineapple, and dates.
Percent Calories From Fat: 55
Fat Grams In 1 Piece: 18

Wheat-Free Carrot Cake: Substitute 3¼ cups whole barley flour for the 3¼ cups whole wheat flour and ¼ cup whole barley flour for the additional ¼ cup whole wheat flour. Or substitute 2½ cups triticale or spelt flour for the 3¼ cups whole wheat flour and 3 tablespoons for the ¼ cup whole wheat flour.

Beth's Jam Cake

I developed this recipe several years ago when I couldn't find a jam cake recipe in any of my natural foods cookbooks. It has become one of my favorite holiday desserts.

¾ cup raw honey
¾ cup oil
3 eggs
10-ounce jar all-fruit jam (black raspberry is my favorite)
2⅔ cups whole wheat pastry flour
1½ teaspoon *Rumford* Baking Powder
¾ teaspoon baking soda
1½ teaspoon cinnamon
¾ teaspoon ground cloves
¾ teaspoon nutmeg
¾ cup buttermilk
1 cup pecan pieces
1 cup currants
3 tablespoons additional whole wheat pastry flour

Preheat oven to 350°. Generously oil Bundt pan or tube pan with *Oil-Lecithin Combination* (p. 205). Beat honey, oil, and eggs together with an electric mixer. Add jam and mix thoroughly. In another bowl, combine 2⅔ cups flour, baking powder, soda, and spices. In a third bowl, mix pecans, currants, and additional flour. Add flour mixture and buttermilk alternately to honey-egg mixture, beginning and ending with flour mixture. Stir in pecan and currants. Pour into pan and bake for 45 to 50 minutes. Cool cake for about 10 minutes in pan. Remove from pan and cool on wire rack. Store in airtight container when cooled. Makes about 24 pieces.

Perfect Whole Foods: No, because of honey, jam, and baking powder.
Percent Calories From Fat: 39
Fat Grams In 1 Piece: 10 when cut into 24 pieces

Wheat-Free Jam Cake: Substitute 2¼ cups spelt flour for the 2⅔ cups whole wheat pastry flour and 2 tablespoons additional spelt flour for the 3 tablespoons additional whole wheat pastry flour.

Prune Cupcakes

I converted this recipe to whole grains and honey from my mother's white flour-white sugar recipe she baked when I was a child. I omitted the frosting since the cupcakes alone are plenty sweet.

¾ cup raw honey
1 cup oil
28 pitted prunes, medium-sized, soaked in 1½ cups water in jar overnight in refrigerator
3 eggs
2½ cups whole wheat pastry flour
1 teaspoon baking soda
2 teaspoons *Rumford* Baking Powder
1 teaspoon *each* of ground nutmeg, allspice, and cinnamon
¼ teaspoon ground ginger
¾ cup buttermilk

Drain prunes and pureé in food processor. Preheat oven to 350°. Cream honey and oil. Add eggs and prunes and mix. Stir together dry ingredients and alternately add to prune mixture with buttermilk, beginning and ending with dry ingredients. Pour into muffin pans lined with papers, filling ¾ full. Bake approximately 25 minutes. Makes 28 to 30 cupcakes.

Perfect Whole Foods: No, because of honey, prunes, and baking powder.
Percent Calories From Fat: 45
Fat Grams In 1 Cupcake: 9 when recipe makes 28 cupcakes

Wheat-Free Prune Cupcakes: Substitute 2½ cups whole barley flour, 1⅞ cups (1¾ cup + 2 tablespoons) triticale or spelt flour, or 1½ cups + 1 tablespoon kamut flour for the whole wheat flour.
Apricot Cupcakes: Substitute 28 medium-sized dried whole apricots for the prunes.

Psalm 118:24
This is the day which the Lord hath made; we will rejoice and be glad in it.

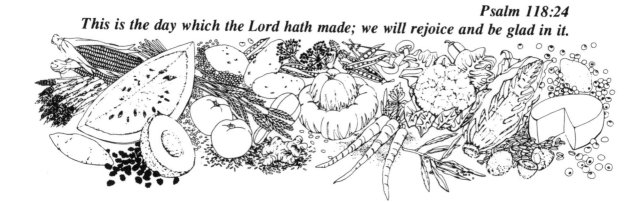

Brownie Surprise Cupcakes

2 eggs
½ cup raw honey
½ teaspoon pure vanilla extract
½ cup oil
¾ cup whole wheat pastry flour
¼ teaspoon *Rumford* Baking Powder
⅓ cup shredded carrots
¼ teaspoon cinnamon
¼ cup carob powder

Preheat oven to 350°. In a small bowl, beat eggs with a mixer. Beat in honey, oil, and vanilla. Combine flour and baking powder, beat into egg mixture. Remove ⅓ cup batter to a small bowl. Stir carrots and cinnamon into the ⅓ cup batter. To the remaining batter, add carob and blend well. Divide carob batter among 12 paper-lined muffin cups. Spoon carrot batter on top, either in the center or off to one side. Bake for 25 minutes and cool on a wire rack. Makes 12 cupcakes.

Perfect Whole Foods: No, because of honey and baking powder.
Percent Calories From Fat: 52
Fat Grams In 1 Cupcake: 10

Wheat-Free Brownie Surprise Cupcakes: Substitute ¾ cup whole barley flour, ½ cup + 1 tablespoon triticale or spelt flour, or 1 cup + 1 tablespoon brown rice flour for the pastry flour.

Cranberry-Pineapple Cupcakes

These cupcakes are good at holiday-time, baked in either the regular-size cupcake papers or the tiny ones. Use the tiny ones when more than one dessert is available. When small servings are offered, guests can sample several items without overeating.

4 eggs
¾ cup oil
¾ cup raw honey
1 teaspoon pure vanilla extract
2 cups whole wheat pastry flour
¼ cup pecan pieces
1 teaspoon baking soda
2 teaspoons *Rumford* Baking Powder
8-ounce can unsweetened, crushed pineapple, drained
1 cup fresh cranberries, washed, dried, and chopped in food processor

Preheat oven to 350°. Beat together eggs, oil, honey, and vanilla extract in a large bowl. Stir together in another bowl the flour, baking powder, and soda, carefully mixing soda in with other dry ingredients. Add dry ingredients to egg mixture and beat well. Stir in fruit and nuts. Pour into paper-lined muffin pans, filling slightly over half full. Bake 12 to 15 minutes, remove from muffin pans, and cool on wire rack. Makes 30 to 36 cupcakes.

Perfect Whole Foods: No, because of honey, baking powder, and canned pineapple.
Percent Calories From Fat: 49
Fat Grams In 1 Cupcake: 7 (when recipe makes 30 cupcakes)

Wheat-Free Cranberry-Pineapple Cupcakes: Substitute 2 cups whole barley flour, 1½ cups triticale or spelt flour, or 1¼ cups kamut for the whole wheat flour.

Crunchy Fudge

½ cup raw honey
½ cup natural peanut butter
½ cup carob powder
1 cup sesame seeds
1 cup raw sunflower seeds
½ cup currants or raisins
¾ cup unsweetened shredded coconut

Oil a 9-inch square pan with *Oil-Lecithin Combination* (p. 205). Heat honey and peanut butter together until hot but not boiling. Stir in carob powder. Quickly add remaining ingredients and stir well. Pour into pan, cover, and refrigerate. Cut into thirty-six 1½-inch squares when cold.

Perfect Whole Foods: No, because of honey and dried fruit.
Percent Calories From Fat: 60
Fat Grams In 1 Piece: 7

Carob Cookies

I developed this recipe after my children, several years ago, discovered some carob cookies at a natural food store. These are just as good-tasting and are much less expensive!

½ cup butter
1 teaspoon pure vanilla extract
⅔ cup raw honey
2⅔ cups whole wheat pastry flour
1 egg
⅔ cup carob powder, sifted

Preheat oven to 350°. Cream together butter and honey. Add egg and vanilla and beat well. Mix together flour and carob powder, then stir gradually into butter mixture. Shape into 1-inch balls and flatten onto ungreased cookie sheet. Bake about 9 minutes and cool on wire rack. Makes about 3½ dozen.

Perfect Whole Foods: No, because of honey.
Percent Calories From Fat: 31
Fat Grams In 1 Cookie: 3

Wheat-Free Carob Cookies: Substitute 2⅔ cups whole barley flour, 2 cups triticale or spelt flour, or 1⅔ cups kamut flour for the whole wheat pastry flour.

Cinnamon-Pecan Cookies

½ cup oil (plus about ½ teaspoon to oil cookie sheet)
2 cups + 2 tablespoons whole wheat pastry flour
½ cup raw honey
1 teaspoon *Rumford* Baking Powder
1 egg
¾ cup pecan meal (finely ground pecans)
1 teaspoon pure vanilla extract
3 teaspoons ground cinnamon

Preheat oven to 375°. Oil cookie sheet. Beat together oil, honey, egg, and vanilla. Mix together flour and baking powder, stirring into oil-honey mixture. Mix nuts and cinnamon together in small bowl and add dough by teaspoons, rolling in mixture. Shape dough into a ball and flatten onto cookie sheet to ⅛-inch thick. Bake 5 to 7 minutes and cool on rack. Makes 4 dozen 2½-inch cookies.

Perfect Whole Foods: No, because of honey and baking powder.
Percent Calories From Fat: 49
Fat Grams In 1 Cookie: 4

Wheat-Free Cinnamon-Pecan Cookies: Substitute 2 cups + 2 tablespoons whole barley flour or 1½ + 1 tablespoon triticale or spelt flour for the whole wheat flour.

Gingersnaps

¼ cup molasses
½ teaspoon ground cinnamon
½ cup raw honey
½ teaspoon ground cloves
¼ cup oil
⅛ teaspoon ground nutmeg
2 tablespoons water
⅛ teaspoon ground allspice
2 cups whole wheat pastry flour
½ teaspoon baking soda
1 teaspoon ground ginger

Combine wet ingredients in bowl. In another bowl combine dry ingredients, mixing in baking soda well. Add dry ingredients to wet ones and mix well. Refrigerate for about 30 minutes. Preheat oven to 375°. Oil cookie sheet with *Oil-Lecithin Combination* (p. 205). Form dough into 1-inch balls with your fingers. Place on cookie sheet and flatten with the side of of your fist to 1/8-inch thick. You may need to oil your fist if dough sticks. Bake for 7 to 9 minutes and cool on wire rack. Makes 3 dozen cookies.

Perfect Whole Foods: No, because of molasses and honey.
Percent Calories From Fat: 25
Fat Grams In 1 Cookie: 2

Wheat-Free Gingersnaps: Substitute 2 cups whole barley flour, 1½ cups + 2 tablespoons triticale or spelt flour, or 1¼ cups kamut flour for the whole wheat pastry flour.

Simple Peanut Butter-Oatmeal Cookies

⅔ cup natural peanut butter (if you are allergic to peanuts, use almond butter or cashew butter)
2 teaspoons pure vanilla extract
½ cup raw honey
2 cups rolled oats

Preheat oven to 350°. Mix peanut butter and honey until smooth. Add vanilla and oatmeal; mix. Form into small balls and place on cookie sheet oiled with *Oil-Lecithin Combination* (p. 205). Flatten. Bake 8 to 9 minutes. Cool on wire rack. Makes about 3 dozen.

Perfect Whole Foods: No, because of honey.
Percent Calories From Fat: 39
Fat Grams In 1 Cookie: 3

Oatmeal Cookies

½ cup oil
½ cup raw honey
1 egg
1¼ cup rolled oats
1½ cup whole wheat pastry flour
½ teaspoon baking soda
¼ cup nuts (pecan, walnut, or peanut pieces), optional

Preheat oven to 350°. Cream together the oil, honey, and egg. Mix dry ingredients together and stir into honey-oil mixture along with pecans. Refrigerate at least 30 minutes. Form into 1-inch balls and flatten on ungreased cookie sheet. Bake 9 to 10 minutes. Cool on wire rack. Makes approximately 3 dozen.

Perfect Whole Foods: No, because of honey.
Percent Calories From Fat: 40
Fat Grams In 1 Cookie: 4

Wheat-Free Oatmeal Cookies: Substitute 1½ cups whole barley flour or 1 cup + 3 tablespoons triticale or spelt flour, or ⅞ cup + 1 tablespoon kamut flour for the whole wheat flour.

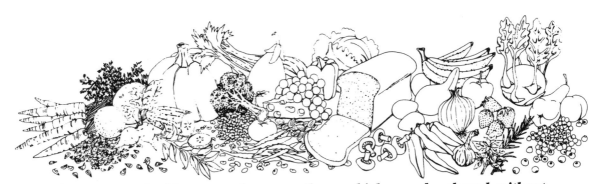

Our most valuable possessions are those which can be shared without lessening, those which, when shared, multiply; our least valuable possessions are those which, when divided, are diminished.   **William H. Danforth**

Oatmeal Fruit Cookies

½ cup oil (plus about ½ teaspoon to oil cookie sheet)
⅓ cup fresh wheat germ
¾ cup raw honey
2 teaspoons *Rumford* Baking Powder
2 eggs
2 teaspoons ground cinnamon
1 cup raisins or currants
¼ teaspoon ground ginger
½ cup chopped dried apples
¼ teaspoon ground cloves
½ cup chopped dates
1 teaspoon ground allspice
½ cup boiling water
1½ cups whole wheat pastry flour
1 cup rolled oats
1 teaspoon pure vanilla extract
⅓ cup nonfat milk powder
1 teaspoon pure almond extract
⅓ cup wheat bran

Soak fruit in the water 10 to 15 minutes. Preheat oven to 375°. Oil cookie sheet. Blend eggs, oil, and honey. Add fruit. Blend in oats and other dry ingredients. Stir in extracts. Drop by teaspoons onto cookie sheet and bake 10 to 13 minutes. Makes about 4 dozen 2½-inch cookies.

Perfect Whole Foods: No, because of honey, baking powder, dried fruit, and extracts with alcohol.
Percent Calories From Fat: 30
Fat Grams In 1 Cookie: 3

Skillet Cookies

My daughter Heather prepared these cookies in a 4-H cooking demonstration competition at school one year. For several weeks, we ate these cookies quite often while she practiced making them. Then after she won the competition in her classroom, we ate them again when she practiced for the next competition. Heather still enjoys making them!

3 tablespoons butter, softened
1 teaspoon *Rumford* baking powder
½ cup raw honey
1 teaspoon ground cinnamon
1 egg, beaten
½ cup dried currants
1½ cups whole wheat pastry or whole barley flour
½ to ¾ cup additional flour
2 tablespoons nonfat milk powder
3 to 4 tablespoons additional butter
½ cup fresh wheat germ

Cream together the 3 tablespoons softened butter, honey, and egg. Mix the 1½ cups flour, milk powder, wheat germ, baking powder, and cinnamon in a separate bowl. Stir these dry ingredients into the creamed mixture. Add currants and mix. Place the additional flour in the bowl you used to mix the dry ingredients. Heat an electric skillet to 325° and melt about 2 teaspoons of the additional butter in it. Drop teaspoon-size pieces of the dough into the flour and shape into balls. Flatten with your hands. Place as many cookies as will fit in the skillet. Cook them until they start to puff up and are brown on the bottom—about 2 or 3 minutes. Turn them over and cook for a minute or two on the other side. Remove and cool on wire rack. Before adding more cookies to the pan, melt 2 teaspoons more butter in it. Makes about 4 dozen cookies.

Perfect Whole Foods: No, because of baking powder, honey, and currants.
Percent Calories From Fat: 31
Fat Grams In 1 Cookie: 2

Humble yourselves therefore under the mightly hand of God, that He may exalt you in due time: casting all your cares upon Him; for He careth for you.   *I Peter 5:6-7*

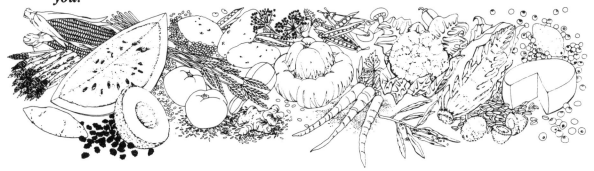

Frozen Strawberry Yogurt

Try this nonfat frozen yogurt recipe that was developed by Anita Courtney, nutritionist at the Lexington-Fayette County Health Department. It's not as creamy as the commercial versions, but it's light and refreshing.

2 cups unsweetened fresh or frozen strawberries
2 to 3 tablespoons raw honey
1 cup plain, nonfat yogurt
2 tablespoons apple juice concentrate

Purée berries, juice concentrate, honey, and yogurt in a blender or food processor. Pour into a shallow 8 or 9-inch metal pan and freeze for about 2 hours. Break the mixture into chunks and purée once again. The mixture should be soft and creamy. Pack it into a one-pint freezer container and freeze. Remove from freezer 10 minutes before serving. Makes about 2 cups.

Perfect Whole Foods: No, because of honey and apple juice concentrate.
Percent Calories From Fat: 3
Fat Grams In 1 Cup: 1

Frozen Yogsicles

Here's another of Anita's ideas for a nonfat frozen treat. It's simple to prepare and so good to eat on a hot, summer day.

¾ cup frozen juice concentrate, such as orange or pineapple
¾ cup plain, nonfat yogurt

Mix ingredients together and pour into molds and freeze. Soften at room temperature for a few minutes before serving. Makes six ¼-cup servings.

Perfect Whole Foods: No, because of fruit juice concentrate.
Percent Calories From Fat: 1
Total Fat Grams In Recipe: 0

Frozen Graham Squares

For each ice cream sandwich use:
  2 100% whole wheat graham cracker squares
  2 teaspoons smooth nut butter (such as peanut or almond butter)
  4 slices ripe banana, each ¾-inch thick

Spread 1 graham cracker square with nut butter, arrange banana slices on top, and add other cracker for lid. Wrap in plastic and freeze. Serve on hot, summery day. Children and adults will like these.

Perfect Whole Foods: No, because of graham crackers.
Percent Calories From Fat: 34
Fat Grams In 1 Sandwich: 7

Strawberry Pie

1 baked and cooled *Whole Grain Pie Crust* (p. 239)
⅓ cup raw honey
1 quart fresh strawberries, washed and hulled:
  1 cup sliced for pie
  2¾ cups whole for pie
  ¼ cup whole for garnish
1 cup water
3 tablespoons arrowroot

Topping:
½ cup whipping cream
¼ teasooon unflavored gelatin

Mix arrowroot and water in 2-quart sauce pan. Add sliced berries. Cook and stir over medium heat until mixture is thick and transparent. Do not bring to a boil or arrowroot will become thin. Cool. Stir in 2¾ cups whole berries and honey. Pour into baked pie crust. Chill until firm or about 3 hours.

Beat whipping cream until it almost holds its shape. Briefly soak gelatin in 1 teaspoon cold water. Warm to dissolve gelatin. Add to cream and beat until it holds its shape. Spread on pie and garnish with remaining berries. Chill until serving time. Serves 6.

Perfect Whole Foods: No, because of honey and arrowroot.
Percent Calories From Fat: 41
Fat Grams In 1 Piece: 18

Pumpkin Pie

1 unbaked *Whole Grain Pie Crust* (p. 239)
½ teaspoon ginger
2 cups cooked, pureed pumpkin
¼ teaspoon cloves
2 eggs, beaten
1 cup plain, nonfat yogurt
¼ to ⅓ cup raw honey
1 teaspoon pure vanilla extract
1 teaspoon ground cinnamon

Blend filling ingredients in food processor or blender. Pour into unbaked crust. Bake at 400° for 45 to 55 minutes or until knife inserted half way between center and crust comes out clean. Cool. Makes 6 servings.

Perfect Whole Foods: No, because of honey.
Percent Calories From Fat: 33
Fat Grams In 1 Piece: 13

Banana-Pineapple Crisp

20½-ounce can crushed or chunk unsweetened pineapple with juice
3 ripe bananas
1 tablespoon cold water
½ teaspoon ground cinnamon
¼ cup unsweetened coconut, flaked
2 teaspoons arrowroot

Topping:
¾ cup raw rolled oats
1 tablespoon oil
1 tablespoon raw honey
¼ cup unsweetened flaked coconut
¼ teaspoon ground cinnamon

Butter a 1½-quart casserole. Preheat oven to 400°. Combine pineapple, juice, and cinnamon in a medium-sized saucepan. Mix arrowroot with water. Stir into pineapple mixture and cook just until thickened, stirring constantly. Remove from heat before mixture boils. Slice bananas into casserole and sprinkle ¼ cup coconut over bananas. Pour pineapple mixture over the bananas and coconut. Prepare topping by mixing all ingredients together. Sprinkle over pineapple mixture. Bake for 12 to 15 minutes. Serve warm or cold. Serves 6.

Perfect Whole Foods: No, because of arrowroot, honey, and dried coconut.
Percent Calories From Fat: 34
Fat Grams In 1 Serving: 10 (when 6 servings)

APPENDIX A: If You Have Candidiasis

Use the *Perfect Whole Foods* diet during *Candida* treatment with just one exception—no fruit for about 3 months. Although many doctors use a more restricted diet (no vinegar, baking yeast, nutritional or brewer's yeast, cheese, mushrooms, tamari, shoyu soy sauce, and sometimes no grains), Dr. Stoll has found that everyone does not need to avoid these foods—only those actually allergic to them. (If you know you're allergic to yeasts and molds or discover you are after treatment begins, see page 333 for help in eliminating yeasts and molds from your diet.)

Diet During *Candida* Treatment

Totally Eliminate
All sugar
All refined complex carbohydrates
All caffeine
All alcohol
All foods to which you know you are allergic or sensitive
All fruit

The only difference between the diet during Candida *treatment and the* **Perfect Whole Foods** *diet is the temporary, total elimination of fruit.*

Most people must eliminate fruit for about three months. Fruit sugar (as well as sugar, refined complex carbohydrates, and alcohol) will feed yeast and prevent its overgrowth from being controlled. If you only restrict these foods (not totally eliminate them), symptoms will decrease, but you're much more likely to have the yeast overgrowth and symptoms return later.

When Eliminating Fruit

- Do not eat any fruit (fresh, canned, frozen, dried, or juiced).
- Do not use lemon or lime juice (even in small quantities).
- Do not use even the small amount of dried fruit in herb tea blends.
- Do not use products containing *natural flavors* unless you are absolutely sure it is not fruit or fruit juice (check with the manufacturer to be certain).

Some Fruit-Derived Products Are Okay

- Apple cider vinegar. In the process of making vinegar, the fruit sugar from the apples changes to an acid. The acid will not feed the yeast.
- Pure citrus oils like lemon oil, lime oil, and orange oil. They provide only oil and flavor, no fruit sugar. Fruit essence and citrus peel or zest are also okay since they provide no fruit sugar.
- Tomatoes, although botanically they are fruits, may be used since they are not sweet.

Try eating fruit again only when your doctor says it's okay—after about 3 months of treatment or after *all* symptoms of *Candida* have disappeared. First test only those fruits grown in the temperate climate, eating them fresh and raw, not canned, frozen, cooked, dried, or juiced. Temperate fruits include apples, pears, peaches, plums, figs, cherries, apricots, grapes, berries of all kinds, melons, and kiwis.

When Adding Fruit Back to the Diet, Try This Test

Eat only one fruit at a time and not too much of it, for example half of an apple. Then observe your body carefully. If you have any symptoms, it is a sign that you are not ready to include either that particular fruit or any fruit in your diet. Symptoms may occur after you've introduced a fruit for the first time or not until you've eaten it a second time. Symptoms vary from person to person. They often include those same symptoms you experienced before treatment. Examples include extreme fatigue, sleepiness, and itching.

Don't get discouraged if you can't tolerate fruit when you first test it. With more time, you will be able to eat it. Wait at least another month before repeating the test if one specific fruit or all fruit should cause symptoms.

You May Find Some of the Following to Be True

• That you can tolerate some fruits, all fruits, or none.
• That you can tolerate specific fruits in small amounts, but not large.
• That you can tolerate only a certain quantity of any fruit.
• That you need to alternate fruits—that is, not have the same fruit every day.

When you can tolerate temperate fruit, it's okay to try fresh lemon and lime juice (they're not as concentrated in natural fruit sugars as are other juices). Don't, however, try any whole citrus fruits, tropical fruits, or other fresh fruit juices for at least another three months since they are more concentrated in fruit sugars. After the *Candida* symptoms have been gone for six months, you might want to try a little dried fruit. Don't make any other changes at the same time so you'll know whether or not you can tolerate it by observing symptoms. Don't try foods containing honey, molasses, white sugar, or any other sugars until you're able to tolerate dried fruit. (Even if you are able to eat foods with sugar with no noticeable symptoms, don't get into the habit of eating them regularly or often!)

It's important to continue eating whole foods after *Candida* treatment, even if you continue to feel well. You should not, however, have to be so perfect with the diet as you were during treatment. Going back to your former eating habits, especially if you had been eating a typical American diet rich in sugar, refined grains, fat, caffeine, or alcohol, will not promote good health and will encourage the return of *Candida* overgrowth. How much you can liberalize your whole foods diet at this point seems to vary with the individual.

APPENDIX B: If You Have Food Allergies

Safe Foods Diet

Individuals with food allergies are *usually* allergic to those foods they eat frequently (this is not *always* true). One way to determine unidentified food allergies is to limit yourself to foods you rarely eat. You will often begin to feel better within a few days of beginning the **Safe Foods Diet**. While continuing to eat those *safe* foods, you can, one by one, add foods you had previously been eating frequently. By carefully observing symptoms, you can often identify food allergies or sensitivities. Omitting those foods that provoke symptoms and including those that don't, you will eventually have a longer list of foods you can tolerate. At this point, to avoid the development of more allergies, many doctors recommend that you rotate the foods you do tolerate—that is, eat as great a variety of foods as possible and not repeat the same foods over and over. Use the **Four-Day Rotation Diet** to accomplish this goal (p. 319).

Important Note: If you have severe symptoms that could be life-threatening, add foods back only under strict medical supervision.

Foods to Totally Avoid in the Beginning

- All grains (members of the grass family including wheat, rye, barley, oats, corn, kamut, millet, rice, triticale, spelt, cane sugar, molasses)
- All dairy (milk, cream, butter, yogurt, cheese, ice cream, etc.)
- All fermented foods (alcohol—beer, wine, and all others; vinegars; and tamari, shoyu, or sauce)
- All yeast and mushrooms
- All eggs, chicken, tomatoes, potatoes, chocolate, coffee, tea, peanuts, oranges, grapefruit, lemons, soybeans and their products, beef, pork, onions, garlic, and all forms of tobacco.

What can you eat? What is safe for you is not necessarily safe for another person. It all depends on what you have been eating regularly. Use the lists of foods that follow and select only those foods you never eat as often as once a week. Plan your diet, temporarily, around those foods. Eat a variety of foods, not the same ones over and over. It's best to eat a larger than normal amount of a few foods at each meal rather than small amounts of many foods. Omit any foods to which you know you are allergic or sensitive. Use organically-grown foods when possible because your sensitivity may be due to the chemicals instead of the food.

Safe Foods From Which to Select

Vegetables: Asparagus, avocado, beet, beet greens, bamboo shoots, broccoli, brussels sprouts, cabbage, carrots, cauliflower, celery, collards, cucumber, eggplant, green beans, green peppers, Jerusalem artichokes, kale, kohlrabi, mustard greens, okra, parsnips, radishes, rutabaga, spinach, sprouts, squash (all kinds), sweet potatoes, turnip greens.

Meats, Fish, Poultry: Clams, crab, duck, deer (venison), fish (fresh or salt water), goose, lamb, lobster, oysters, quail, rabbit, sardines, scallops, salmon, shrimp, squirrel, turkey (fresh or frozen without additives; read label carefully), tuna (fresh or canned in water without vegetable broth or hydrolyzed vegetable protein).

Beans: Any dried beans or peas except soybeans.

Grain-Like Foods (but not members of the grain family): Amaranth (omit if you have allergies to pollen), buckwheat (do not eat often since those with food allergies seem to develop allergies to this food easily), quinoa.

Fruit: (Eliminate fruit temporarily if you are being treated for *Candida*.)   Include fresh, unsweetened frozen, or dried. Select from apples, apricots, bananas, blackberries, blueberries, boysenberries, cantaloupe, cherries, coconut, cranberries, currants, dates, dewberries, figs, grapes, kiwi, loganberries, mangos, nectarines, papaya, peaches, pears, persimmons, pineapple, plums, prunes, raisins, raspberries, strawberries, and watermelon. Totally eliminate fruit juice and dried fruit if you are following the **Perfect Whole Foods** diet.

Nuts, Seeds, Nut Butters, Oil: Almonds, almond butter, almond oil, apricot kernel oil, Brazil nuts, butternuts, canola oil (unrefined or expeller-pressed), cashews, cashew butter, chestnuts, flaxseeds, fresh flax oil, hazel nuts, hickory nuts, macadamia nuts, olives, olive oil, pinenuts, pecans, pistachios, pumpkin seeds, pumpkin seed oil, safflower oil (unrefined or expeller-pressed), sesame seeds, tahini, sesame oil, sunflower seeds, sunflower butter, sunflower oil, walnuts (English and black), walnut oil.

Seasoning: Mineral or sea salt (not iodized sea salt).

Sweeteners: None.

Water: Spring water, preferably glass bottled.

You may experience withdrawal symptoms for the first few days and, therefore, feel worse.

If you eat only the foods previously listed and do not feel considerably better in 10 days to 2 weeks, then suspect allergies to a rare food you are currently eating, environmental allergies, or a medical problem other than or in addition to allergies.

Adding New Foods to the Safe Diet

- Add food in pure form only. For example, try cooked organic wheat berries, not whole wheat bread made of flour, yeast, oil, and sweetener.
- If you have severe symptoms that could be life-threatening, add foods back *only* under strict medical supervision.
- Wait at least 5 days between trying new foods.
- Grains to try adding first include brown rice, millet, teff, spelt, and kamut. These are less allergenic than wheat and rye.

Four-Day Rotation Diet

A four-day rotation diet can be helpful when you have multiple food allergies since it encourages you to eat a greater variety of foods and not repeat the same foods over and over. You can often prevent additional allergies from developing while you use the **Perfect Whole Foods** diet to improve your health. Although the rotation diet may seem complicated at first, it gets easier with time. Remember to eat simply. Don't expect traditional meals or mixed dishes. As with the perfect diet, it's best to work with your doctor when using the rotation diet.

General Information for Rotation

- Prepare all foods simply and nutritiously. Avoid mixed dishes at first since you should limit the number of food items at each meal and since it's easy to make mistakes with mixed dishes.
- In order to improve your health, the rules for the **Perfect Whole Foods** diet still apply. Eat *only* unrefined foods. Foods not used on the **Perfect Whole Foods** diet are printed in italics.
- Totally eliminate any food to which you know you react for at least 3 months and wait up to 6 months before trying it again. With your doctor's approval, you can then test each food individually and try rotating it into your diet if it causes no symptoms.
- Keep your environment as *chemically clean* as possible. Avoid perfumes, hair sprays, fabric softeners, tobacco smoke, paint fumes, etc.
- It is preferable (sometimes necessary) to use preservative-free foods grown without pesticides, hormones, and antibiotics. Use pure, uncontaminated water for drinking and cooking.
- You may use mineral or sea salt (not the iodized variety) daily unless you are also on a low sodium diet.
- I have listed foods on the **Four-Day Perfect Whole Foods Rotation Diet** (p. 320) according to categories (**Animal Foods, Vegetables, Grains and Grain-Like Foods, Herbs/Spices, Fruits, Teas**, and **Other Foods**). Use these categories to help plan your menus.
- Many foods are related to each other. I have identified foods in a given category according to their food families by beginning each family list with an bold, upper case letter and on a new line. The foods are separated by commas and each family list ends with a number. The only significance of the number is to help you find that same family listed under more than one food category.
- In most cases, use larger than normal serving sizes so you'll get enough to eat. Take a hypo-allergenic multi-vitamin and mineral supplement, if tolerated.
- It's helpful to keep a notebook listing your meals and snacks.

Four-Day *Perfect Whole Foods* Rotation Diet

Category	Day 1	Day 2	Day 3	Day 4
Animal Foods Preferably organically grown, fresh. No cured meats, no commercially frozen turkeys. Read labels.	Chicken, chicken eggs(151) **V**enison(159) **S**almon, trout(170) **C**od, scrod, haddock, pollack, hoki(172)	**B**eef, veal, cow's milk, cheese, yogurt, goat's milk, goat's cheese, lamb(152) **T**una, mackerel, albacore(175) **S**hark(176)	Fresh pork(155) **D**uck, goose, duck eggs, goose eggs(158) **G**rouper(185) **O**cean perch(178) **C**rab, lobster, shrimp(179)	**T**urkey(156) **R**abbit(157) Flounder, halibut, sole, turbot(180) **O**range roughy(183) **C**lam, oyster, scallop(182)
Vegetables Fresh, frozen, or dried; no canned; preferably organically grown.	**C**arrot, celery, celeriac, parsley, parsnip(1) **A**loe, asparagus, chives, garlic, leek, onion, shallot(2) **S**weet potato(8) **S**weet corn, bamboo shoots(61) **M**ushroom(9) **K**elp, kombu, arame, kijiki, wakame(10)	**L**ettuce, all leaf & head, globe & sunchoke artichokes(3) **C**ucumber, pumpkin, all squash, chayote(4) **B**eet, chard, spinach(5) **D**ulse, nori, laver, irish moss, carrageen(11)	**A**ll dried beans & peas, alfalfa sprouts, mung sprouts(15) **B**ok choy, broccoli, brussels sprouts, cabbage, cauliflower, Chinese cabbage, collards, cress, horseradish, kale, kohlrabi, mustard greens, napa, radish, rutabaga, turnip(6) **A**vocado(17)	**T**omato, unpeeled potato, sweet or bell pepper, chili pepper, pimento, eggplant, ground cherry(7) New Zealand spinach(9) **O**kra(10) **S**pirulina(12) **C**hlorella, sea lettuce(13)
Grains & Grain-Like Foods *Do not use foods shown in italics on the Perfect Whole Foods diet. They are refined.*	**W**hole wheat, rye, triticale, barley, oats, job's tears, teff, millet, spelt, corn, kamut, brown rice, wild rice, sorghum grain(61) **B**uckwheat(66) *Arrowroot(64)*	**Q**uinoa(5) **J**erusalem artichoke flour(3)	*Tapioca(70)* Garbanzo flour, *kuzu or kudzu(15)*	**A**maranth(63) *Potato starch(7)*

Category	Day 1	Day 2	Day 3	Day 4
Fruits *Use only fresh or unsweetened frozen (no juice, canned, or dried fruit) on the* **Perfect Whole Foods** *diet.*	Grape, fresh currant, muscadine(34) Peach, apricot, cherry, plum, nectarine(32) Pawpaw(41) Pomegranate (42)	All melons(4) Pineapple(40) Papaya(43) Fresh dates, fresh coconut(44) Mango(45) Starfruit(46) Prickly pear(47) Gooseberry(48)	Apple, pear, quince(31) Banana, plantain(49) Fig(50) Kiwi(51) Blueberry, cranberry, huckleberry(52) Persimmon(53)	Grapefruit, orange, lemon, lime, tangelo, tangerine, ugli, kumquat(35) Blackberry, black & red raspberry, strawberry(33) Passion fruit(54)
Nuts/Seeds/ Oils/Fats Fresh, not rancid. Read labels carefully.	Macadamia(97) Chinese water chestnuts(101) Pinenut(102) Poppyseed(95) Corn oil(61)	Cashew, pistachio(91) Sunflower seeds(3) Olive, olive oil(92) Dairy butter(152) Safflower, sunflower oils, psyllium seeds(3)	Peanut & oil(15) Black walnut, english walnut, hickory nut, pecan(93) Almond & oil(31) Soy oil, peanut oil(15) Canola oil(6) Walnut oil(93)	Flaxseed (100) Filbert, hazelnut(94) Brazil nut(103) Sesame seed(96) Chia seed(104) Sesame oil(96) Cottonseed oil(99)
Herbs/ Spices/ Flavorings	Caraway, dill, cumin, anise, chervil, cilantro, coriander(1) Ginger, turmeric, cardamon(64)	Peppercorn(25) Tarragon(3)	Cinnamon, bay leaf(17) Nutmeg(122) Allspice, cloves(123) Mustard seed(6)	Paprika, cayenne pepper(7) Basil, marjoram, oregano, savory, rosemary, sage, thyme(104) Saffron(125)
Teas	Fennel, gotu kola(1) Lemon grass, citronella(61) Ginseng(141)	Chamomile(3) *Decaffeinated coffee*(145) Comfrey(149)	Rosehip(31) Red clover, fenugreek(15)	Peppermint, spearmint(104) Lemon verbena(143) Elderberry flower(144) Goldenseal(62) Raspberry leaf(33)
Other Foods *Do not use foods in italics on the* **Perfect Whole Foods** *diet. They are refined.*	Baker's and nutritional yeast(9) Cream of tartar(34) *Molasses(61)*	*Date sugar(44)* *Beet sugar(5)*	Apple cider vinegar(31) Carob powder, *clover honey,* gums: acacia, guar, tragacanth(15)	Vanilla bean(140) *Maple syrup(60)* Stevia(104)

Specific Rules for Rotation

- Do not repeat an individual food more often than every four days.
- Do not repeat an individual family (foods with the same number) more often than every two days.
- You can have more than one form of the same food at a meal (dairy butter and milk; corn and corn oil; almonds and almond butter).
- You do not need to select a food from each category at each meal.
- At the beginning, select only 3 different foods at a meal. For example, on Day 1, at breakfast, eat grapes (family #34), brown rice (family #61), and pinenuts ((family #102). When you're feeling better, you can gradually add more items at each meal.
- At the beginning, you should not have two different foods from one family at a meal or during the day. For example, on Day 1, eat carrots *or* celery (family #1), not carrots *and* celery. You may try two foods from one family at the same meal or during the same day later when you have felt well for a while.
- For your preference and convenience, you may permanently transfer any entire food family (*all* foods in that family or *all* foods with the same number) to a different day. Don't make temporary transfers since it's easy to make mistakes.

Exceptions to the Rules

- Cereal Grains (family #61): Since gluten-containing foods are highly allergenic, it's best to eat *only one* food containing gluten every four days. This includes wheat, rye, triticale, oats and barley. Grains with only trace amounts of gluten or a kind of gluten that is less likely to provoke allergy symptoms include spelt, kamut, millet, quinoa, job's tears, teff, buckwheat, and amaranth. After you are feeling well, you can experiment to see if you tolerate them and treat them like gluten-free grains if you do. Gluten-free grains such as brown rice and corn can be rotated on the two day schedule as long as you don't repeat any individual food more often than every four days.
- The Fungi family(9) of yeasts, molds, and mushrooms are also present in aged cheeses and yogurt(152), apple cider vinegar(31), and leftover foods. Consider this when planning your food rotations and include this type of food only every four days.

Some doctors recommend other instructions or rules for rotation diets. You can adapt the *Four-Day Perfect Whole Foods Rotation Diet* to any set of rules. Since it includes a greater variety of foods than we normally eat, you'll find this helpful if you have multiple food allergies.

APPENDIX C: If You Have Food Sensitivities

If you're on the *Perfect Whole Foods* diet yet continue to have puzzling symptoms, be aware of the possibility of food sensitivities. Various food additives as well as natural substances in foods can cause reactions in sensitive people. Some reactions are more serious than others. In this section, I will discuss a few additives (MSG, sulfites, and aspartame) as well as some natural substances that can cause problems (gluten, nightshade plants, and tyramines). Note that you might be sensitive to these or any of the scores of other additives, contaminants, and natural substances in foods and in the environment (like artificial coloring, artificial flavoring, pesticide residues, fungicides, waxes, antibiotics, hormones, and chlorine).

MSG

MSG (monosodium glutamate) is a flavor enhancer that is often added to processed foods. Simply looking for the name on ingredient lists is not enough if you happen to be very sensitive to MSG. Foods not listing MSG as an ingredient may still contain it since MSG is naturally occurring in hydrolyzed vegetable protein (hydrolyzed vegetable protein is 12 to 20% MSG). Hydrolyzed vegetable protein is commonly used in processed foods as a flavor enhancer.

Some people are more sensitive than others to MSG. Almost one-third of the American population reacts to five grams of MSG; some react to as little as one gram. Symptoms vary greatly from one person to another. The classical symptoms of a headache, a tightness in the chest and a burning sensation in the forearms and back of the neck are often identified as the *Chinese Restaurant Syndrome*. Many people who eat food containing large amounts of MSG, especially soup in Chinese restaurants, complain of these symptoms. The fact that soup is often eaten on an empty stomach makes MSG more quickly absorbed into the bloodstream. Also, many people find that their reaction is more severe if they include an aspartame or *NutraSweet-*containing food at the same meal.

Since I'm very sensitive to MSG (I get a headache almost every time I eat out or eat foods containing hydrolyzed vegetable protein or natural flavoring), several years ago I took advice I read to take a 50 mg. B-6 supplement with food that might contain MSG (most restaurant meals and processed foods). Since it works for me (no headache), I take one of these supplements anytime I go out to eat. I still avoid foods that I know contain MSG, but it's nice to know that I can eat out occasionally without having a headache later. If you plan to try this, please note that you should not take single B vitamins without taking the whole B-complex. If you aren't already taking a supplement containing the whole B-complex, then do so if you try the B-6 for MSG sensitivity. (Check with your doctor for further advice.)

Possible Symptoms of MSG Sensitivity

Arthritis-like symptoms of joints	Mental confusion
Asthma	Moodiness
Chest pain and pressure	Nerve cell degenerative diseases
Depression	Pressure around the eyes
Diarrhea and cramps	Restlessness
Dizziness	Skin rash
Headache	Sneezing
Hyperactivity	Tingling of face or fingers
Insomnia	Vision problems
Mild nausea	Worsening of PMS

Beware of These Ingredients If You Are Sensitive to MSG

Accent	Kombu extract
Autolyzed yeast	Monosodium glutamate
Beef broth*	MSG
Chicken broth*	Natural flavoring*
Chinese seasoning*	Protein hydrolysate
Flavorings*	Spices*
Hydrolyzed plant protein	Vegetable broth*
Hydrolyzed vegetable protein	Vegetable powder*
HVP	Zest

These terms may or may not indicate that hydrolyzed vegetable protein, a source of MSG, is present.

There are several less common terms for MSG sources including Ajinomote, Glutacyl, Glutavene, Mei-jing, RL-50, Subu, Vetsin, and Wei-jing. If you are sensitive to MSG, be aware that other flavor enhancers such as disodium guanylate, disodium inosinate, and monopotassium glutamate may cause the same reactions as MSG.

Common Food Sources of MSG

Bacon	Frozen dinners
Bouillon	Frozen entrees
Canned gravies and meats	Ground beef and poultry with flavorings added
Canned soups	
Canned tuna	Meat tenderizers
Convenience foods with flavor packets	Salad dressings
Deli foods	Sauces, especially spaghetti
Dry soup mixes	Sausages
Fast food restaurants products including breading	Seasoning salts
	Turkeys injected with broth

Sulfites

Although sulfur is a mineral required by the body, the sulfur-based chemicals called sulfites cause adverse reactions in certain individuals. These reactions are usually acute and sometimes severe, especially in those with a history of asthma. Some with asthma even have anaphylactic shock when exposed to sulfites! If you are sensitive to sulfites or have asthma (many people with asthma also react to MSG, aspartame, and aspirin), beware of the many foods that might contain sulfites.

Since 1985, the FDA has required the food industry to label foods with more than 10 parts per million of sulfites. This means, therefore, that foods with less than 10 parts per million of sulfites are not required to be labeled. Although sulfites are banned on raw produce like lettuce and other raw vegetables in salad bars, sulfites can still be present in salad bars in dishes like potato salad, shrimp salad, and salad dressings. If you react severely to sulfites, be extremely cautious about questioning restaurant employees regarding ingredients since you may not always get a correct answer.

Possible Sources of Sulfites

Asparagus, fresh
Baked goods (dough conditioners)
Beer
Cake mixes
Campden tablets used in making wine
Cheese, some (check labels)
Cider
Cider vinegar
Cod fish
Coffee, instant
Colas
Coleslaw
Cookies
Cooking sherry
Corn products like cornmeal, cornstarch, corn flour, corn syrup, corn sugar, and corn oil (sulfur dioxide may be used in separating the parts of the corn kernel)
Drugs like antibiotics, asthma drugs, IV solutions, Novocaine, and steroids
Fruit (dried, fresh, or frozen, cut up, juices, purees, fillings)
Gelatin
Ginger ale
Guacamole (avocado dip)

Maraschino and glacé cherries
Mushrooms, fresh and canned
Pancake syrup
Pickles
Pie dough
Potatoes (cut up, fresh, frozen, dried, salad, or canned)
Potato chips
Salad dressing (especially the dry mix)
Salad bar items (not raw vegetables)
Sauces and gravies
Sausages
Sauerkraut
Seafoods including cod, shrimp, clams, lobster, scallops, and crab (fresh, frozen, canned, or dried)
Soups, canned or dried
Sugar
Tea, instant
Vegetables (cut up, fresh, frozen, canned, or dried)
Wine vinegar
Wine
Wine coolers

Terms on Labels' Ingredient Lists Indicating Sulfites Are Present

Potassium or sodium bisulfite
Potassium or sodium metabisulfite
Potassium, sodium or calcium sulfite
Sulfites
Sulfur dioxide*

*Dried fruit is usually treated with sulfur dioxide. This treatment does not have to be stated on the label. Untreated dried fruit will usually be labeled as unsulphured. Note that unsulfured dried fruits can also cause problems in very sensitive individuals since they are usually contaminated with other chemical residues like pesticides and fumigants.

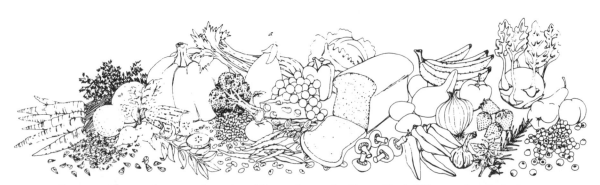

I carry hope in my heart. Hope is a feeling that life and work have meaning, whatever the state of the world around you. I am thankful to God for the gift of hope. It is as big a gift as life itself.   **Vaclav Havel**

Tyramines

If you have migraine headaches, see your doctor to make certain your headaches are actually migraine-related. In many cases, treatment for *Candida* will eliminate migraines. If it doesn't, then try to discover what triggers your migraines and avoid them. Possible triggers include foods rich in the amino acid tyramine; certain odors like cigarette smoke, perfume, gasoline, cleaning supplies, and new carpets; bright lights; a drop in blood sugar level (the ***Perfect Whole Foods*** diet will control this); stress; food additives; and several other foods.

Foods Rich in the Amino Acid Tyramine

Avocados	Dried or pickled fish
Bananas	Wild game
Beans, fava	Liver
Beef	Nuts
Beer	Soy sauce
Cheeses, aged (brie, camembert, cheddar, gouda, gruyere, mozzarella, Parmesan, provolone, romano, roquefort, stilton, and emmentaler)	Smoked meats
	Tea
	Vanilla
	Vinegar
Chocolate	Red wine
Coffee	Yeast and yeast extract
Sour cream	Yogurt

Typical additives that are known to trigger migraines in susceptible people include monosodium glutamate or MSG (see previous discussion of MSG beginning on page 323), sodium nitrite (in cured meats), sulfites (see previous discussion on page 325), and tartrazine (yellow dye # 5). Typical foods (other than those rich in tyramines) that are known to trigger migraines in susceptible people include cane sugar, canned figs, citrus fruits, corn, eggs, fried foods, milk, peas (including split peas and black-eyed peas), pork, and seafood.

Since the problem is often dose related, you might get by with a small amount of the triggering agent. A lot of any one agent or a small amount of several might lead to a headache. Also, stress might play a part with other triggers. You may be able to tolerate certain triggers unless you are under more than normal stress. If you keep a food diary with a detailed list of foods you eat, stresses in your life, and your symptoms, you may be able to determine what your migraine triggers are.

Aspartame

The Food and Drug Administration has received a number of complaints about aspartame, the artificial sweetener in diet drinks, sugar-free chewing gum, frozen desserts, and almost 4,000 other products. Aspartame (the chemical name) or *NutraSweet* (the trade name) is made of two naturally occurring amino acids, aspartic acid and phenylalanine. Although aspartame sounds innocent, each amino acid has specific functions in the brain just as do other amino acids. When specific amino acids are consumed in a greater proportion than is normally eaten, they can compete with other amino acids and possibly alter the function of neurotransmitters in the brain. Aspartame has another component, methanol, which is a toxic poison when it is converted in the body to formaldehyde and formic acid.

Some Common Reactions to Aspartame

Allergic symptoms such as itching, rashes, and asthmatic breathing	Memory loss
	Muscle weakness
Anxiety attacks	Personality changes
Depression	Seizures
Dizziness	Sleepiness
Headaches	Stomach pain
Hyperactivity	Tremors
Insomnia	Visual disturbances
Irritability	

In the first printing of this book, I reluctantly said that aspartame, *NutraSweet*, and *Equal* (as it's called when sold separately as an artificial sweetener) were okay to use as long as the products themselves and foods containing them contained no refined carbohydrates. I suggested that you totally eliminate aspartame if you had any of the above reactions. Today, I am increasingly concerned about aspartame's effect on health and, therefore, cannot recommend it at all.

Nightshades

If you have arthritis (including osteoarthritis and rheumatoid arthritis), your symptoms might be diminished or relieved if you eliminate foods to which you are allergic or sensitive. This could be any food or additive. People with arthritis are particularly sensitive to the group of alkaloid chemicals that are present in *nightshade* plants. Solanine in potatoes, nicotine in tobacco, and other alkaloids in the additional nightshade plants interfere with certain enzymes in the muscles of sensitive individuals. Although eliminating nightshades does not cure arthritis, it keeps it under control in some individuals.

Eliminate nightshades strictly for three to twelve months to determine if you are sensitive. Some people must also eliminate milk products that are fortified with vitamin D3.

Nightshade Plants

Tomatoes
Potatoes including potato starch (not sweet potatoes or yams)
Peppers including green, red, and yellow peppers, paprika, chili peppers, and cayenne
  pepper, but not black and white pepper. (An ingredient list could read *spice* and be paprika.)
Eggplant
Tobacco

If you are typical of others with arthritis, you might also be sensitive to chemical additives including artificial colorings, flavorings, preservatives, and emulsifiers as well as pesticides, herbicides, fungicides, and other chemical pollutants. Also, losing excessive weight usually helps control some of the symptoms. Remember, a whole foods diet can help you lose weight as well as improve your general health.

Gluten

Gluten intolerance is a condition in which even a small amount of gluten naturally present in wheat, rye, triticale, barley, and oats will result in health problems. If you are truly gluten-intolerant, you will need to eliminate gluten from your diet for the rest of your life since your body can't digest gluten properly. Gluten actually injures the lining of your small intestine. When you totally eliminate gluten from your diet, the lining repairs itself. While the intestine is damaged, you may be sensitive to other foods—especially dairy products and possibly soy products, eggs, and sugar.

Although improvement occurs in a few days after eliminating gluten, total recovery may take up to 6 months. In some cases, failure to respond may indicate the presence of gluten still in the diet or a wrong diagnosis.

It is believed by some that, of the several gluten fractions, only one, called *gliadin*, causes symptoms in those with gluten intolerance. Since the word gluten is a general term, foods may contain gluten but not the culprit, *gliadin*. The gluten fraction in buckwheat (not related to wheat), millet, teff, job's tears, amaranth, and quinoa apparently is not the type to cause problems in most persons. Due to many contradictions about this information in medical literature and by various celiac societies, check with your physician about the possibility of trying gliadin-free foods if you are gluten intolerant. Totally eliminate all sources of gluten for at least six months. If you no longer have symptoms, then cautiously try the gliadin-free foods one at a time, in small amounts at first (one tablespoon or less), noting any symptoms and waiting several weeks before trying a different gliadin-free food. It seems that each person is different in tolerance to these foods. If you can tolerate even a few of these foods, your diet will have greater variety.

Remember This When Reading Labels

Wheat-free is not gluten-free!
Low gluten is not gluten-free!

Two grains are completely free of all gluten and are, therefore, from the very beginning of the diet, safe for all who must eliminate gluten. The two grains are corn and rice.

Gluten-Free Grain Products

Corn Products
Corn bran
Corn fiber
Corn germ
Corn pasta
Cornstarch
High-lysine cornmeal
Hominy grits
Masa corn flour
Popcorn
White or yellow corn grits
Yellow, white, or blue corn meal

Rice Products
Basmati rice
Brown rice
Rice Bran
Rice flour
Rice pasta
Rice polish
Wild rice

*If you are on the **Perfect Whole Foods** diet, make certain you select only whole corn and rice products. For more information, read about corn on page 123 and see the typical terms and sources for refined corn and rice products on page 27.*

Food products made with wheat, rye, barley, and oats are extremely common in the American diet. Triticale is less common. If you need to eliminate gliadin (the usual gluten culprit), memorize or carry with you the following list of terms found on labels and ingredient lists that indicate its presence.

Beware of These Terms If You Must Eliminate Gluten (Gliadin) From Your Diet

Bran (unless it is corn, rice, or soy bran)
Breaded
Barley
Barley malt
Bulgur
Couscous
Cracked wheat
Cracker crumbs
Durum
Farina
Flour
Graham flour
Gluten flour
Malt
Oat bran
Pasta (unless it is corn or rice pasta)

Rye
Semolina
Starch
Thickener (unless a non-gluten source is specified)
Wheat berries
Wheat flakes
Wheat germ
Wheat germ oil
Wheat berries
Wheat flakes
Wheat starch
Whole grain (unless non-gluten source is specified)
Whole rye
Whole wheat

To avoid gluten sources, carefully read all ingredient lists. Write or call companies to find out the source of ingredients in question. To obtain toll-free numbers, call the toll-free operator at 1-800-555-1212. The following may be unsuspected sources of gluten (gliadin).

Unsuspected Sources of Gluten (Gliadin)

- Alcoholic beverages made with gluten-containing grains (grain alcohol, ale, beer, cordials, liqueurs, gin, malt beverages, aquavit, vodka, whiskey, vermouth).
- Candy—sometimes candy is made gluten-free, but often the conveyor belt in the candy factory is dusted with wheat flour so candy will not stick. In this case, wheat will not be listed on the label.
- Caramel color—usually made from dextrose (corn), invert sugar, molasses, sucrose (beet or cane). May be made from gluten-containing malt syrup or starch hydrolysates which can include wheat.
- Chewing gum.
- Communion bread or wafers at church.
- Denture adhesives.
- Dextrin—is made from corn, potato, tapioca, rice, or *wheat*. Malto-dextrin is always made from corn.
- Distilled vinegar—can be distilled from either wood or grain (usually, but not always, corn). Check with company of products made with distilled vinegar. Wine vinegar, cider, and rice vinegars are free of gluten.
- Flavorings and extracts—if they contain alcohol, it is usually made from a gluten-containing grain. Select alcohol-free flavorings and extracts.
- Flour from wheat may be a hidden ingredient in ice cream, catsup, mayonnaise, self-rising corn meal, and instant coffee.
- Hydrolyzed vegetable protein (or HVP), hydrolyzed plant protein (or HPP)—could be wheat, soy, corn, rice, peanuts, or casein.
- Imitation cheese.
- Imitation seafood (called sirimi)—contains starch from corn or wheat. Beware of restaurants who use a combination of imitation and real seafood.
- Luncheon meat, ham, frozen turkeys, canned meat based foods—read labels carefully.
- Malt, malt extract—if source is not identified, avoid the product or call the company.
- Medicines—check with your pharmacist about gluten content.
- Modified food starch—it could be wheat; if the ingredient list says just *starch*, it will be corn.
- Rice syrup—often contains barley malt, a source of gluten.
- Vegetable gum—if source is not identified, may be oat gum.
- Wheat germ oil in shampoos.

Yeasts and Molds

If you are allergic or sensitive to yeasts and molds, then beware of the foods, medicines, and vitamins that are sources of them.

Sources of Yeasts and Molds

Alcoholic beverages (like beer, wine, and whiskey)
Antibiotics
Baking yeast
Brewer's yeast
Buttermilk
Cheese, including cottage
Citric acid
Coffee
Dried fruits
Fermented foods
Foods enriched with vitamins
Fruit juice (unless freshly homemade)
Herb tea
Hydrolyzed vegetable protein (HVP)
Leftover foods
Malt
Many fresh fruits (especially grapes, oranges & melons)
Meat from animals fed antibiotics
Mineral supplements (especially selenium & chromium)
Miso
Monosodium Glutamate (MSG)
Morels

Mushrooms
Nutritional yeast
Nuts and nut butter
Peanuts and peanut butter
Pepper
Products with vinegar (like mayonnaise, dressings, catsup, mustard, pickles, kraut, and olives)
Shoyu soy sauce
Sour cream
Sourdough bread
Sprouts
Tamari soy sauce
Tea
Tempeh
Tobacco
Tomato sauce
Torula yeast
Truffles
Vinegars
Vitamins, especially B vitamins, unless labeled as *yeast free*
Xantham gum (fermented from corn)
Yogurt

Sometimes individuals allergic to yeast can tolerate yogurt, buttermilk, and natual sourdough bread (with no baking yeast added).

APPENDIX D: If You Need a Soft Diet

If you have problems swallowing, dental problems, or intestinal disorders that require soft or fairly smooth food, use the following list to help you select foods that you can tolerate. If necessary, use a baby food grinder or food processor to make foods smooth.

Fairly Smooth Foods From Which to Choose

Cereals: quick rolled oats (oatmeal), oat bran, Wheatena, Cream of Buckwheat, short grain brown rice, whole grain corn grits (all grains well-cooked).

Potatoes: *Whole Mashed Potatoes* and *Golden Potatoes* (p. 171 and 173).

Dairy: plain, nonfat yogurt with optional ingredients added–natural peanut butter or other nut butter, or a drop of lemon oil; mashed or puréed cottage cheese. (Read ingredient list carefully if you are on the perfect diet.)

Vegetables: fresh, raw vegetable juice (limit carrot juice to a 1 cup serving per day on the perfect diet); very soft steamed vegetables; shredded raw vegetables like carrots, if tolerated.

Fruit: ripe banana, or other fresh, ripe fruit run through a baby food grinder.

Main Dishes: *Black Bean Soup* (puree all, not just part of the soup), *Split Pea Soup*, *Navy Bean Soup* (puree all, not just the vegetables), canned tuna mixed with nonfat yogurt and unsweetened mayonnaise. (The main dish soup recipes are located on pages 78 to 81.)

When you are able to advance to more textured foods, there are many foods and recipes in this book from which to select. Consider some of the following.

Soft But Not Smooth Whole Foods and Recipes

Scrambled eggs
Lentil Stew (p. 82)
Vegetable Barley Soup (p. 186)
Whole wheat spaghetti with unsweetened pasta sauce
Macaroni-O's (p. 98)
Fish (p. 109 to 113)
Country Garden Rice (p. 139)
Gooey Brown Rice (p. 138)

APPENDIX E: If You Need to Reduce Fat

The Low Fat Diet (15 to 25 Percent Calories from Fat)

The low fat diet described below is used primarily for lowering blood cholesterol and for weight control. It varies from fifteen to twenty-five percent calories from fat, depending on your doctor's recommendation. (For a Pritikin or Ornish-type diet that's ten percent calories from fat and based on the perfect diet, see page 341.) The low fat diet explained here is based on fat grams. Since each person varies according to calories required and what percent calories should derive from fat, the exact number of daily fat grams will vary from person to person.

If you are just beginning to make changes in your diet, I hope you will incorporate the whole foods principles that are presented throughout this book. I have seen a number of people count fat grams faithfully without getting the results they expected. They were concerned with fat only—not with the rest of their diet. They didn't eat whole grains; they didn't restrict their sugar intake; they didn't eat a variety of vegetables; and they weren't concerned with avoiding saturated fat and incorporating essential fatty acids in their diet. They were only concerned with not exceeding a specific number of grams of fat that had been calculated for them. Don't simply count fat grams without an overall awareness of good nutrition. You won't get the best results if you do.

Since *The Healing Power of Whole Foods* was not written primarily for those counting fat grams, you will probably want to purchase a book listing foods along with their fat grams. Although I've included the amount of fat in most foods recommended in this book, a small reference book might be handy. For your convenience, most recipes in this book include either the total fat grams in the recipe or fat grams in a specified amount.

Before Determining the Number of Fat Grams to Include in Your Daily Diet

You should determine
• Approximately how many calories you need each day
• The percentage of calories from fat that's appropriate for you

If you do not know approximately how many calories you need to maintain your weight or to lose undesirable excess weight safely, use the chart that follows for calculating it. Check with your doctor about the percentage of calories from fat that's right for you.

To Calculate Approximate Caloric Needs

Your current weight: _____

Multiply by the factor based on how active you are:
  Women, 12 to 15; Men, 14 to 17
  (Select the appropriate number based on your sex and
  level of activity. For example, if you are a very
  sedentary woman, use the factor 12; if you are a
  fairly active man, use the factor 16.)   × _____

Calories needed to maintain weight: = _____

If you are overweight, subtract 500 calories per day to lose
1 pound per week. Exercise will help speed the loss. − _____

Approximate Daily Calorie Requirement   = _____
Women should not go below 1200 to 1500 calories per day.
Men should not go below 1500 to 1800 calories per day.

Check with your doctor about the appropriate percentage of fat in your diet and calculate the exact fat grams from the chart that follows. Although some medical authorities still recommend thirty percent calories from fat, many have come to the agreement that, to lose weight and decrease the risk of heart disease, the percentage should be less than thirty.

C. Norman Shealy, M.D., Ph.D.
The three major determinants of health are proper nutrition, physical exercise and mental attitude, including spiritual attunement.

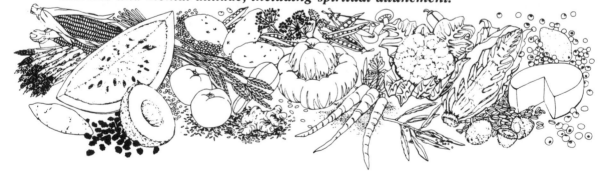

To Determine Daily Fat Allowance

Select the caloric level nearest your Approximate Daily Calorie Requirement as determined above. Use the total calories and percent calories from fat that your doctor recommends for you to determine your daily fat allowance. The Daily Fat Allowance calculated below is in grams of fat. (One gram of fat equals nine fat calories.)

	Percent Calories From Fat			
	15%	20%	25%	30%
Total Calories	Daily Fat Allowance (in grams)			
1200	20	27	33	40
1500	25	33	42	50
1800	30	40	50	60
2000	33	44	56	67
2400	40	53	67	80
3000	50	67	83	100

A low fat diet should not only restrict total fat, but should also limit total dietary cholesterol and saturated fat. If you simply reduce your fat intake, you'll also cut down on cholesterol-containing and saturated-fat-containing foods. However, be aware of the foods that are especially high in cholesterol and replace most of them with foods that contain polyunsaturated and monounsaturated fats.

Limit Cholesterol-Rich Foods

Egg yolks (no more than 3 or 4 per week)
Organ meats like liver, kidney, and brains
Certain shell fish—shrimp, oysters, mussels, and lobster (no more than 1 serving a week)
Caviar

Note that only animal products contain cholesterol.

Eliminate or Limit All Saturated Fats

Beef tallow
Butter
Cheese
Cocoa butter (chocolate)
Coconut and coconut oil
Cream, sour cream, and ice cream
Desserts like cakes, pies and cookies
Fatty and marbled meats like bacon, ribs, and most steaks, roasts, and ground beef
Fried foods
Gravies, sauces, and toppings (most)

Hydrogenated and partially-hydrogenated oils
Lard
Luncheon meats (hot dogs, bologna, salami)
Margarine
Palm and palm kernel oil
Poultry skin and fat
Sausages
Shortening
Whole milk

Choose Polyunsaturated and Monounsaturated Fats

Polyunsaturated fats
Flaxseed oil*
Fish and fish oil*
Grains
Corn oil
Safflower oil (regular, not high-oleic)
Sunflower oil (regular, not high-oleic)
Walnuts*

Monounsaturated fats
Canola oil
Safflower oil (high-oleic)
Sunflower oil (high-oleic)
Olives and olive oil
Peanuts, peanut butter, and peanut oil
Avocados
Nuts like cashews, almonds, pecans, and filberts

*Sources of the beneficial essential fatty acid linolenic acid (Omega-3). For more information about fats, see page 44.

Tips for Lowering Your Fat Intake

• Select only lean cuts of beef. Trim away visible fat from all meat before you cook it.
• Choose white meat of poultry rather than dark meat and remove skin and fat before cooking it.
• Roast, broil or bake meats. Cook meat or poultry on a rack so the fat can drain off.
• Chill meat or poultry broth until the fat hardens. Discard the fat before using the broth.
• Use nonstick *SilverStone* pans so you won't have to add fat when you sauté or pan-fry.
• Choose low-fat and nonfat varieties of dairy products (read labels carefully to eliminate undesirable ingredients).
• Use mustard instead of mayonnaise on sandwiches.
• Dilute mayonnaise with nonfat, plain yogurt for coleslaw and potato salads.
• Steam, bake, braise, or stir-fry vegetables in a very small amount of oil or water.

The Very Low Fat Diet (10 Percent Calories from Fat)

This Pritikin or Ornish-type diet provides no more than ten percent of calories from fat and no more than 100 milligrams of cholesterol each day. It also conforms to the *Perfect Whole Foods* diet discussed throughout this book. Note that you should use the *Very Low Fat* diet only under the direction of your doctor and for a limited time only since long term use will result in an essential fatty acid deficiency unless supplemental essential fatty acids are used.

While on the *Very Low Fat, Perfect Whole Food* Diet

Totally Eliminate
All sugars
All refined complex carbohydrates
All alcohol
All dried fruits and fruit juices*
All caffeine
All very high fat foods
Most canned foods

Avoid
Dry cereals
Most additives

*Freshly squeezed vegetable juices are okay (limit carrot juice to 1 cup serving per day); canned tomato juice and V-8 juice are okay to use in cooking, not as beverages. **Totally Eliminate** means that you should not eat these while on the perfect diet. **Avoid** means that you should try to refrain from using these or use them only in very small amounts.*

High Fat Foods to Eliminate on the *Very Low Fat* Diet

- All pure fats like butter, margarine, oil, lecithin, shortening, and lard
- Very high fat meats like bacon, sausage, marbled steaks, fatty hamburger, spareribs, hot dogs, luncheon meat, duck, goose, poultry skin, organ meats like liver and kidney, fish canned in oil, pre-basted turkey or chicken
- Egg yolks, fish eggs like caviar
- Dairy products like cream, half-and-half, whole milk, 2% milk, sour cream, and low fat yogurt
- Nuts and seeds (chestnuts are okay and seeds in small amounts in seasonings)
- Avocados
- Olives
- Wheat germ
- Coconut
- Products prepared with any of the above ingredients like mayonnaise, salad dressings, sauces, and gravies

Foods to Eat on the *Very Low Fat, Perfect Whole Foods* Diet

Vegetables: all kinds if fresh or frozen, raw or cooked like broccoli, carrots, celery, corn, mushrooms, parsley, spinach, tomatoes, lettuce, cauliflower, kale, onions, garlic, squash, peas, beets, and small potatoes including the skin (unlimited amounts).

Whole grains: brown rice, rolled oats (oatmeal), oat bran, millet, hulled barley, popcorn, whole grain corn grits, whole grain cornmeal, whole wheat flour, whole grain pasta (with no eggs added), and unsweetened 100% whole grain bread and crackers if no fat is added (unlimited amounts).

Dried Beans: dried beans and peas like pintos, navy beans, split peas, lentils, and black beans (limit to 5 to 7 cups per week unless more is substituted for the meat allowance).

Dairy products: 1 cup plain, nonfat yogurt; 1 cup skim milk; 1 cup buttermilk (no more than 1% fat); 1 cup reconstituted nonfat dry milk; or 2 ounces of 100% skim milk cheese like dry cottage cheese (2 servings daily maximum).

Fruit: all whole fruit if fresh or frozen without sugar (5 per day maximum).

Condiments and seasonings: fresh and dried herbs and spices, apple cider vinegar, mineral or sea salt (not iodized sea salt), unsweetened canned tomato products, carob powder, and baking yeast and baking soda for leavening.

Beverages: spring water, peppermint tea, camomile tea, ginger tea.

Meat, fish, poultry: fish, canned tuna in spring water, skinned chicken (white meat only), skinned fresh turkey (white meat only), lean beef trimmed of visible fat (round and flank cuts), lean game (limit meat, fish, and poultry to 3½ ounces per day). If you wish to omit these meat products, you can substitute 1 cup cooked beans in place of the 3½-ounce serving.

Eggs: egg whites only (7 per week maximum).

Nuts, seeds, and nut butters: none other than seeds (small amounts in seasonings only, less than ⅛ teaspoon per day) and chestnuts (unlimited).

Fats: none.

Determine which recipes are okay on the *Very Low Fat* diet by checking the *Percent Calories From Fat* listed at the end of most recipes in this book. If the percentage is less than ten and the recipe contains no oil, cheese, or other ingredients eliminated from your diet, then you may use the recipe as is. Many of the foods you will be eating (grains, vegetables, nonfat dairy products, and fruits) provide less than ten percent and a few foods will provide more than ten percent. The average percentage will equal less than ten since the foods providing more than ten percent are allowed in limited amounts. Even if the recipe has fewer than ten percent calories from fat yet includes a small amount of oil, alter the recipe according to the description that follows.

You can often alter recipes in this book and other cookbooks to make them compatible with the **Very Low Fat** diet. However, not all recipes can be changed. Read each recipe's ingredients and instructions carefully to determine if high fat ingredients can be omitted or if they are necessary in the recipe. Here are some helpful hints on making recipe changes.

Altering Recipes

- In soups, stews, other main dishes, and grain dishes, sauté vegetables in a few drops of water or broth rather than oil or use a *SilverStone* pan (if all other ingredients are appropriate for the diet).
- In some recipes, omitting the cheese will not greatly change the dish. Make certain other ingredients are appropriate for the **Very Low Fat** diet.
- In quick breads, two egg whites can often be substituted for 1 whole egg. Prepare muffins without oil by substituting unsweetened applesauce (homemade on the perfect diet) for the oil. A little more applesauce is needed to replace the oil. Eliminate high fat nuts and seeds.

Other Foods That May Be Used on the *Very Low Fat* Diet

Sapsago (green) cheese, a very strong-flavored cheese than is almost free of fat: 1 to 2 tablespoons per week maximum

Gelatin, plain: 1 ounce per week (9 teaspoons or 4 envelopes) maximum

Soybeans, tofu, and tempeh: 2-ounce serving in place of 3½-ounce meat serving due to fat

Shrimp: 2-ounce serving in place of 3½-ounce meat serving due to cholesterol

Salt and salty foods: in moderation

APPENDIX F: If You Need to Lose Weight

Most people automatically lose weight when they follow the *Perfect Whole Foods* diet. Simply eliminating all processed foods containing sugar, refined complex carbohydrates, caffeine, and alcohol often will make weight loss possible. Eliminating these foods will control fluctuating blood sugar levels that can trigger hunger and cravings. Excluding processed foods from the diet also usually decreases the amount of fat eaten. Not all people, however, lose weight this easily. Use the following information if you need more help.

For years, medical science thought that the best way to lose weight was to restrict calories, often to very low levels. Unfortunately, if you lose weight on a very low calorie diet, you will probably gain it back (plus some extra weight) after the diet is over. Several diets later, you will weigh more than ever. This process of losing, gaining, losing, and gaining has become known as yo-yo dieting. It gets progressively harder to lose weight as a result of very low calorie diets. When calories are severely restricted, your body thinks it is being starved. In an attempt to survive, its metabolic rate (speed at which calories are burned) slows down. Lean muscle is lost. These two factors promote weight gain after the diet is over. Since the weight gain is in the form of fat, your body becomes fatter. Very low calorie dieting is not the answer to losing weight, so don't let anyone talk you into following one. To maintain your metabolic rate and muscle mass, don't diet below 1200 to 1500 calories if you are a woman or 1500 to 1800 if you are a man. (These are general guidelines; if you are already very active or have greater muscle mass than most, then you should include more calories in your weight loss diet.)

If the very low calorie diet is not the answer to overweight, what is? It is important *to strictly avoid refined carbohydrates* (keep following the *Perfect Whole Foods* diet), *have a moderate amount of protein and a littte fat with each meal, eat lots of vegetables, get more exercise*, and *learn to control your response to stress*. We know that refined carbohydrates trigger you to crave more carbohydrates and perhaps even lose control of what you're eating, while protein and fat help keep you satisfied. Since a diet of excessively high in protein and fat does not promote good health, there is yet another option. Since you shouldn't reduce your total calories too much, simply add to your moderate protein portion, a small amount of fat, and lots of vegetables, a *moderate* portion of a whole grain or starchy vegetable and a serving of whole, fresh fruit to each meal. This meal plan, along with an increase in exercise should allow you to gradually weight loss.

With your doctor's approval, get involved in some kind of exercise, doing something that you enjoy and will continue. Exercise helps you lose body fat, not simply pounds. It helps you burn more calories as well as speeds the rate at which your body uses calories when the exercise period is over. Walking is an excellent way to begin if you have not been active for a while. Gradually increase the time and speed you walk each day. Start out walking slowly and increase your speed only when your body has warmed up to prevent injuries. Exercise, especially aerobic exercise (only if you have your doctor's okay) is an important key to both losing weight and maintaining your loss.

I highly recommend that anyone beginning a weight loss program first study the book *The Ultimate Fit or Fat* by Covert Bailey (Houghton Mifflin Company, 1999) to become convinced that diets without exercise don't work and to discover valuable fitness guidelines.

Keep These Hints in Mind

- Don't attempt to lose more than 1 to 2 pounds per week. You're more likely to maintain your weight loss if you lose weight gradually. Fast weight loss means you're losing lean muscle mass and water rather than fat. Weigh only once a week, not every day, since normal daily fluctuations are often discouraging.
- Include a moderate-size portion of a good protein source at each meal.
- Have small to moderate-size portions of unrefined complex carbohydrates (see page 18).
- Greatly increase the amount of raw and cooked vegetables you eat. Also eat plenty of fresh, whole fruit, but make certain that you eat more vegetables than fruit.
- Include a small amount of good quality fat at each meal to help with satiety. Make a point of including Omega-3 essential fatty acids daily (p. 47).
- Sauté foods in water or a small amount of butter or olive oil.
- Never skip a meal or go more than 4 or 5 hours without a meal or light snack. Eat three planned meals every day.
- Take a good multiple vitamin-mineral supplement daily. Brands from health food stores and natural food stores usually contain better quality ingredients than the less expensive one-a-day type brands from discount stores and drug stores.
- Drink 6 to 8 glasses of clean water each day.
- Plan your meals carefully so you won't find yourself in a situations where you eat refined foods. Often as little as one bite of refined foods will make you crave more.
- Learn to control your response to stress.
- Vary your food and habits. Don't eat the same foods each day.
- Consider whole foods a permanent new way of eating, not a temporary diet. This program will not only help you lose weight but will help you develop habits that will be beneficial to your health.

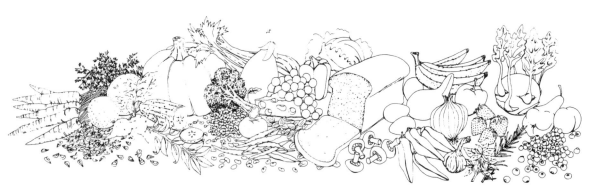

The journey of a thousand miles begins with one step.   *Lao-Tsze*

APPENDIX G: If You Need Quick References

Use these convenient guides to help you determine which foods, ingredients, additives, and name brands you may use on the *Perfect Whole Foods* diet. Although I have not attempted to investigate all foods, additives, and brands, the list is complete enough so that, with the information I have given you throughout the book and with the **Quick References** themselves, you'll be able to make decisions concerning foods and brand names not included.

If you're looking for a specific item in question, refer to either the **Quick Reference for Foods** or the **Quick Reference for Additives**. In general, foods containing additives should be consumed less often than those without additives. Use the **Quick Reference for Brand Names** to discover specific brands of foods to enjoy and to get ideas for similar brands not listed. Since common products like aspirin and mouthwash products include refined carbohydrates, I've included a **Quick Reference for Minor Remedies**. Don't, however, attempt to self-medicate serious problems. Check with your doctor.

My decisions for determining what is acceptable and what is not are based on the guidelines of the *Perfect Whole Foods* diet as listed below.

Guidelines for the *Perfect Whole Foods* Diet

Totally Eliminate	**Avoid**
All sugars	Excessive fat
All refined complex carbohydrates	Hydrogenated fats including margarine
All alcohol	Refined oils
All dried fruit	Most canned foods
Most juices	Dry cereals
All caffeine	Most additives
	Tap water

Totally Eliminate means that you should not eat these while on the perfect diet. Avoid means that you should try to refrain from using them or use them only in very small amounts.

Occasionally a food or additive is derived from sugar, starch, or alcohol but has been changed chemically and is no longer a sugar, starch, or alcohol. In this case, the resulting food or additive may be used on the perfect diet. For example, the refined sugar in apple juice (the fruit sugar became refined when the fiber was removed in the juicing process) is converted into an acid when apple cider vinegar is produced. Vinegar is, therefore, appropriate for the *Perfect Whole Foods* diet since it is not a source of refined carbohydrate.

Explanation of Quick References

Yes: You may use this item on the *Perfect Whole Foods* diet.

No: Totally eliminate this item while on *Perfect Whole Foods*.

Avoid: Use occasionally, if necessary. These foods will not interfere with the *Perfect Whole Foods* diet but should not be used regularly for one reason or other. In most cases, they include an ingredient that is not health-promoting. In small amounts occasionally, they should not be a problem. But regular use is not wise.

Maybe: Before using this product, determine what is in it by very carefully reading the ingredient list, and in a few cases you may need to find out from the manufacturer how an ingredient is made. For example, natural lemon flavor might be lemon juice, lemon peel, or lemon oil. Only the manufacturer knows which it is when the term *natural lemon flavor* is used on the ingredient list.

Quick Reference for Foods

Since there are so many fruits and vegetables available, it is unlikely that this list will cover them all. If you don't find something listed, you may have it on the perfect diet, as long as it is fresh or frozen with no added sugar or starch. It may be eaten raw or lightly cooked.

Quick Reference for Foods

Food or Ingredient	Used on Perfect Diet	Food/Ingredient	Used on Perfect Diet
Acidophilus (bacteria culture)	yes	Arrowroot	no
Acorn squash	yes	Arrowroot flour	no
Aduki beans, fresh or dried	yes	Arrowroot starch	no
Agar or agar-agar	yes	Artichokes, globe (canned)	no
Alfalfa sprouts	yes	Artichokes, globe (fresh or frozen)	yes
All-purpose flour	no	Artichokes, Jerusalem	yes
Almond butter	yes	Artichoke Flour, Jerusalem	yes
Almonds, raw or toasted	yes	Artificial sweetener products, granulated or powdered	no
Aloe vera juice	yes	Asparagus, canned	no
Amaranth flour	yes	Asparagus, fresh	yes
Amaranth grain	yes	Asparagus, frozen	yes
Amasake	no	Avocado, fresh	yes
Anasazi beans, fresh or dried	yes		
Apple, canned	no	Bacon (sugar)	no
Apple cider	no	Baking powder	no
Apple cider vinegar (preferably raw or unpasteurized)	yes	Baking soda	yes
Apple, dried	no	Baking yeast	yes
Apple, fresh	yes	Banana, dried	no
Apple juice, fresh or canned	no	Banana, fresh	yes
Applesauce, canned	no	Balsamic vinegar	yes
Applesauce, homemade	yes	Bancha tea (caffeine)	no
Apricot, canned	no	Barley flakes (refined)	no
Apricot, fresh	yes	Barley flour (from pearled barley)	no
Apricot, dried	no	Barley flour (from hulled barley)	yes
Arame	yes	Barley grits (if whole)	yes

Food or Ingredient	Used on Perfect Diet
Barley, hulled (whole)	yes
Barley malt (sweetener)	no
Barley, pearled (refined)	no
Barley, pot (lightly refined)	no
Barley, scotch (lightly refined)	no
Barley syrup	no
Basmati brown rice	yes
Basmati white rice	no
Basil, fresh or dried	yes
Beans, dried (canned)	no
Beans, dried (cooked or sprouted)	yes
Beans, green (canned)	no
Beans, green (fresh)	yes
Beans, green (frozen)	yes
Bee pollen	yes
Bee propolis (if no honey is added)	yes
Beef, deli-style sliced (sugar)	no
Beef-flavored broth powder (starch)	no
Beef, fresh or frozen (lean is preferable)	yes
Bell pepper	yes
Beer	no
Beer, non-alcoholic	no
Beet, canned	no
Beet, fresh	yes
Beet sugar	no
Black beans, canned	no
Black beans, dried (cooked or sprouted)	yes
Black olives	yes
Black tea (caffeine)	no
Blackstrap molasses	no
Bleached wheat flour	no
Blue corn (if whole grain)	yes
Blue corn, treated with lime, lye, or wood ash (if whole grain)	yes
Blueberry, canned	no
Blueberry, fresh	yes
Blueberry, frozen	yes
Bologna	no
Bolted cornmeal (refined)	no
Bouillon cubes (sugar)	no
Bran (wheat, corn, oat, or rice)	yes
Bread crumbs (refined)	no
Bread, 100% whole grain, unsweetened	yes
Bread, sourdough, 100% whole grain, unsweetened	yes
Brewer's yeast	yes
Broccoli, fresh	yes
Broccoli, frozen (plain, no sauce)	yes
Broth powders (contains starch or sugar)	no
Brown rice	yes
Brown rice, partially milled	no
Brown rice syrup	no
Brown sugar	no
Brussels sprouts, fresh	yes
Brussels sprouts, frozen	yes
Buckwheat	yes
Buckwheat flour	yes
Buckwheat groats	yes
Bulgur	yes
Bulgur wheat	yes
Butter Buds	no
Butter, salted	yes
Butter, unsalted or sweet	yes

Food or Ingredient	Used on Perfect Diet
Buttermilk, commercial	maybe
Buttermilk, homemade	yes
Buttermilk powder (added whey)	no
Cabbage, fresh	yes
Cake flour	no
Cane juice, granulated	no
Cane sugar	no
Candy, sugar-free (contains sorbitol)	no
Canola oil, expeller-pressed	yes
Cantaloupe, fresh	yes
Capers, canned	yes
Caramel	no
Caramel coloring (from sugar)	no
Caramel flavoring (from sugar)	no
Carob candy	no
Carob candy, unsweetened (contains malt)	no
Carob chips, unsweetened (contains malt)	no
Carob flour	yes
Carob powder	yes
Carrot, canned	no
Carrot, fresh	yes
Carrot juice, fresh (1 cup only per day)	yes
Carrot juice, canned	no
Cashew butter	yes
Cashews, raw or toasted	yes
Cauliflower, fresh or frozen	yes
Celery, fresh	yes
Chamomile tea	yes
Chapattis, 100% whole wheat (if no baking powder or sweetener added)	yes
Cheese, natural	yes
Cheese, low-fat	maybe
Cheese, shredded artificial (contains starch)	no
Cherries, canned	no
Cherries, dried	no
Cherries, fresh	yes
Chestnuts, water, canned	yes
Chewing gum, sugar-free (contains sorbitol)	no
Chicken-flavored broth powder (contains starch)	no
Chicken, fresh or frozen	yes
Chicken eggs, preferably farm, not factory	yes
Chickory	yes
Chickpeas, canned	no
Chickpeas, dried (cooked or sprouted)	yes
Chickpea or garbanzo flour	yes
Chile peppers, dried	yes
Chocolate	no
Chocolate chips	no
Cider	no
Cocoa	no
Coconut (sweetened)	no
Coconut, dried	no
Coconut, fresh (unsweetened)	yes
Coconut milk (fresh)	avoid
Coconut oil	avoid
Coffee (contains caffeine)	no
Confectioner's sugar	no
Converted rice	no
Corn, canned	no
Corn chips, baked (if whole grain)	yes
Corn chips, whole grain, no hydrogenated oil, sugar,	

Food or Ingredient	Used on Perfect Diet
or starch added	yes
Corn, cracked & degerminated	no
Corn flour (refined)	no
Corn, fresh	yes
Corn, frozen (whole kernel, not cream-style)	yes
Corn fructose	no
Corn oil, expeller-pressed	avoid
Corn oil, refined	avoid
Corn oil, unrefined	yes
Corn pasta (refined)	no
Corn sugar	no
Corn sweetener	no
Corn syrup (sugar)	no
Corn tortillas (if whole grain)	yes
Corn, treated with lime, lye, or wood ash (if whole grain)	yes
Cornmeal (check with manufacturer)	maybe
Cornmeal, bolted (refined)	no
Cornmeal, degerminated (refined)	no
Cornmeal, enriched	no
Cornmeal, stone ground (only if whole grain)	yes
Cornmeal, unbolted (only if germ is present)	yes
Cornmeal, whole grain	yes
Cornstarch	no
Cottage cheese	maybe
Couscous (most is refined)	no
Couscous, whole wheat	yes
Cracked wheat	yes
Cranberry juice	no
Cranberries, canned	no
Cranberries, fresh	yes
Cranberries, frozen (if sugar-free)	yes
Cream of tartar	yes
Cucumbers	yes
Currants, dried	no
Dark rye flour (whole grain)	yes
Date sugar	no
Dates, dried	no
Dates, fresh	yes
Decaffeinated coffee	no
Decaffeinated tea	no
Degerminated corn	no
Demerar sugar	no
Dextrin	no
Dextran	no
Dextrose (sugar)	no
Diastatic malt (sprouted, dried, and ground grain)	yes
Diet soft drinks, decaffeinated	maybe
Dried beans, canned	no
Dried beans, cooked	yes
Dried beans, sprouted & cooked	yes
Dried fruit	no
Durum	no
Durum flour	no
Durum pasta	no
Durum, whole	yes
Egg white powder (if no other ingredients)	yes
Eggs, preferably farm, not factory	yes
Enriched cornmeal (denotes refined)	no
Enriched flour (denotes refined)	no

Food or Ingredient	Used on Perfect Diet
Enriched pasta	no
Enriched rice	no
Farina (refined wheat)	no
Fish, fresh	yes
Fish, frozen (no breading)	yes
Flax seeds	yes
Flour (denotes refined)	no
Fortified grain	no
FOS (fructo-oligosaccharides)	no
Fructose	no
Fruit, canned	no
Fruit, cooked from fresh	yes
Fruit, dried	no
Fruit, fresh or frozen (unsweetened)	yes
Fruit juice concentrate	no
Fruit juice, fresh or canned	no
Fruit sugar	no
Galactose	no
Garbanzo beans, dried	yes
Garbanzo or chickpea flour	yes
Garlic, fresh	yes
Garlic oil	yes
Garlic powder	yes
Garlic salt (powder is preferred)	yes
Gelatin	yes
Germinated barley	yes
Glaze (if sugar)	no
Gluten (contains some starch)	no
Gluten flour (contains some starch)	no
Granulated artificial sweeteners (contain sugars)	no
Granulated cane juice	no
Granulated garlic	yes
Granulated onion	yes
Granulated rice	no
Grapes, canned	no
Grapes, fresh	yes
Grape juice	no
Grape sugar	no
Grape sweetener	no
Grapefruit, fresh	yes
Green olives	yes
Green tea (contains caffeine)	no
Greens, fresh or frozen	yes
Grits, corn, most commercial (if refined)	no
Grits, corn, whole grain	yes
Grits, wheat	no
Grits, whole wheat	yes
Ground beef (lean is preferred)	yes
Ham (contains sugar)	no
Hard whole wheat berries	yes
Hard whole wheat flour	yes
Herb tea, caffeine-free (read ingredient list to avoid those with malt or other sweeteners)	maybe
Herb blends (read ingredient list)	maybe
Herbs, fresh or dried	yes
High-fructose corn syrup	no
High gluten flour	no
Hominy (refined)	no
Hominy grits (refined)	no

Food or Ingredient	Used on Perfect Diet
Honey (sugar)	no
Honey, raw (sugar)	no
Hulled barley	yes
Hulled oats (hull is not edible)	yes
Hydrolyzed cereal solids	no
Hydrogenated starch hydrolysate (sweetener)	no
Instant brown rice	yes
Instant rice (refined)	no
Instantized flour	no
Invert sugar	no
Jam, no sugar added (made with juice)	no
Jelly, no sugar added (made with juice	no
Job's tears	yes
Kale, canned	no
Kale, fresh	yes
Kale, frozen	yes
Kamut flour (whole grain)	yes
Kamut whole grain	yes
Kanten	yes
Kelp	yes
Koji	yes
Kombu	yes
Kraut	yes
Kudzu (starch)	no
Kukicha tea (caffeine)	no
Kuzu (starch)	no
Lamb	yes
Lactose (as an added ingredient)	no
Lactose (as naturally present in dairy products)	yes
Lecithin, liquid	yes
Lecithin, granules	yes
Leeks, fresh	yes
Legumes, all dried	yes
Lemon, fresh (only if pulp is included)	yes
Lemon juice, canned in bottle	no
Lemon juice, fresh or frozen	no
Lemon oil	yes
Lemon peel, dried or fresh	yes
Lemon powder (contains added sugar)	no
Lentils, green or red	yes
Lettuce	yes
Lime, fresh (pulp included)	yes
Lime juice, canned	no
Lime juice, fresh	no
Lime oil	yes
Lime peel	yes
Lime, used to treat corn (not a fruit)	yes
Light rye flour (is refined)	no
Long grain brown rice	yes
Long grain rice (is refined)	no
Luncheon meat	no
Macaroni (is refined)	no
Macaroni, enriched	no
Macaroni, 100% whole grain	yes
Macaroni, semolina	no
Malt (unless you know it is diastatic malt or sprouted grains, dried, and ground)	no

Food or Ingredient	Used on Perfect Diet
Malt extract	no
Malted barley syrup	no
Malted grain syrup	no
Maltodextrin	no
Maltol	no
Maltose	no
Mango, fresh	yes
Mannitol (sweetener)	no
Maple sugar	no
Maple syrup	no
Margarine	avoid
Masa (refined)	no
Masa corn flour (refined)	no
Masa harina (refined)	no
Mayonnaise, most commercial	no
Mayonnaise, sugar and starch-free	yes
Medium grain brown rice	yes
Medium grain rice (is refined)	no
Medium rye flour (is refined)	no
Melon, fresh or frozen	yes
Milk, chocolate	no
Milk sugar	no
Milk, whole, 2%, 1% 1/2%, skim	yes
Milled corn (is refined)	no
Miller's bran	yes
Millet	yes
Millet flour	yes
Milo (sorghum grain)	yes
Mirin (alcohol)	no
Miso, white (contains refined rice)	no
Miso, (if made without grains or with whole grains)	yes
Mixed vegetables, canned	no
Mixed vegetables, frozen (if no potatoes added)	yes
Mochi	yes
Mochi rice flour (sweet brown rice flour)	yes
Modified food starch	no
Molasses	no
Mouthwash (contains alcohol)	no
Mustard (if no sweetener, starch or wine)	yes
Mustard, dried	yes
Mustard flour	yes
Mustard powder	yes
Mustard seeds	yes
Natural flavor	maybe
Natural sweetener	no
Nightingale flour (refined wheat)	no
Nigari	yes
Noodles (term denotes refined noodles)	no
Nonfat milk solids	yes
Nonstick cooking sprays (contain alcohol)	no
Nutritional yeast	yes
Nut milk (if no sugar or starch added)	yes
Nuts, fresh, raw	yes
Nuts, roasted (if no sugar or starch added)	yes
Oat bran	yes
Oat flour (if bran is removed)	no
Oat flour (if whole)	yes
Oat groats	yes
Oats, hulled	yes
Oatmeal, instant (if it contains sugar, starch, or	

Food or Ingredient	Used on Perfect Diet
dried fruit)	no
Oatmeal, quick	yes
Oats, rolled	yes
Oats, steel cut	yes
"ol," words ending in (are sugars or alcohol)	no
Olives, black and green	yes
Oolong tea (contains caffeine)	no
Orange flavor (if oil or peel, not juice)	maybe
Orange, fresh	yes
Orange juice	no
Orange oil	yes
Orange peel	yes
Orange Pekoe tea (contains caffeine)	no
Orange powder (contains sugar)	no
Oregano, fresh or dried	yes
Orzo (refined rice-shaped pasta)	no
"Ose," words ending in (are sugars except for cellulose)	no
Palm kernel oil	avoid
Palm oil	avoid
Pam (contains alcohol)	no
Pancakes, commercial	no
Pancakes, homemade, allowed ingredients	yes
Panocha (flour from sprouted wheat)	yes
Paprika (flavor, coloring)	yes
Parboiled rice	no
Partially hydrogenated oil	avoid
Partially milled brown rice (is refined)	no
Partially polished brown rice (is refined)	no
Pasta (term denotes that it is refined)	no
Pasta, 100% whole grain	yes
Pastry flour	no
Patent flour	no
Peach, canned	no
Peach, dried	no
Peach, fresh	yes
Peach, unsweetened and frozen	yes
Peanut butter, most commercial brands	no
Peanut butter, natural style, no sugar added	yes
Peanuts (if no sugar or starch added)	yes
Pearled barley	no
Pearled wheat	no
Peas, split and dried	yes
Pecan meal	yes
Pecans	yes
Pectin (fiber)	yes
Peeled potatoes	no
Pentose	no
Peppermint oil (flavor)	yes
Pepper, bell	yes
Pepper, black, white and red	yes
Pickles, dill or sour (if no sugar added)	yes
Pickles, sweet	no
Pimento	yes
Pineapple, canned	no
Pineapple, dried with sugar added	no
Pineapple, dried without sugar	no
Pineapple, fresh	yes
Pineapple juice, fresh or canned	no
Plum, fresh	yes
Poi (from starchy taro root)	no

Food or Ingredient	Used on Perfect Diet
Polished rice	no
Polydextrose	no
Popcorn, home popped	yes
Pork, fresh (lean)	yes
Pot barley (lightly refined)	no
Potato chips	no
Potato, dried (peeled)	no
Potato flour	no
Potato, mashed (if peeled)	no
Potato, mashed (if not peeled)	yes
Potato, peeled	no
Potato, small and with skin	yes
Potato starch	no
Potato, sweet	yes
Powdered sugar	no
Processed cornmeal	no
Protein powder (if powdered milk)	yes
Prune (dried plum)	no
Prune juice	no
Puffed cereal, refined grains	no
Puffed cereal, whole grain	avoid
Pumpkin, canned	no
Pumpkin, fresh cooked	yes
Quinoa flour	yes
Quinoa grain	yes
Quinoa pasta (contains partially refined corn)	no
Raisins	no
Raw honey	no
Raw sugar	no
Reduced lactose whey	no
Refined sugar	no
Rice (term for refined rice)	no
Rice, Basmati, brown	yes
Rice, Basmati, white	no
Rice, brown, short, medium, or long grain	yes
Rice, brown, partially milled	no
Rice cakes with degerminated corn	no
Rice cakes without refined grains such as degerminated corn	avoid
Rice flour (is refined)	no
Rice flour, brown	yes
Rice, long grain	no
Rice pasta if 100% whole grain	yes
Rice syrup	no
Rice, white	no
Rice, white Basmati	no
Rice, wild, pure	yes
Rice, wild, blend of white and wild rice and labeled *wild rice*	no
Roast beef (cooked at home, not from deli)	yes
Roasted malt	no
Rolled oats	yes
Rose hips	yes
Rusk flour (refined)	no
Rye (term for refined rye)	no
Rye berries	yes
Rye flour (term for refined rye flour)	no
Rye flour, dark (if whole grain)	yes
Rye flour, light (refined)	no
Rye flour, medium (partially refined)	no

Food or Ingredient	Used on Perfect Diet
Rye flour, pumpernickel	yes
Rye flour, sifted (refined)	no
Rye flour, stone ground	no
Rye flour, whole or whole grain	yes
Rye, light (refined)	no
Rye meal (refined)	no
Rye meal, whole	yes
Rye, sprouted	yes
Rye, whole grain	yes
Rye, whole	yes
Saccharin, liquid	avoid
Saccharin, powder & tablets	avoid
Safflower oil, expeller-pressed	avoid
Safflower oil, refined	avoid
Safflower oil, unrefined	yes
Salt, iodized (contains dextrose)	no
Salt, mineral	yes
Salt, rock	yes
Salt, sea (if not iodized with sugar added)	yes
Salted processed foods that contain no sugar, starch, alcohol, or caffeine (processors use the least expenxive salt or non-iodized)	yes
Samp (coarse hominy grits)	no
Sausage (if it contains sugar or starch)	no
Scotch barley (lightly refined)	no
Sea vegetables	yes
Seitan (contains some starch)	no
Self-rising flour	no
Semolina (refined flour used in pasta)	no
Semolina flour	no
Sesame butter	yes
Sesame oil	yes
Sesame seeds, whole	yes
Sesame seeds, hulled	yes
Sesame tahini	yes
Shortening	avoid
Shoyu soy sauce (if no alcohol added)	yes
Shrimp, no breading	yes
Sifted flour (refined)	no
Sifted rye flour (refined)	no
Sifted whole rye flour (refined)	no
Sifted whole wheat flour (refined)	no
Soba (if 100% buckwheat)	yes
Soft whole wheat berries	yes
Soft whole wheat flour	yes
Sorbo (sweetener)	no
Sorbitol (sweetener)	no
Sorghum (sweetener)	no
Sorghum, whole grain	yes
Soup, canned	no
Soup, homemade with allowed ingredients	yes
Soup, dehydrated mix with allowed ingredients	yes
Soy milk, with sweetener added	no
Soy milk powder	yes
Soy oil, refined	avoid
Soy sauce powder (contains dextrin)	no
Spaghetti (refined grain)	no
Spaghetti sauce, most commercial brands	no
Spaghetti sauce, no sugar or starch added	yes
Spaghetti, whole wheat	yes
Spelt berries	yes

Food or Ingredient	Used on Perfect Diet
Spelt flakes	yes
Spelt flour	no
Spelt flour, whole	yes
Spelt pasta (if from whole spelt flour)	yes
Spelt, whole grain	yes
Spices, pure (ingredient lists must name them specifically, not just say "spices"	yes
Spinach, canned	no
Spinach, fresh or frozen	yes
Split peas, dried	yes
Squash, fresh or frozen	yes
Steel-cut oats	yes
Stevia Rebaudiana, pure (herbal sweetener)	yes
Stone ground rye flour (is refined)	no
Stone ground wheat flour (is refined)	no
Stone ground whole wheat flour	yes
Strawberry, fresh	yes
Strawberry, frozen, no sugar added	yes
Sucanat (evaporated cane juice)	no
Sugar, any kind	no
Sugar cane	no
Sunflower seeds, raw or roasted	yes
Sweet brown rice (a variety of brown rice)	yes
Sweetleaf (herbal sweetener, if pure)	yes
Syrup	no
Tahini	yes
Tamari soy sauce (if no alcohol is added)	yes
Tap water	avoid
Tapioca (thickener)	no
Taro root (starch)	no
Tea, black or green	no
Tea, decaffeinated	no
Tea, herb with no caffeine (read ingredient list carefully to avoid malt and dried fruit)	maybe
Teff	yes
Teff flour	yes
Textured vegetable protein (TVP)	yes
Tofu, fresh	yes
Tofu, silken	yes
Tomato juice, canned, for cooking, not drinking	yes
Tomato juice, fresh	yes
Tomato paste	yes
Tomato puree	yes
Tomato sauce, canned, if no sugar or starch added	yes
Tomatoes, canned	yes
Tomatoes, dried	yes
Tomatoes, fresh	yes
Tortillas, corn (if treated with lime, lye, or wood ash)	no
Tortillas, corn (if from whole grain corn)	yes
Tuna, canned in water	yes
Turbinado sugar	no
Turkey, deli-style (contains sugar or starch)	no
Turkey, fresh	yes
Turkey, frozen (if without sugar or starch)	yes
Turkey, ground (lean is better than 15% fat)	yes
Turmeric	yes
Unbleached flour (refined)	no
Unbleached whole wheat flour	yes

Food or Ingredient	Used on Perfect Diet
Vanilla bean	yes
Vanilla extract, containing alcohol	no
Vanilla extract, containing glycerine	yes
Vanilla oleoresin (contains alcohol)	no
Vegetables, canned, commercial or home canned (Tomatoes used in cooking are an exception.)	no
Vegetable food starch	no
Vegetable shortening	avoid
Vegetables, fresh	yes
Venison	yes
Vermicelli (a refined grain)	no
Vinegar, Balsamic	yes
Vinegar, distilled	avoid
Vinegar, pasteurized	avoid
Vinegar, raw cider	yes
Vinegar, raw wine	yes
Walnuts	yes
Water chestnuts	yes
Water, tap	avoid
Wheat (term for refined product)	no
Wheat bran	yes
Wheat, cracked	yes
Wheat farina	no
Wheat flour	no
Wheat flour, enriched	no
Wheat germ, defatted	yes
Wheat germ flour (white flour + wheat germ)	no
Wheat germ, fresh and refrigerated	yes
Wheat malt (if sprouted wheat, dried, and ground)	yes
Wheat, pearled	no
Whey (source of lactose)	no

Food or Ingredient	Used on Perfect Diet
Whey protein concentrate (source of lactose)	no
Whey, reduced lactose	no
White flour	no
White sugar	no
White rice	no
White rice flour	no
White rye flour	no
White spelt flour	no
Whole durum flour	yes
Whole durum wheat flour	yes
Whole meal flour	yes
Whole rye flour	yes
Whole rye meal	yes
Whole wheat berries	yes
Whole wheat pastry flour	yes
Whole wheat flour	yes
Wild rice blend with white rice	no
Wild rice, pure	yes
Wine	no
Winter squash	yes
Xylitol (sweetener)	no
Yeast, baking	yes
Yeast, brewer's or nutritional	yes
Yogurt, fruit-flavored (contains sugar)	no
Yogurt, plain (read label to avoid starches)	yes
Yogurt, vanilla-flavored (contains sugar)	no
Zest, citrus (peel)	yes

Explanation of Quick References

Yes: You may use this item on the **Perfect Whole Foods** diet.

No: Totally eliminate this item while on **Perfect Whole Foods**.

Avoid: Use occasionally, if necessary, but not regularly or in large amounts.

Maybe: Before using this product, determine what is in it by reading the ingredient list very carefully and, in a few cases, find out from the manufacturer how an ingredient is made. For example, natural lemon flavor might be lemon juice, lemon peel, or lemon oil. Only the manufacturer knows which it is when the term *natural lemon flavor* is used on the ingredient list.

Quick Reference for Additives

Since most foods on the **Perfect Whole Foods** diet are simple and minimally processed, your intake of additives will automatically be restricted. Although many additives are allowed in the chart that follows, I do not encourage you to use them often. I'm listing them only because I have been asked about many specific additives in the past and want to help you as much as possible with questions I can anticipate.

I would urge you to avoid whenever possible additives such as artificial coloring, artificial flavoring, phosphates, sulfites, MSG, nitrites, nitrates, and aluminum-containing products. These additives are associated with health problems I have mentioned elsewhere in this book.

You may use artificial sweeteners like aspartame (the brand name is *NutraSweet*) and saccharin but I don't encouraged them since most have not been shown to be 100 percent safe. Also, some people continue craving sweets as long as they continue to eat anything sweet-tasting including artificial sweeteners. And finally, there are some who respond to aspartame with such reactions as rashes, headaches, stomachaches, and even seizures. Before using any such products, pay close attention to the ingredient list to avoid those products with added ingredients such as lactose, dextrose, sorbitol, maltodextrin, dextrin, and other ingredients not allowed on the perfect diet. Liquid saccharin and tablets are more likely to be acceptable than powdered artificial sweeteners.

The success of the perfect diet is not dependent on the total elimination of many additives. If you happen to be sensitive to any, then eliminate them from your diet. Refer to **Appendix C** beginning on page 323 for information to help you eliminate MSG, sulfites, and aspartame.

The chemical structure determines whether or not an additive may be included on the **Perfect Whole Foods** diet. If an additive is a sugar, starch, alcohol, or caffeine or if an additive contains one of these, that additive should be eliminated from the perfect diet.

Quick Reference for Additives

Additive	Used on Perfect Diet
Acacia (gum arabic)	yes
Acetates	yes
Acetic acid	yes
Acid modified starch	no
Agar-agar (seaweed extract)	yes
Alcohol	no
Alum or kasal (firming agent)	yes
Algin (thickener, from seaweed)	yes
Algin gum	yes
Ammonium salts	yes
Annatto extract (coloring)	yes
Ascorbic acid (nutrition, curing meats)	yes
Artificial color	yes
Artificial flavor	yes
Aspartame (if no sugar or starch added)	avoid
Autolyzed yeast (flavoring)	yes
Baking powder (contains starch)	no
Baking soda (leavening)	yes
Barley malt (sweetener)	no
Benzoate of soda	yes
Benzoic acid	yes
Benzoyl peroxide	yes
Beta carotene (coloring, nutrition)	yes
Beet powder	yes
BHA (antioxidant)	yes
BHT (antioxidant)	yes
Bicarbonate of soda (leavening)	yes
Bran (nutrition)	yes
Bromines	yes
Butyl paraben (preservative)	yes
Caffeine	no
Calcium acid phosphate (baking acid)	yes
Calcium bromate (oxidizing agent)	yes
Calcium carbonate	yes
Calcium caseinate (nutrition and flavoring)	yes
Calcium chloride (firming agent)	yes
Calcium citrate	yes
Calcium disodium EDTA	yes
Calcium iodate (oxidizing agent in bread)	yes
Calcium lactate (batter conditioner)	yes
Calcium oxide (acidity regulator)	yes
Calcium peroxide (dough conditioner)	yes
Calcium propionate (preservative)	yes
Calcium salts (firming agent)	yes
Calcium stearoyl-2-lactylate (dough conditioner)	yes
Calcium sulfate (firming agent, conditioner)	yes
Caramel (coloring or flavoring from sugar)	no
Carob bean gum (thickener)	yes
Carotene (color)	yes
Carrageenan (thickener)	yes
Casein (thickener, whitening agent)	yes
Cellulose (fiber)	yes
Cellulose gum (thickener)	yes
Char-smoke flavor	yes
Cinnamaldehyde (flavor)	yes
Citric acid (acidifier)	yes
Cornstarch	no
Cream of tartar	yes

Additive	Used on Perfect Diet
Dextran (sweetener)	no
Dextrin (product of starch)	no
Dicalcium phosphate (dough conditioner)	yes
Diethyl pyrocarbonate	yes
Diglycerides (emulsifier)	yes
Disodium guanylate (flavor enhancer)	yes
Disodium inosinate (flavor enhancer)	yes
EDTA (preservative)	yes
Enzymes	yes
Equal (contains dextrose and maltodextrose)	no
Erythorbic acid (antioxidant)	yes
Essence of fruit (flavor)	yes
Essential oils (flavor)	yes
Ester gum (thickener)	yes
Ethyl alcohol (solvent)	no
Ethyl maltol (flavor enhancer)	no
Ethyl vanillin (contains alcohol)	no
Ethylene dibromide	yes
Ethylene oxide	yes
Ferrous gluconate (coloring, nutrient)	yes
Ferrous sulfate (nutrition)	yes
Fig pep (sweetener made from fig extract)	no
Fumaric acid (acid and antioxidant)	yes
Gelatin (gelling agent)	yes
Gelatinized wheat starch (thickener)	no
Gluconolactone (acid)	yes
Gluten (protein of wheat containing starch)	no
Gluten flour (contains starch)	no
Glycerin	yes
Green tea extract (contains caffeine)	no
Guar gum (fiber thickener)	yes
Gum gluten	no
Gums (arabic, cellulose, ghatti, karaya, tragacanth, xanthan)	yes
Gypsum	yes
Heptyl paraben (preservative)	yes
Hydrochloric acid (acidifier)	yes
Hydrogen peroxide (bleaching agent)	yes
Hydrolyzed plant protein or HPP (seasoning)	yes
Hydrolyzed vegetable protein or HVP	yes
Hydroxylated lecithin (emulsifier)	yes
Imitation flavoring (if not alcohol-based)	yes
Irish moss	yes
Irish moss extract	yes
Lactic acid (acidifier)	yes
Lactalbumin (protein from milk)	yes
Lecithin (emulsifier)	yes
Lime used to soften corn hull (not a fruit)	yes
Liquid smoke	yes
Locust bean	yes
Locust bean gum	yes
Lye used to soften corn hull	yes
Magnesium silicate	yes

Additive	Used on Perfect Diet
Magnesium stearate	yes
Malic acid (acidifier from apples)	yes
Malt	no
Malt, diastatic	yes
Malt extract	no
Malt, wheat (if diastatic malt)	yes
Maltodextrin	no
Maltol	no
Menthol	no
Methyl paraben (preservative)	yes
Milk serum (contains lactose)	no
Modified food starch (thickener)	no
Modified starch	no
Monocalcium phosphate (dough conditioner)	yes
Monoglycerides (emulsifier)	yes
Monosodium glutamate or MSG (flavor enhancer)	yes
Monostearate	yes
Natural flavor	maybe
Natural smoke flavors (flavoring)	yes
Niacin (enrichment)	yes
Nigari	yes
Nitrates	yes
Nitrites	yes
NutraSweet	avoid
Nutritional yeast	yes
Oleic acid	yes
Oleoresin paprika (coloring)	yes
Oleoresin turmeric (coloring)	yes
Orange powder (contains sugar)	no
Oxystearin (prevents fat crystallization)	yes
Palmitic acid	yes
Papain (enzyme)	yes
Paprika (flavor, coloring)	yes
Pectin (fiber which sets fruit jelly)	yes
Peppermint oil (flavor)	yes
Phosphoric acid (acidifier)	yes
Polysorbate 60, 65, 80 (emulsifier)	yes
Potassium alum (firming agent)	yes
Potassium bicarbonate (leavening)	yes
Potassium bromate (oxidizing agent)	yes
Potassium citrate (acidity control)	yes
Potassium iodate (oxidizing agent)	yes
Potassium sorbate (preservative)	yes
Potassium sulfite (preservative)	yes
Propyl gallate (antioxidant)	yes
Propyl paraben (preservative)	yes
Propylene glycol (flavor solvent)	yes
Propylene glycol alginate (thickener)	yes
Propylene glycol monostearate	yes
Propylene oxide	yes
Quinine (flavoring)	yes
Reduced iron (nutrition)	yes
Rennet (enzyme that causes milk curdling)	yes
Rennin (enzyme that causes milk curdling)	yes
Riboflavin (nutrition)	yes
Rye-sour flavor	no

Additive	Used on Perfect Diet
Salt (if not iodized)	yes
Saccharin, liquid	avoid
Saccharin, tablets or powder	avoid
Salicylic acid	yes
Saltpeter (curing agent)	yes
Silicon dioxide (anticaking agent)	yes
Smoke flavoring	yes
Smoked yeast	yes
Sodium alginate (thickener)	yes
Sodium aluminum phosphate (leavening)	yes
Sodium ascorbate (nutrition, curing of meats)	yes
Sodium benzoate (preservative)	yes
Sodium bicarbonate (leavening)	yes
Sodium bisulfite (preservative)	yes
Sodium carboxymethyl cellulose (thickener)	yes
Sodium caseinate (thickener, whitening agent)	yes
Sodium citrate (controls acidity)	yes
Sodium chloride (table salt)	yes
Sodium chloride, if iodized	no
Sodium diacetate (preservative)	yes
Sodium erythorbate (curing agent)	yes
Sodium hexametaphosphate (texture modifier)	yes
Sodium metabisulfite (preservative)	yes
Sodium nitrate (curing agent)	yes
Sodium nitrite (curing agent)	yes
Sodium phosphate (consistency regulator)	yes
Sodium propionate (preservative)	yes
Sodium pyrophosphate (firms meat when water is added)	yes
Sodium saccharin	avoid
Sodium stearoyl-2-lactylate (dough conditioner)	yes
Sodium sulfite, sodium bisulfite	yes
Sorbic acid (mold inhibitor)	yes
Sorbitol (sweetener)	no
Soy lecithin	yes
Soy-protein concentrate (seasoning)	yes
Soy protein isolate (TVP)	yes
Starch	no
Stearic acid	yes
Stevia (herbal sweetener)	yes
Sucanat (granulated cane juice)	no
Succinic acid	yes
Sucrose (sugar)	no
Sugar, any kind	no
Sulfur dioxide (preservative)	yes
Sweetleaf (herbal sweetener)	yes
Sweet One packet (artificial sweetener contains dextrose)	no
Sweet'n Low (contains dextrose)	no
Talc (filler in tablets and capsules)	yes
Tannin (tannic acid)	yes
Tapioca (thickener)	no
Tartaric acid (baking acid, from grapes)	yes
TBHQ or tertiary butylhydroquinone (antioxidant)	yes
Textured vegetable protein (TVP)	yes
Thiamine/mononitrate (nutrition)	yes
Titanium dioxide (coloring)	yes
Torula yeast	yes
Tricalcium phosphate (prevents lumping)	yes
Turmeric (coloring)	yes

Additive	Used on Perfect Diet
Ultramarine blue (coloring)	yes
Unmodified starch	no
Vanilla bean	yes
Vanilla extract, with alcohol	no
Vanilla extract, with glycerine	yes
Vinegar	yes
Vitamin C (if tablets are sugar and starch-free)	yes
Whey (milk component, includes lactose)	no

Additive	Used on Perfect Diet
Whey protein concentrate (includes lactose)	no
Wood ash used to soften corn	yes
Xanthan gum (thickener)	yes
Xylitol	no
Xylose (wood sugar)	no
Yeast, baker's (leavening)	yes
Yeast, brewer's or nutritional (nutrition)	yes
Yeast, torula	yes

Quick Reference for Brand Names

As I have repeated over and over in this book, pay close attention to the ingredient lists of commercial products if you're on the perfect diet. The products listed below are sugar-free and starch-free at the time of printing this book. However, the ingredients of all commercial products are subject to change. It is also possible that name brand products differ in various parts of the country.

Because there are thousands of food products on the market today, with many regional items, it is impossible to list them all. Use this guide to get started, making your own list of additional products as you discover them.

Quick Reference for Brand Name Products

Name of Product	Used on Perfect Diet
Beverages (Some companies would not give details)	
All diet colas (caramel color)	no
Celestial Seasonings Herb Teas (if it contains natural flavors)	no
Bengal Spice (dates)	no
Chamomile	yes
Ginseng Plus (barley malt)	no
Grandma's Tummy Mint	yes
Mama Bear's Cold Care (dates)	no
Mint Magic	yes
Peppermint	yes
Roastaroma (barley malt)	no
Sleepytime	yes
Spearmint	yes
Clearly Canadian (contains sugar)	no
Crystal Geyser Sparkling Mineral Water, Fruit Flavored (fruit essence)	yes
Diet *Crystal Clear*	no
Diet *7-Up* (flavor from oil)	avoid
Diet *Sprite* (flavor from oil)	avoid
La Croix Fruit-Flavored Water (fruit essence)	yes
Perrier Fruit-Flavored Water (flavor from oil)	yes
Poland Spring Sparkling water, Fruit Flavored (fruit essence)	yes
Postum Coffee Substitute (refined wheat and molasses)	no
Sanka Decaffeinated Coffee (very small amount of caffeine)	no

Name of Product	Used on Perfect Diet
7 Sprouted Grain Bread (honey & molasses)	no
Sprouted Whole Grain Bread (malted barley)	no
French Meadow Spelt Bread and Buns	yes
Garden of Eatin' Corntillas	yes
Great Harvest Unsweetened Bread (contains [diastatic] wheat malt)	yes
International Mr. Pita 100% Whole Wheat Pocket Bread	yes
Manna Sprouted Rye Bread	yes
Sprouted Wheat Bread	yes
Sprouted Bread with Dried Fruit	no
Nature's Garden Bakery Bavarian Sour Dough Rye Bread (refined rye flour and rye meal)	no
Macrobiotic Brown Rice Bread (rye flour)	no
Macrobiotic Wheat Bread (rye flour)	no
Spelt Bread (barley malt)	no
Wheat-Free Millet Bread (rye flour & barley malt)	no
Nokomis Farms Bakery Sour Dough Breads (those without unbleached wheat flour and refined rye flour)	yes
Oasis Flourless Sprouted 7-Grain Bread (honey)	no
Kamut Sprouted Egyptian Wheat Bread (contains honey & gluten)	no
Rudi's Spelt Burger Buns (honey)	no
Spelt Pita Bread	yes
Toufayan 100% Whole Wheat Pita	yes
Tyson Mexican Original Enchilada Style Corn Tortillas	yes

Breads

Name of Product	Used on Perfect Diet
Alvarado St. Bakery Sprouted Sourdough French Bread (gluten & honey)	no
Berlin Spelt Bread (contains honey)	no
Breads for Life Seven Grain Bread	no
Essene Sprouted Rye Bread	yes
Sprouted Wheat Bread	yes
Sprouted Bread with Dried Fruit	no
Food for Life Ezekiel 4:9 Bread (malted barley)	no

Crackers, Rice Cakes, and Chips

Name of Product	Used on Perfect Diet
Barbara's Corn Chips (corn is whole grain, check other ingredients)	maybe
Edward & Sons Baked Brown Rice Snaps Onion-Garlic	yes
No Salt-Sesame	yes
Buckwheat-No Salt	yes
Guiltless Gourmet Baked Chips (whole grain)	yes
Hol.Grain Whole Wheat Crackers	yes
Brown Rice Crackers	yes
Kavli Crispy Thin All Natural Whole Grain Crispbread	yes
Lifestream Wheat & Rye Krispbread	yes
Lifestream Whole Rye Krispbread (made of organically grown rye flour which is refined)	no
Lundberg Mochi Sweet Rice Cakes	yes
Popcorn Rice Cakes	yes

Name of Product	Used on Perfect Diet
Rye with Caraway Rice Cakes	yes
Wehani Rice Cakes	yes
Wild Rice Rice Cakes	yes
Manischewitz Whole Wheat Matzo Cracker with Bran	yes
Mother's Barley & Oat Rice Cakes (pearled barley)	no
Multigrain Rice Cakes	yes
Natural Butter Popped Corn Cakes (degerminated corn)	no
Plain Rice Cakes	yes
Sesame Rice Cakes	yes
Pritikin Multigrain Rice Cakes	yes
Plain Rice Cakes	yes
Sesame Rice Cakes	yes
Ralston Purina RyKrisp, Natural	yes
RyKrisp, other varieties	no
Ryvita Whole Grain Crisp Breads:	
Toasted Sesame Rye	yes
Flavorful High Fiber	yes
Tasty Light Rye (the *light* is whole grain)	yes
Tasty Dark Rye Whole Grain Crisp Bread (malt)	no
Wasa Crispbread: Hearty-Rye	yes
Sesame-Rye	yes
Light Rye (the *light* is whole grain)	yes

Dairy Products

Name of Product	Used on Perfect Diet
Alta Dena Plain Nonfat Yogurt (milk protein is nonfat dry milk)	yes
Kefir Cheese	yes
Light Sour Cream	yes
Bowman Buttermilk (whey)	no
Breakstone's Dry Curd Cottage Cheese	yes
Low Fat Cottage Cheese	yes
Dannon Plain Nonfat Yogurt	yes
Kroger Plain Nonfat Yogurt	yes
Lactaid Lactose-Reduced Milk	yes
Mountain High Natural Plain Yoghurt (tapioca)	no
SouthernBelle Buttermilk	yes
Stonyfield Farm Plain Nonfat Yogurt (whey protein concentrate)	no

Egg Whites and Egg Substitutes

Name of Product	Used on Perfect Diet
EnerG Egg Replacer	no
Natural Choice Egg Product (whey and starch)	no
Now Eggwhite Powder	yes
Eggwhite Protein	yes

Flours, Meals, and Baking Mixes

Name of Product	Used on Perfect Diet
Arrowhead Mills	
Barley Flour (refined)	no
Hi-Lysine Cornmeal	yes
Kamut Flour	yes
Millet Flour	yes
Multi Blend Flour	yes
Oat Flour	yes
Stone Ground Whole Wheat Flour	yes
Teff Flour	yes
Toasted Garbanzo Flour	yes
Triticale Flour	yes
Unbleached White Flour (refined)	no
Wheat Gluten	no
Whole Grain Brown Rice Flour	yes
Whole Grain Buckwheat Flour	yes

Name of Product	Used on Perfect Diet
Whole Grain Durum Flour	yes
Whole Grain Millet Flour	yes
Whole Grain Pastry Flour	yes
Whole Grain Yellow Cornmeal	yes
Whole Rye Flour	yes
Deaf Smith Whole Wheat Flour	yes
EnerG	
Barley Mix	no
Corn Mix	no
Oat Mix	no
Potato Mix	no
Pure Potato Flour	no
Pure Potato Starch	no
Pure Rice Flour	no
Pure Rice Polish	yes
Rice 'N Rye Bread Mix	no
Rice Mix	no
Fearn Brown Rice Baking Mix	no
Gold Medal Whole Wheat Flour	yes
Hodgson Mill Oat Bran Flour	yes
Oat Bran Flour Blend	no
Yellow Cornmeal (from Unenriched Whole Grain Corn)	yes
Now Whole Grain Triticale Flour	yes
Vita-Spelt Whole Spelt Flour	yes
Walnut Acres Buckwheat Flour	yes
Whole Wheat Bread Flour	yes
Whole Wheat Flour	yes
Graham Flour (some bran is removed)	no
Corn Flour	yes
Millet Flour	yes
Whole Rye Flour	yes
Whole Barley Flour	yes
Ezekiel Flour	no
Brown Rice Flour	yes
Cornell Bread Flour	yes
Whole Corn Meal	yes
Weisenberger	
Soft Whole Wheat Pastry Flour	yes
Hard Whole Wheat Bread Flour	yes

Grains and Cereals

Name of Product	Used on Perfect Diet
American Prairie	
Creamy Rye & Rice	no
Arrowhead Mills	
Bear Mush (refined wheat)	no
Bulgur Wheat	yes
Corn Grits (corn is degerminated)	no
Cracked Wheat Cereal	yes
Four Grain Cereal (barley is refined)	no
Kamut Flakes	yes
Oat Bran	yes
Oat Flakes	yes
Oat Groats	yes
Puffed Brown Rice, Whole Corn, Millet, and Whole Wheat (all are highly processed)	avoid
Quick Brown Rice	yes
Quinoa	yes
Rice and Shine	yes
Seven Grain Cereal (wheat and corn are refined)	no
White Corn Grits (degerminated)	no
Whole Grain Kamut	yes

Name of Product	Used on Perfect Diet
Whole Grain Rye	yes
Whole Grain Teff	yes
Whole Rye Flakes	yes
Yellow Corn Grits (degerminated)	no
Casbah Whole Wheat Couscous	yes
Country Grown Golden Kamut Flakes	yes
Earth's Best Brown Rice Baby Cereal	yes
Baby Oatmeal Cereal	yes
Eden Quinoa	yes
Erewhon Barley Plus	no
Brown Rice Cream	yes
Hodgson Mill Cracked Wheat Cereal	yes
Oat Bran	yes
Malt-O-Meal	no
Mother's Oat Bran	yes
Quick Barley (refined)	no
Nabisco Cream of Wheat cereal (refined)	no
Corn Grits	no
Shredded Wheat (highly processed)	avoid
Now Barley Grits	no
Buckwheat Grits	yes
Hominy Grits	no
Whole Grain Triticale	yes
Pacific Rice Products, Inc. Quick 'N Creamy	yes
Pocono Cream of Buckwheat cereal	yes
Quaker Old Fashioned Oats	yes
One Minute Quick	yes
Instant Oatmeal	no
Grits	no
Roman Meal Cream of Rye	yes
Original Wheat, Rice, Bran, Flax Cereal	yes
Kashi 7 Whole Grains & Sesame	yes
Wheatena Toasted Wheat Cereal	yes
Weisenberger Bolted White Corn Meal	no

Meat, Poultry, Fish

Any frozen hen with sugar or starch added	no
Any frozen turkey with sugar or starch added	no
Butterball (hydrogenated oil added)	avoid
Louis Rich Fresh Turkeys and parts	yes
Lean Ground Turkey	yes
Perdue Fresh Turkeys and parts	yes
Lean Ground Turkey	yes
Shelton's Cooked Uncured Chicken Franks	yes
Uncured Turkey Bologna	yes

Nut Butters

Arrowhead Mills Peanut Butter (creamy or crunchy)	yes
Sesame Tahini	yes
Co-op Old Fashioned Peanut Butter (smooth or crunchy)	yes
East Wind Almond Butter (smooth or crunchy)	yes
Cashew Butter (roasted or raw)	yes
Peanut Butter	yes
Roasted Tahini	yes
Erewhon Sesame Butter	yes
Sunflower Butter	yes
Kroger All Natural Peanut Butter	yes
Roddenbery's Old Fashioned Creamy Natural Peanut Butter	yes
Smucker's Natural Peanut Butter	yes

Name of Product	Use on Perfect Diet

Oils and Related Products

Arrowhead Mills Unrefined Oils	
Canola Oil	yes
Hazelnut Oil	yes
Olive Oil	yes
Sesame Oil	yes
Sunflower Oil	yes
Fresh Flax Oil	yes
Barlean's Fresh Flax Oil	yes
Eden Unrefined Extra Virgin Olive Oil	yes
Unrefined Safflower Oil	yes
Spectrum Naturals Unrefined Corn Oil	yes
Unrefined High Oleic Safflower Oil	yes
Unrefined Safflower Oil	yes

Pasta

Ancient Harvest Quinoa Pasta (refined corn)	no
DeBole's Corn Pasta (corn flour is refined)	no
American Artichoke Pasta (semolina)	no
Eden 100% Soba, Buckwheat Pasta	yes
Soba Japanese Buckwheat Pasta (refined wheat)	no
Ener-G Rice Lasagna (refined rice flour)	no
Rice Vermicelli (refined rice flour)	no
Florence Whole Wheat Sesame Rice Spiral Pasta (brown rice)	yes
Hodgson Mills Whole Wheat Lasagna	yes
Whole Wheat Spaghetti	yes
Pastariso 100% Brown Rice Pasta	yes
Purity Foods Vita Whole Grain Spelt Pasta	yes
Westbrae Corn Spaghetti (refined)	no

Personal Care Products

Most Toothpaste (contains sorbitol)	no
Nature's Gate Toothpaste (read ingredient list carefully)	maybe
Oxyfresh Mouthrinse	yes

Salad Dressings

Duke's Mayonnaise	yes
Duke's Light Mayonnaise	no
La Martinique True French Vinaigrette	yes
Mrs. Clark's Mayonnaise	yes
Newman's Olive Oil & Vinegar Dressing (contains lemon juice)	no
Pritikin Fat Free, Sodium Free Dressings (fruit juice)	no

Seasonings/Flavorings/Condiments

Accent (contains sugar)	no
Bragg Liquid Aminos	yes
Butter Buds Butter Flavored Mix (maltodextrin)	no
Butter-Flavored Sprinkles (maltodextrin)	no
Aura Cacia Lemon Oil	yes
DeSouza Solar Sea Salt	yes
Dr. Bronner's Balanced-Mineral Bouillon (molasses, orange juice solids)	no
Balanced-Mineral Seasoning	no
Durkee Red Hot Cayenne Pepper Sauce	yes
Eden Raw Apple Cider Vinegar	yes
Raw Red Wine Vinegar	yes
Miso: Soybeans	yes

Name of Product	Used on Perfect Diet
Miso: Soybeans and Barley (pearled barley)	no
Miso: Soybeans and Brown Rice	yes
Shoyu Soy Sauce (no alcohol added)	yes
Shoyu Soy Sauce, Reduced Sodium (alcohol)	no
Tamari Soy Sauce, Wheat-Free (alcohol)	no
Fakin' Bacon Bits (barley malt)	no
Frontier (company would not give information on some of these flavorings)	
Alcohol-Free Almond Flavoring	yes
Alcohol-Free Brandy Flavoring	no
Alcohol-Free Butter Flavoring	no
Alcohol-Free Butterscotch Flavoring	no
Alcohol-Free Coconut Flavoring	no
Alcohol-Free Pineapple Flavoring	no
Alcohol-Free Walnut Flavoring	no
Broth Powders (contain starch)	no
Gayelord Hauser's All Natural Vegetable Broth	yes
Hain Iodized Sea Salt (dextrose)	no
Hormel Real Bacon Bits (sugar)	no
Kikkoman Soy Sauce (refined wheat)	no
Lima Atlantic Sea Salt	yes
Louisiana Hot Sauce	yes
McCormick's Parsley Patch	
All-Purpose Seasoning	yes
Garlicsaltless	yes
Italian Blend	yes
It's a Dilly Seasoning	yes
Lemon Pepper	yes
Popcorn Blend	yes
Seafoodsaltless	yes
Sesame All-Purpose Seasoning	yes
Miso Master Chickpeas Miso (partially polished brown rice)	no
Mellow White Miso (partially polished brown rice) . . .	no
Traditional Country Barley Miso (pearled barley)	no
Molly McButter All Natural Dairy Sprinkles (contain maltodextrin)	no
Now Lemon Oil	yes
Poppa Dash Seasoning (contains maltodextrin)	no
San-J Shoyu Soy Sauce (alcohol)	no
Tamari Soy Sauce (alcohol)	no
Tamari Lite, Low Sodium (alcohol)	no
Spike All Purpose Seasoning (orange powder)	no
Salt-Free Seasoning (orange crystals)	no
Tobasco Pepper Sauce	yes
Westbrae Mellow White Miso (white rice)	no

Soups

Name of Product	Used on Perfect Diet
Edward & Sons Miso Cup:	
Golden Light Soup (rice)	no
Rich, Savory Soup with Seaweeds (rice)	no
Mayacamas Soup, Dip & Recipe Mixes (unbleached flour)	no
Pritikin Chicken Broth (canned)	no
Taste Adventure Black Bean Chili (dried)	yes
Black Bean Soup (dried)	yes
Curry Lentil Soup (dried)	yes
Lentil Chili (dried)	yes
Red Bean Chili (dried)	yes
Westbrae Natural Whole Wheat Ramen	yes
All varieties with sifted wheat flour	no

Name of Product	Used on Perfect Diet
Soy Milk	
WestSoy Westbrae Natural Unsweetened Non-Dairy Beverage	yes
EnerG Pure SoyQuik, A Soy Based Imitation Milk Mix	yes
Soy Cheese	
Soya Kaas American Cheddar Style Natural Cheese Alternative	yes
Jalapeno Mexi-Kaas	yes
Mozzarella Style	yes
Soymage Cheddar Style	yes
Mozzarella Style	yes
Tofu Rella Mozzarella Style Cheese Alternative . . .	yes
Mild Cheddar	yes
Soy Tempeh	
White Wave Tempeh	
Brown Rice	yes
Five Grain (some refined grains)	no
Sweeteners	
Equal Artificial Sweetener Tablets (lactose & maltodextrin)	no
Artificial Sweetener Packets (lactose & maltodextrin) .	no
Kroger No Calorie Liquid Sweetener	avoid
Now Stevia Powder or Extract	yes
Now Stevia Liquid Extract (contains alcohol)	no
NutraSweet Spoonful (maltodextrin)	no
Sweet'n Low Granulated Sugar Substitute (dextrose) . .	no
Low Calorie Liquid Sweetener	avoid
Powdered Sugar Substitute (contains dextrose)	no
Sugar Substitute Tablets	avoid
Superose Liquid Sugar Substitute	avoid
Tofu	
Mori-Nu Silken Tofu	yes
Spring Creek Tofu	yes

Tomato Products, Canned

Check your favorite brands of crushed tomatoes in tomato pureé, diced tomatoes, tomato juice, tomato paste, tomato pureé, tomato sauce, and whole tomatoes. Some brands contain sugar or starch so read ingredient lists carefully.

Name of Product	Used on Perfect Diet
Catsup	
Westbrae Un-Ketchup (unsweetened)	yes
Juices	
Campbell's V-8 100% Vegetable Juice	yes
Knudsen's Very Veggie Juice (contains lemon concentrate)	no
Mexican Sauces	
Chi-Chi's Salsa (Mild, Medium, and Hot)	yes
Picante Sauce (sugar)	no
Enrico's Chunky Style Salsa (Mild and Medium)	yes
Old El Paso Mild Thick 'n Chunky Salsa	yes
Pace Picante Sauce (Mild, Medium, and Hot)	yes
Chunky Salsa Dip (Mild or Medium)	yes
Pizza Sauces	
Enrico's All Natural Pizza Sauce	yes
Ragu 100% Natural Pizza Sauce	yes

Name of Product	Used on Perfect Diet
Pizza Quick Sauce (contains sugar)	no

Spaghetti Sauces

Ci'Bella Pasta Sauce	yes
Pasta Sauce Marinara Style	yes
Classico Di Napoli Tomato & Basil Pasta Sauce	yes
Ripe Olives & Mushrooms Pasta Sauce	no
Enrico's Spaghetti Sauce	yes
Spaghetti Sauce with Mushrooms	yes
Spaghetti Sauce with Mushrooms and Green Peppers	yes
Pritikin Chunky Garden Style Spaghetti Sauce (fruit juice concentrate)	no
Ragu Today's Recipe Spaghetti Sauces	yes

Vegetarian Convenience Foods

Arrowhead Mills Seitan Quick Mix (contains gluten which includes some starch)	no
Casbah Greek Classics Gyros	yes
Falafil Mix	yes
Fantastic Foods Falafil Mix	yes
Instant Refried Beans Mix	yes
Tofu Burger Mix (arrowroot)	no
Jerusalem Falafil Vegetable Burger Mix	yes

Name of Product	Use on Perfect Diet
Grainburger Mix, Wheat-free & Salt Free	yes
Grainburger Mix, Bar-B-Que (refined *wheat flour*)	no
Lightlife Tofu Pups	yes
Loveburger (potato flour)	no
Spring Creek Soysage	yes

Other Products

All Sugar-free Chewing Gum (contains sorbitol or sorbo)	no
Adolph's Meat Tenderizers	no
Fruit Fresh Fruit Protector (sugar)	no
Grey Poupon Dijon Mustard (wine)	no
I Can't Believe It's Yogurt Sugar-Free Frozen Yogurt (maltodextrin, polydextrose, and sorbitol)	no
Kraft Prepared Mustard	yes
Nabisco Shredded Wheat (highly processed)	avoid
Pam Baking Spray (contains alcohol)	no
Plochman's Prepared Mustard	yes
Promise Ultra Fat Free Nonfat Margarine (contains rice starch and lactose)	no
Rice Dream Non-Dairy Dessert (contains partially-milled brown rice plus starch	no

Quick Reference for Minor Remedies

Since many over-the-counter remedies contain sugar, starch, or alcohol, I've provided a few home remedy suggestions if you are on the *Perfect Whole Foods* diet. Use them for temporary relief for minor problems only if you are an adult, not pregnant and not nursing. Never use these remedies when medical treatment is needed.

Quick References for Minor Remedies

Breath Fresheners: Chew on a sprig of fresh parley. For an alcohol-free mouth wash, mix ½ cup food grade hydrogen peroxide with ½ cup purified water. Add one drop of peppermint oil and mix. Store in an air-tight bottle. Also freshen breath with a toothpick dipped quickly in peppermint or spearmint oil.

Colds and Flu: Try fresh ginger tea for temporary relief of cold and flu symptoms (use 1 to 2 teaspoons grated root per cup of tea and steep for 4 to 6 minutes).

Cough: Try slippery elm tea for relief of a cough (no more than 3 cups per day). To prepare, steep 1½ teaspoons of the herb in 1 cup of almost boiling water for 4 to 6 minutes. See your doctor if cough persists.

Digestive Aid: Use one of the following teas to help with minor digestive problems— peppermint (1½ teaspoons dried mint leaves per cup of almost boiling water, steeped 4 to 6 minutes), fresh ginger (1 to 2 teaspoons grated root per cup of almost boiling water, steeped 4 or 6 minutes) or caraway tea (2 to 3 teaspoons bruised seeds per cup of almost boiling water, steep 10 to 20 minutes). Check with your doctor if digestive problems are more than minor and occasional.

Headache: Boil a handful of mint leaves in a quart of water for about 10 minutes. Strain and cool slightly. Dip a towel into the mint solution and lay this warm compress on your forehead.
Also, for simple headaches (not migraine-type) and with your doctor's approval, use white willow bark capsules. This is a mild pain-reliever that's similar to aspirin but without starch fillers.

Sore throat: Salt water gargle using ¼ teaspoon sea or mineral salt in 1 cup warm water (as warm as you can tolerate). Gargle every hour or two to soothe and enhance healing. Another helpful gargle is a mixture of ½ cup raw apple cider vinegar and ½ cup warm water (again as warm as you can tolerate). If you don't get relief in a couple of days, make certain you seek medical advice for diagnosis and treatment.

Stress: Practice deep breathing with air moving the abdomen outward as air enters it. Avoid shallow or chest breathing. Also, learn and practice daily some kind of skilled relaxation. This will help you better handle the stresses of life.

REFERENCES

Ballentine, Rudolph, M.D., *Transition to Vegetarianism: An Evolutionary Step.* Honesdale, Pennsylvania: The Himalayan International Institute of Yoga Science and Philosophy of the U.S.A., 1987.

Block, Zenas. *It's All on the Label: Understanding Food, Additives, and Nutrition.* Boston: Little, Brown and Company, 1981.

Brostoff, Jr. Jonathan and Linda Gamlin. *The Complete Guide to Food Allergy and Intolerance.* New York: Crown Publishers, Inc., 1989.

Chaitow, Leon, D.O., N.D. *Candida Albicans: Could Yeast Be Your Problem?* Rochester, Vermont: Healing Arts Press, 1985.

Cheraskin, Emanuel, Dr., Dr. W. Marshall Ringsdorf, Jr., and Dr. Emily L. Sisley. *The Vitamin C Connection: Getting Well and Staying Well with Vitamin C.* New York: Harper & Row, Publishers, 1983.

Crook, William G., M.D. and Marjorie Hurt Jones, R.N. *The Yeast Connection Cookbook.* Jackson, Tennessee: Professional Books, 1989.

Erasmus, Udo. *Fats and Oils: The Complete Guide to Fats and Oils in Health and Nutrition.* Vancouver, Canada: Alive Books, 1986.

Finnegan, John. *The Facts About Fats: A Consumer's Guide to Good Oils.* Malibu, CA: Elysian Arts, 1992.

Fisher, Jeffrey A., M.D. *The Chromium Program.* New York: Harper and Row, Publishers, 1990.

Galland, Leo, M.D. *Superimmunity for Kids.* New York: Bantam Doubleday Dell Publishing Group, Inc., New York, 1988.

Garland, Cedric, Dr., and Dr. Frank Garland. *The Calcium Connection.* New York: G.P. Putnam's Sons, 1988.

Giller, Robert M., M.D., and Kathy Matthews. *Maximum Metabolism: The Diet Breakthrough for Permanent Weight Loss.* New York: G.P. Putnam's Sons, 1989.

Giller, Robert M., M.D., and Kathy Matthews. *Medical Makeover: The Revolutionary No-Willpower Program for Lifetime Health.* New York: Beech Tree Books, 1986

Goldbeck, Nikki and David. *The Goldbecks' Guide to Good Food.* New York: New American Library, 1987.

Golos, Natalie and Frances Golos Golbitz. *Coping with Your Allergies.* New York: Simon & Schuster, Inc., 1986.

Goulart, Frances Sheridan. *The Caffeine Book: A User's and Abuser's Guide.* New York: Dodd, Mead & Company, 1984.

"Great Grilling with Soyfoods," *Delicous!*, Vol. 9, No. 5, July/August, 1993, pp. 54-56.

Greenberg, Ron, M.D. and Angela Nori. *Freedom from Allergy Cookbook.* Vancouver, B.C.: Blue Poppy Press, 1988.

Hass, Elson M., M.D. *Staying Healthy with Nutrition: The Complete Guide to Diet and Nutritional Medicine.* Berkeley, California: Celestial Arts, 1992.

Hoffman, Mark S., Editor. *The World Almanac and Book of Facts.* New York: Pharos Books, 1990.

Hunt, Goudlas, M.D. *No More Cravings.* New York: Warner Communications Company, 1987.

Jacobson, Michael F., Ph.D., Lisa Y. Lefferts, and Anne Witte Garland. *Safe Food: Eating Wisely in a Risky World.* Los Angeles, Living Planet Press, 1991.

Johnson, Otto, Editor. *The 1990 Information Please Almanac.* Boston: Houghton Mifflin Company, 1990.

Johnston, Ingeborg M., C.N. and James R. Johnston, PhD. *Flaxseed (Linseed) Oil and the Power of Omega-3: How to Make Nature's Cholesterol Fighters Work for You.* New Canaan, Connecticut: Keats Publishing, Inc., 1990.

Kamen, Betty, Ph.D, and Si Kamen. *Osteoporosis: What It Is, How to Prevent It, How to Stop It.* New York: Pinnacle Books, Inc., 1984.

Kane, Patricia, Ph.D. *Food Makes the Difference: A Parent's Guide to Raising a Healthy Child.* New York: Simon and Schuster, 1985.

Krohn, Jacqueline, M.D. *The Whole Way to Allergy Relief and Prevention.* Point Roberts, Washington: Hartley & Marks, Inc., 1991.

Lines, Anni Airola, R.D. *Vitamins & Minerals: The Health Connection.* Phoenix: Health Plus Publishers, 1985.

Null, Gary. *No More Allergies: Identifying and Eliminating Allergies and Sensitivity Reactions to Everything in Your Environment.* New York: Villard Books, 1992.

Ornish, Dean, M.D. *Dr. Dean Ornish's Program for Reversing Heart Disease.* New York: Random House, 1990.

Philpott, William H., M.D. and Dwight K. Kalita, PhD. *Brain Allergies: The Psychonutrient Connection.* New Canaan, Connecticut: Keats Publishing, Inc., 1980.

Pritikin, Nathan. *The Pritikin Program for Diet and Exercise.* New York: Bantam Books, 1979.

Pritikin, Robert. *The New Pritikin Program.* New York: Pocket Books, a division of Simon & Schuster, 1990.

Quillin, Patrick, Ph.D., R.D. *Healing Nutrients.* New York: Vintage Books, 1987.

Quillin, Patrick, Ph.D., R.D., and A. Gordon Reynolds, M.D. *Nutrition Encyclopedia.* San Diego: Nutrex Enterprises, 1984.

Randolph, Theron G., M.D., and Ralph W. Moss, Ph.D. *An Alternative Approach to Allergies.* New York: Harper Row, Publishers, 1989.

Rodale, J.I. and Staff. *Complete Book of Minerals for Health.* Emmaus, PA: Rodale Books, Inc., 1977.

Rohé, Fred. *The Complete Book of Natural Foods.* Boulder: Shambhala Publications, Inc., 1983.

Rudin, Donald O., M.D. and Clara Felix. *The Omega-3 Phenomenon: The Nutrition Breakthrough of the '80s.* New York: Rawson Associates, 1987.

Shannon, Marilyn M. *Fertility, Cycles, and Nutrition: Can What You Eat Affect Your Menstrual Cycles and Your Fertility?* Cincinnati: The Couple to Couple League, Inc., 1990.

Schwartz, George R. *In Bad Taste: The MSG Syndrome.* Sante Fe: Health Press, 1988.

Smedley, Lydia and Agatha Thrash, M.D. *Special Food for Special People: Celiac and Allergy Diets—Food Rotation.* Kamloops, BC, Canada: Lydia Smedley Publisher, 1985.

Thrash, Agatha M., M.D and Calvin L. Thrash, Jr., M.D. *Poison With A Capital C: A Case Against Coffee and Other Brown Drinks.* Seale, AL: New LifeStyle Books, 1991.

Wood, Rebecca. *The Whole Foods Encyclopedia: A Shopper's Guide.* New York: Prentice Hall Press, 1988.

Wright, John W., Editor. *The Universal Almanac.* Kansas City: Andrews and McMeel, 1991.

Yudkin, John, M.D. *Sweet and Dangerous.* New York: Bantam Book, 1972.

INDEX

ABOUT THE AUTHOR

Beginning in 1977, Beth Loiselle saw her own health as well as her family's improve when she changed their diet from typical American food to whole foods. She is now dedicated to teaching others about the benefits of whole foods as well as how to incorporate them into their lifestyles. Beth believes that whole foods nutrition is a critical key to good health, both in the treatment and prevention of disease.

Beth works at Good Foods Co-op in Lexington, Kentucky where she helps customers shop for their special needs and diets, counsels them to help them improve their diets, answers questions about whole foods cooking and nutrition, and consults with clients upon physician referral. She is founder of *HealthWays* Weight Control Program in which she helps her clients not only achieve a healthy body weight through a lifestyle change, but also improve their health. Through her *Nutrition Mission* program, Beth presents motivational and educational talks to classrooms, church, scout, and neighborhood groups, homemaker clubs, support groups, and employee meetings. Her goal is to spark an interest in health and nutrition in those she meets.

Beth received a Bachelor of Science Degree from the University of Tennessee in Foods Science and Institution Management and is a registered dietitian. She lives in Nicholasville, Kentucky with her husband Jim, daughter Heather, and son Keith.

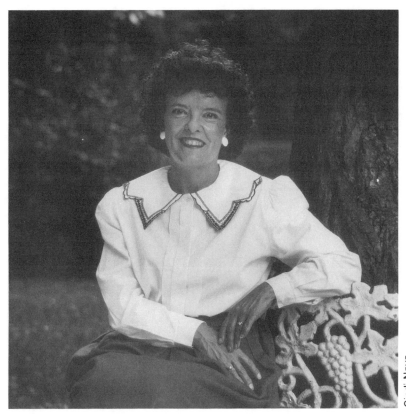

Cindi Nave

BOOK ORDER FORM

Please send me:

_____ copies of *The Healing Power of Whole Foods* [ISBN 0-9637478-0-0]

@ $24.95 each. . . . . $_____

KY residents, please add 6% tax . . . . _____

Postage and handling . . . . _____

___Book Rate: $3.00 for first book and $2.00 for each additional book

___Priority Mail: $ 5.00 for one book

(For more than one book, please call us for UPS shipping information.)

Total: $_____

Please print:

Name_____

Address_____

City_____ State_____ Zip Code_____

Make checks or money orders (U.S. funds only) payable to *Healthways Nutrition*.

Mail to:

Healthways Nutrition
93 Summertree Drive
Nicholasville, KY 40356-9190

• Order with credit card by calling (800) 870-5378 or (859) 223-2270. *MasterCard*, *Visa*, and *Discover* are accepted.

• Order online at www.wholefoodsforlife.com

• Call to inquire about quantity discounts for businesses.

WHAT OTHERS ARE SAYING

From an Internet Holistic Health Bulletin Board:

Have just read most of The Healing Power of Whole Foods *by Beth Loiselle. She deserves a lot of credit for the most complete coverage in the fewest words. She has separate lists for food sensitivities involved in migraine, MSG, gluten, and others. The print is large, descriptions clear as for omega 3 and 6 essential fatty acids. I have never seen a better listing of hidden sugars. The introduction from Dr. Stoll is very motivating. The necessary info is there, it is up to us readers to use it!*

Martha Kent, Columbus, OH

From an unsolicited letter:

...The education I learned from this book has helped me so much in controlling my appetite...I am totally amazed at how my cravings have diminished. I can remain calm throughout the day. I no longer have the sugar highs and lows. When I get hungry, it's a manageable hunger. I'm not starved. I can't say enough about how good I feel and how excited I am about my new eating habits.

P.A., NY

From Dr. Walt Stoll, Introduction:

...Only your own personal experience will ever let you find out if the results (of a whole foods diet) are worth the effort. The Healing Power of Whole Foods *gives the most practical set of tools I know of to learn that for yourself.*

Dr. Walt Stoll, Panama City, FL

From Grocery Manager of Washoe Zephyr Food Co-op:

This book - The Healing Power of Whole Foods *- is one of the best I've seen. The recipes are easy to follow; the ingredients are easy to find in Natural Food Stores, like Co-ops. Congratulations to Beth on a great book! I highly recommend this book to anyone interested in improving their eating habits and health!*

Mya Robertshaw, Reno, NV

From a local chiropractor (an unsolicited letter):

This is just a brief note to tell you how very much I have enjoyed your book. This great nutritional resource has everything! You have included excellent recipes, complete information for the new whole foods consumer, and the detailed physiological benefits of the program for those of us who really get excited about superior health. All in all, Beth, you produced an outstanding product that I will recommend highly to my patients!

Dr. Kathryn A. Bolton, Lexington, KY

From owner of Georgetown Health Foods:

The Healing Power of Whole Foods *is excellent and a must for anyone who really wants to understand the value of foods....If a person asks me to recommend a book on learning about eating right, recipes, etc., this is the first book that I show them.*

Richard Montieth, Indianapolis, IN

From a satisfied follower of *The Healing Power of Whole Foods*:

I just can't believe how much better I'm feeling now that I've followed your book for less than a month. And I thought I was already making good food choices! As a side benefit of whole foods, I've begun to lose weight! Needless to say, I'm thrilled!

T.J., Lexington, KY

The book that can change your health!!

The whole foods diet described in this book has helped these conditions:

Allergies
Arthritis
Behavior problems in
  children
Candida albicans
  overgrowth
Chronic muscle aches
Chronic fatigue syndrome
Constipation
Cravings for sweets
Depression
Diabetes (see caution)
Digestive disorders
Elevated triglycerides

Elevated cholesterol
Environmental illness
Fatigue
Headaches
Hypertension
Hypoglycemia
Learning disabilities
Overweight
Panic attacks
Poor health in general
Premenstrual syndrome
  (PMS)
Weakened immune system
...plus many others

If you'd like to feel better, why not give whole foods a try? It just may be the best money, time, and effort you've ever spent!